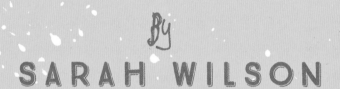

I QUIT SUGAR
SIMPLICIOUS

By

SARAH WILSON

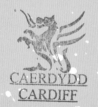

Llyfrgelloedd Caerdydd
www.caerdydd.gov.uk/llyfrgelloedd
Cardiff Libraries
www.cardiff.gov.uk/libraries

CAERDYDD
CARDIFF

bluebird
books for life

When my seriously lovely publisher Ingrid "invited" me to write this book, I said, "Only if we can make it fun." → this meant doing meetings over breakfast or martinis at my favourite (like-minded) cafes

I also added that it would have to be really AUTHENTIC.

We'd have to cook with SCRAPS, grow leftovers, enlist community + be TRANSPARENT.

WHICH is why the props in the photographs are actually my daggy things, the garnishes and offcuts from other shoots + this messy handwriting + the "naive" illustrations are mine. To keep things real(ish).

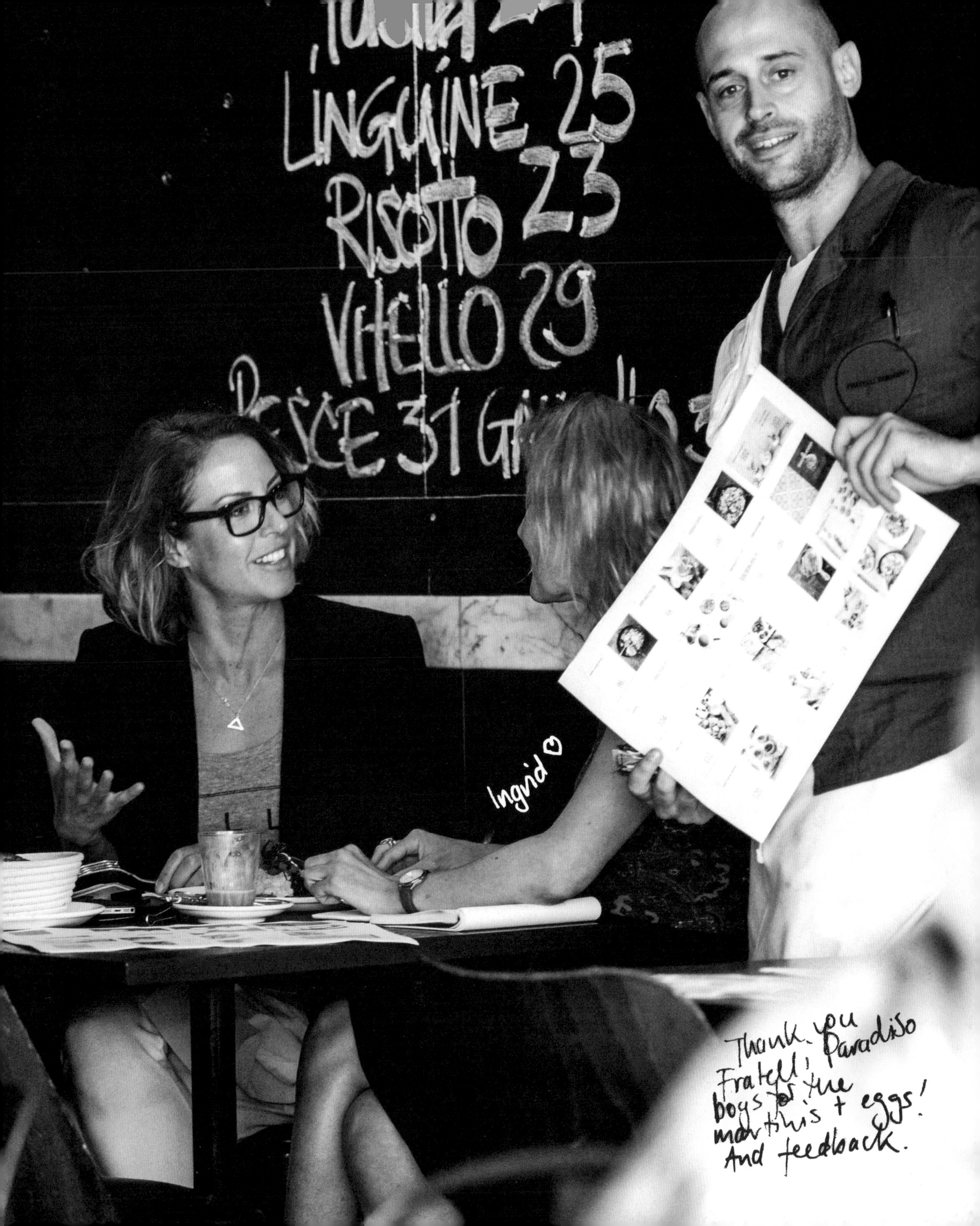
LINGUINE 25
RISOTTO 23
VITELLO 29
Ingrid ♡
Thank you Fratelli Paradiso boys for the martinis + eggs! And feedback.

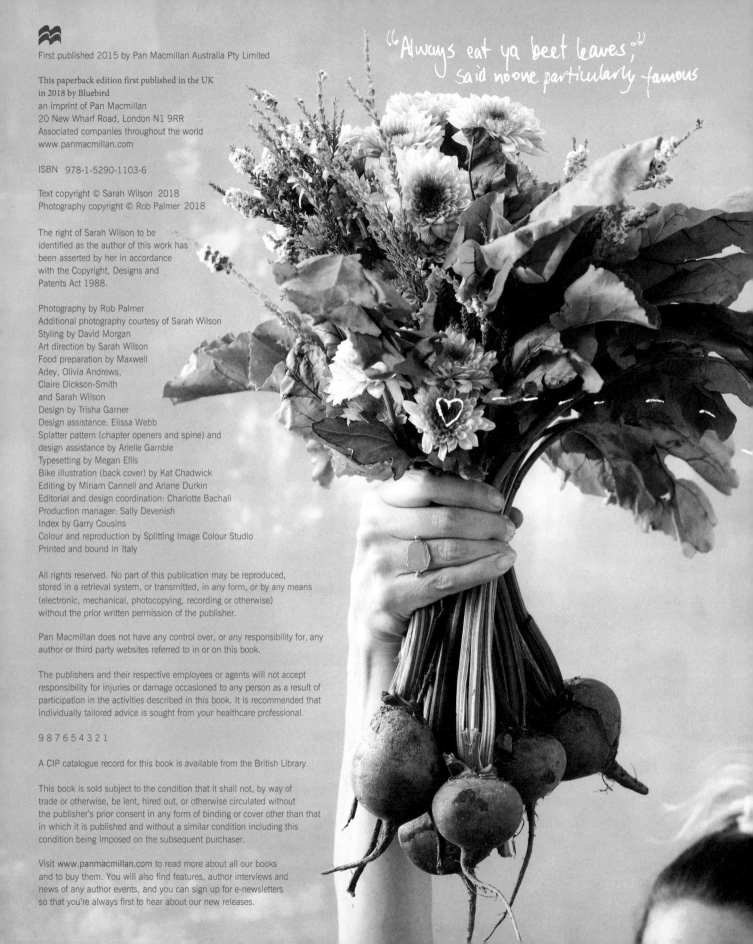

First published 2015 by Pan Macmillan Australia Pty Limited

This paperback edition first published in the UK
in 2018 by Bluebird
an imprint of Pan Macmillan
20 New Wharf Road, London N1 9RR
Associated companies throughout the world
www.panmacmillan.com

ISBN 978-1-5290-1103-6

Photography by Rob Palmer
Additional photography courtesy of Sarah Wilson
Styling by David Morgan
Art direction by Sarah Wilson
Food preparation by Maxwell
Adey, Olivia Andrews,
Claire Dickson-Smith
and Sarah Wilson
Design by Trisha Garner
Design assistance: Elissa Webb
Splatter pattern (chapter openers and spine) and
design assistance by Arielle Gamble
Typesetting by Megan Ellis
Bike illustration (back cover) by Kat Chadwick
Editing by Miriam Cannell and Ariane Durkin
Editorial and design coordination: Charlotte Bachali
Production manager: Sally Devenish
Index by Garry Cousins
Colour and reproduction by Splitting Image Colour Studio
Printed and bound in Italy

Visit www.panmacmillan.com to read more about all our books
and to buy them. You will also find features, author interviews and
news of any author events, and you can sign up for e-newsletters
so that you're always first to hear about our new releases.

*"Always eat ya beet leaves,"
said no one particularly famous*

The bit where I place a quote
that sums up where we're about to head:

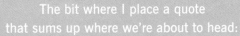

"Each of us is responsible for everything
and to every human being."

DOSTOYEVSKY

(upfront, before I forget)

The bit where I thank those who inspired me to love food more
Mum (always), Michael Pollan, and my first boyfriend, George.

The bit where I thank my crew, the *I Quit Sugar* team.
Especially Jo Foster who made sure this book didn't veer
into a compost heap.

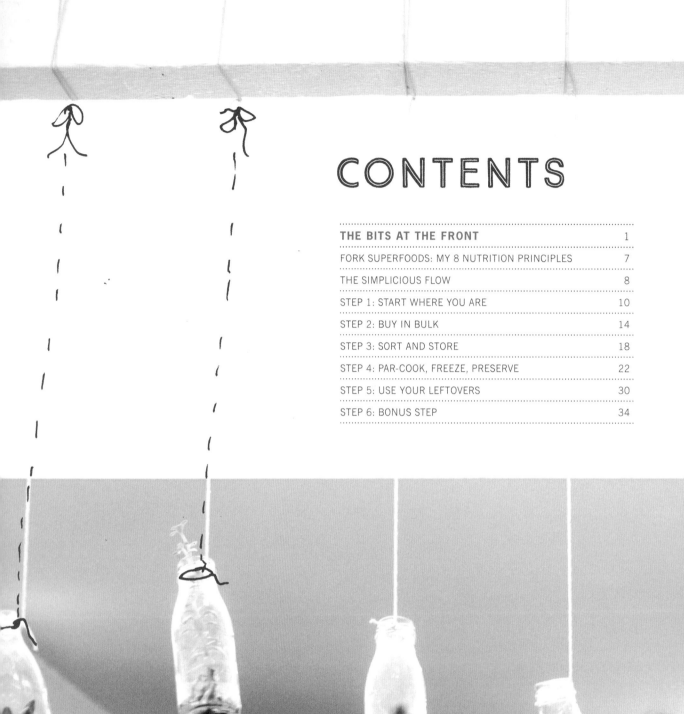

CONTENTS

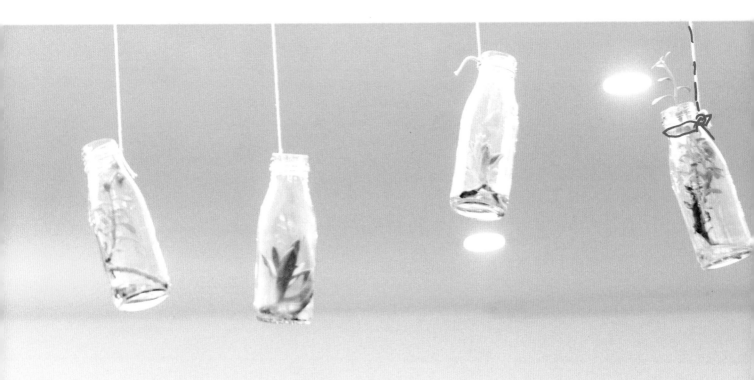

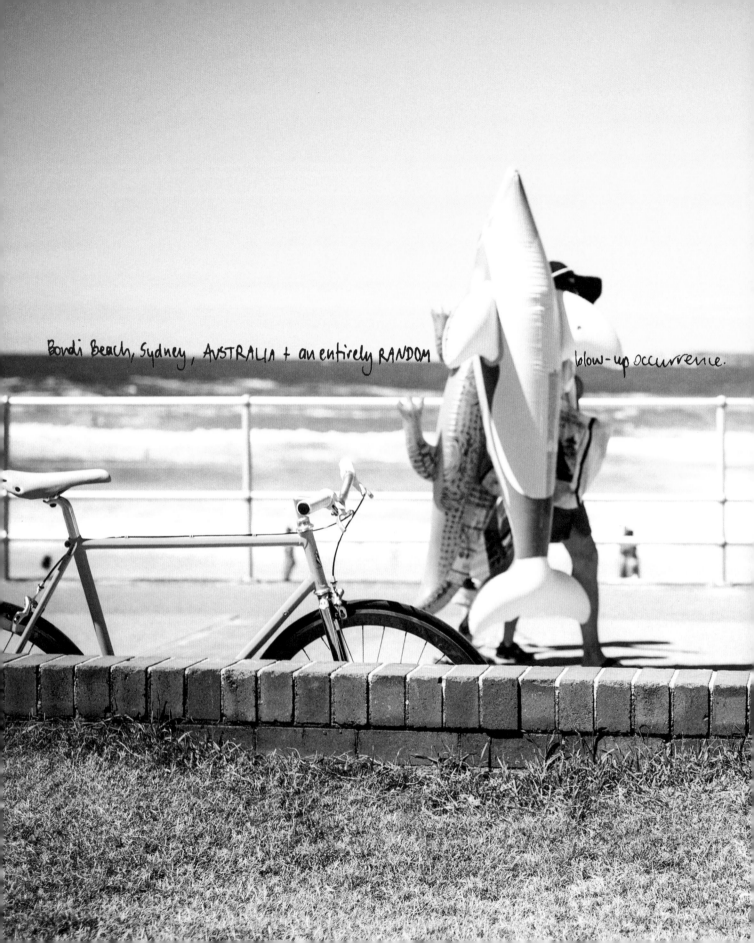

Bondi Beach, Sydney, AUSTRALIA + an entirely RANDOM blow-up occurrence.

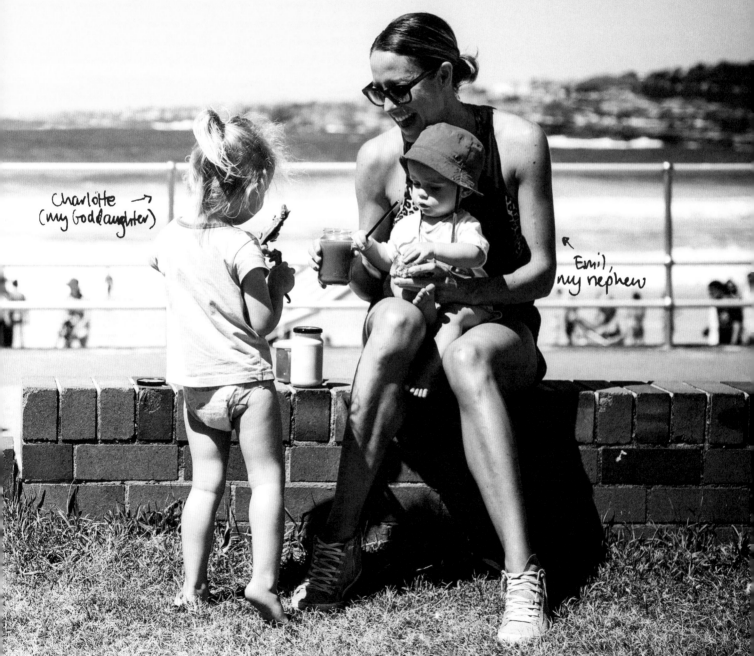

THE BITS AT THE FRONT

Charlotte →
(my Goddaughter)

Emil,
my nephew

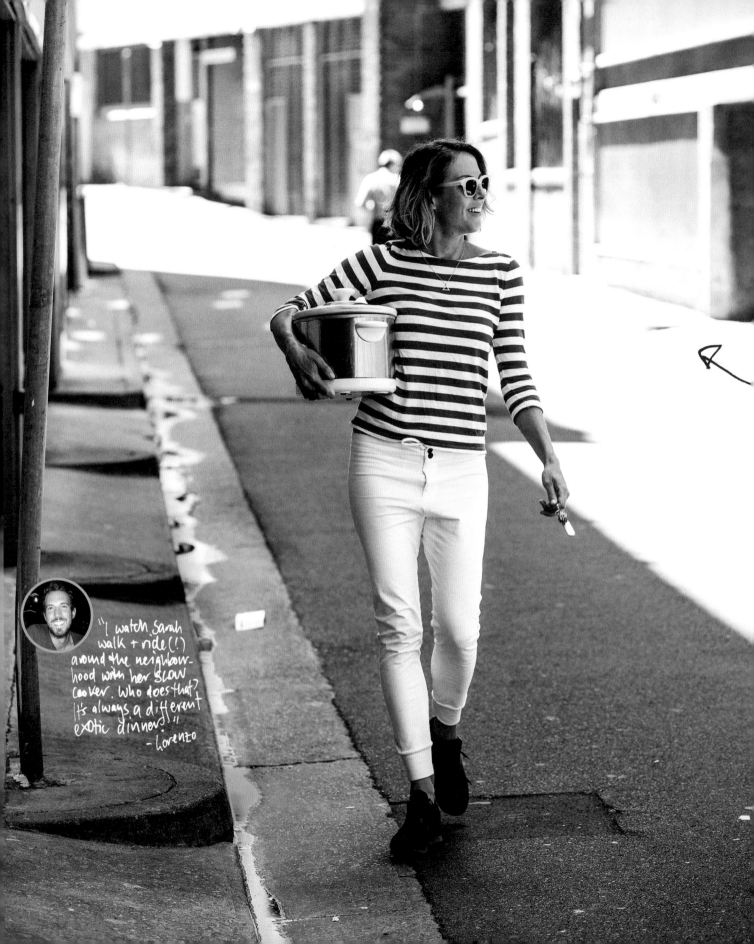

"I watch Sarah walk + ride (!) around the neighbourhood with her slow cooker. Who does that? Its always a different exotic dinner."
— Lorenzo

Dear Reader,

I'd like to take a few moments to justify the next 373 pages.

I've always eaten the whole apple, core and all. My tiny apartment kitchen is littered with recycled jars filled with the drippings from last night's chops (which I use to sweat my veggies, thus adding the right fats for absorbing the essential vitamins), the water from steaming my chard (perfect for padding out soup) and the olive oil from the marinated feta my friend was going to chuck when I was at her place for lunch last weekend (ready-made salad dressing, people!).

My fridge is a rainbow of fermented vegetables made from the 'ugly' veggies my local markets can't sell on. My freezer boasts a plastic bucket containing three fish carcasses that I retrieved from guests' plates at a friend's dinner party a few weeks back. They'll be turned into fish stock shortly, a litre of which I'll send back to said friend as a thankyou gift. And I should mention the carcass haul came *after* I'd been through my friend's bin and pulled out a bag of still-sprightly celery leaves and asked if I could keep them . . . for making my Leftovers Pesto (page 55).

If she's lucky she'll get a batch of that, too.

I should also mention I've been known to ask strangers at the restaurant table next to me if I can take home their leftovers (well, they had no intention of doing so themselves); they acquiesced and I turned their indulgent angus beef strips into a Vietnamese soup. Aren't you just glad you only know me from a distance!

All of which I share here to explain why I've decided to write a book about how to eat your scraps. Sustainability has always been at the guts of my books, albeit camouflaged behind pretty recipes and shiny, smiley pictures of myself. My recipes use leftovers and secondary cuts of meat. I've used my sugar-free platform to promote doggie bags and, um, cauliflower, to the masses.

Plus, there's this: where do you go after you've written I Quit Sugar *and* I Quit Sugar for Life? I Quit Sugar in the Afterlife?!

As many of you know, I first quit sugar back in January 2011 because I had an autoimmune disease that seriously mucked with my ability to enjoy life. I wanted a better life, a richer life, a well life, so I tried going sugar-free. It worked a treat and so I continued with the experiment a little longer. But along the way, several bigger, deeper themes emerged. I realised food wastage mattered. More than anything else, actually. I also realised it shouldn't just be the quirky obsession of earnest types with black-framed glasses, farmers' market satchels and single-speed bikes. Ha! Hello!

sustainable
Other Things I Do (as collated by my oft-bewildered friends and family):

* 'She once retrieved sardine heads left over from a book shoot on my rooftop. She made them into a pizza topper for her dinner.' – Joice

* 'Coming over to cook dinner at my place, going through my veg drawer and turning all my old stuff into our dinner. She does this every Sunday night.' – Ricky G

* 'I once witnessed her fishing a tea bag out of the office bin because "it had only been used once".' – Zoe

* 'Eating everyone's fish skins and heads at our local fish restaurant. We now know to dump all bones and bits on her plate straight up.' – Brad

Friends tell me they
don't cook because it's
too complicated and
time-consuming. But
I've conducted tests.
I have timed friends as
they got takeaway while
I cooked my beef stew
for myself (with six
portions of leftovers).
My friends took *37
minutes* (finding
car keys, driving
there, waiting in line,
reheating each dish
separately) while I
took *11 minutes*.
Divide that by six and,
well . . . you can work
it out.

versus

You see, it goes like this: the biggest source of CO_2 emissions on
the planet is food waste (not cars, not factories). The biggest food
wasters are consumers (us!), not farmers or Big Food. Indeed, we
toss out up to 50 per cent of our groceries every week.

must

I'll say it straight – this is unconscionable and the change we seek
so deeply in life (to the planet, to our being) can come from each of
us. Each of us is responsible. For everything. And to every human
being.

And BTW, recycling and composting doesn't cut it. Not buying
and wasting it in the first place does. That is, using what we have,
cooking our leftovers, eating the whole food – pith, peel, stalks,
stems, leaves, bones, brine, fat, skin and all. This is the future,
my dear friends.

I soon realised that buying, cooking and eating this way made life
better. Because when you learn to eat your scraps and consume
less, life begins to flow. Things become simpler, more elegant;
everything falls into place and makes sustainable sense. You don't
have to worry whether local or organic or egg-yolk-free is better, or
whether your dinner classifies as a superfood. Nope, you simply find
yourself flowing to the 'right' outcome. Without the palaver.

For example:
When you quit sugar, you essentially quit processed food and all its
associated nasty additives. Which means you benefit not only from
the absence of sugar, but also from eliminating a stack of other toxic
chemicals, crappy fats and low-brow carbs. Quitting sugar,
by necessity, steers you to the right outcome.

**Plus, when you quit processed food you're left with real, whole
food only – which you have to cook, right?** This means you're
motivated (forced?) to cook, which means you save money and
time, plus your health improves with exponential flourish. Which
in turn means you stick to this way of eating and living because it
feels so good. And on and on the sustainable vibe flows.

Another example:
When you eat secondary cuts of meat you save money (they're
much cheaper), plus you tick ethical and environmental boxes too,
as you're contributing to more of the beast being eaten (or less of it
being wasted). Secondary cuts are best slow-cooked, which requires
less electricity (saving you even more), and they are more densely
nutritious – even more so when cooked slowly. Plus, as the slow-
cooked flavour is richer, you can use less meat, saving money and
the environment and . . . oh, you get the point! Needless to say, this
book celebrates the secondary cut.

*Slow cookers use
less power than a
light bulb! And they
never break . . .
which is why you
don't see them
advertised!*

*Slow-and-
low cooking
preserves
the meat's
enzymes and
also releases
wonderful gut-
healing gelatine
and minerals.*

*True story! It's also why
you always find them in
mint condition at every
Garage Sale around
town.*

And one more:

Ever gone to make a recipe, realised you're missing an ingredient or two so improvised with what you've got . . . and found it tasted better? My favourite meals are the ones I've made when camping and I've used leftover trail mix to flavour the evening stew. Or when I've created a fridge surprise (check out my creations on Instagram at #fridgesurprise) from a dearth of talent in my crisper.

I believe we like to fend, to create from what we have. We actually *like* living without. We are most creative in these situations. Also, we like it when we don't have corner cupboards bulging with waffle-makers. Or mouldy lettuce at the bottom of the crisper.

So. We cook with what we've got, with scraps and leftovers, and we become happier and more creative. We also stop going to the shops as often to pick up a lone chicory bulb or carton of cream or whatever, which saves time, petrol and money, and prevents processed-food temptation at the checkout. All of which sees us get happier and scrappier. And on we flow.

This book elevates leftovers to the main attraction, saving money, time, nutrients, scraps, energy, pans, washing up and all those random ingredients that usually sit at the back of the pantry after a single use.

I don't start and finish with a recipe. A meal never should. It should keep going and going – a perpetual recipe – the juices, scraps and leftovers all repurposed into further meals. The recipes in this book, right from the get-go, are orchestrated to work to a magnificent, elegant flow where we take an ingredient and use every last bit of it. A chicken can spread to 13 meals, 1.5 kg of cheap stewing steak to 14.

I cheat, take shortcuts and do stuff my culinary peers no doubt frown upon. I use my fingers to test the readiness of food, skip pointless steps, toss salads with my hands and feature fridge dregs in my ingredients lists. I improvise, fend, get loose, get responsible . . . and I encourage you all to do the same.

This is simplicious. This is what makes life better.

Where's the proof?
I haven't bogged this book down in data. However, all claims, factlets etc are backed with science or my own research and a simple search on iquitsugar.com or sarahwilson.com will deliver the data you're after. Also head to sarahwilson.com and click on **The Kit**, where much background guff will be housed for your deeper reading pleasure.

Sarah xxxxxxxxxxxxx

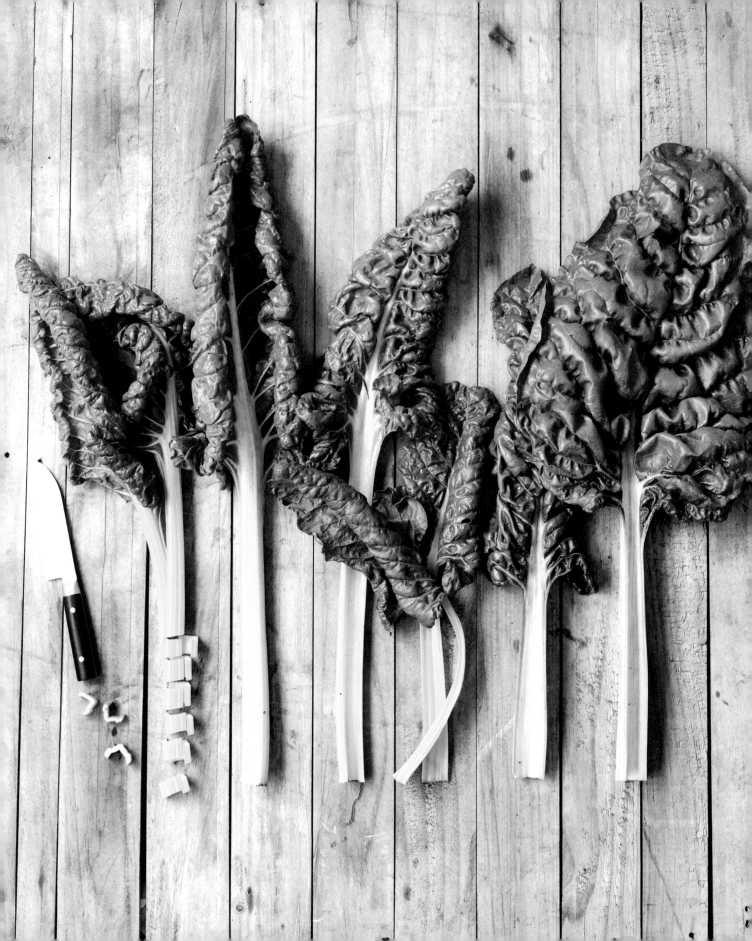

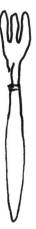

MY 8 FAD-FREE!! NUTRITION PRINCIPLES

For the past 50 years we've made a clusterfork of our dinner. 'Nutritionism' has complicated things to the point where most of us have no idea what we're meant to eat. In this book I avoid referring to superfoods and have left off vegan and paleo considerations (many recipes will suit both, as well as those with lactose, nut and dairy intolerances) because I want to keep my message 'simplicious'. That said, there are a few mantras I work to:

1. Eat for gut health
The gut is where it's at. More than one-third of us have an inflammation-related disease (including obesity, arthritis, fatty liver, allergies and high cholesterol), stemming from poor bacteria in the large intestine. I focus on food-prep techniques that assist in building the gut microbiome and aid digestion, primarily fermenting, sprouting, preserving enzymes and minimising toxins.

2. Opt for the most nutrient-dense option
And steer away from toxins. Where possible. My recipes include carbs and legumes and soy, which contain anti-nutrients. But rather than eliminating these foods, I focus on preparing them properly and veering towards more nutritious options.

3. Eat like your grandmother (or great-grandmother) used to
Sixty years ago we ate an appropriate amount of sugar and metabolic diseases were almost unheard of. My offal recipes are a homage to All Of The Nanas. 'Cos they had it going on.

4. Less is more
Partly for gut health reasons, partly for simplicious reasons, having too many ingredients in a dish causes unnecessary angst.

5. The French are right to be arrogant
About food, that is. After spending time in France over the past few years, I've come to admire the Francophile way of eating. They eat proper meals and don't snack; they 'eat like they mean it'. They've also made an art of using leftovers. Lots of my recipes draw on their techniques.

6. Go slow and low
Cook slow and at a low temperature to preserve enzymes and maximise nutrients. Eat slow to maintain mindfulness and elegance and good gut health.

7. Try some Ayurvedic balance
I have a lot of time for this Indian approach to wellness. It's about (among many things) using food to maintain balance. Which is not quite the same as using food as medicine. According to Ayurveda, we don't need to fix or reverse anything; we balance dis-ease or wobbliness using certain foods. For more, see page 362.

8. And, yes, JERF
Just Eat Real Food, people.

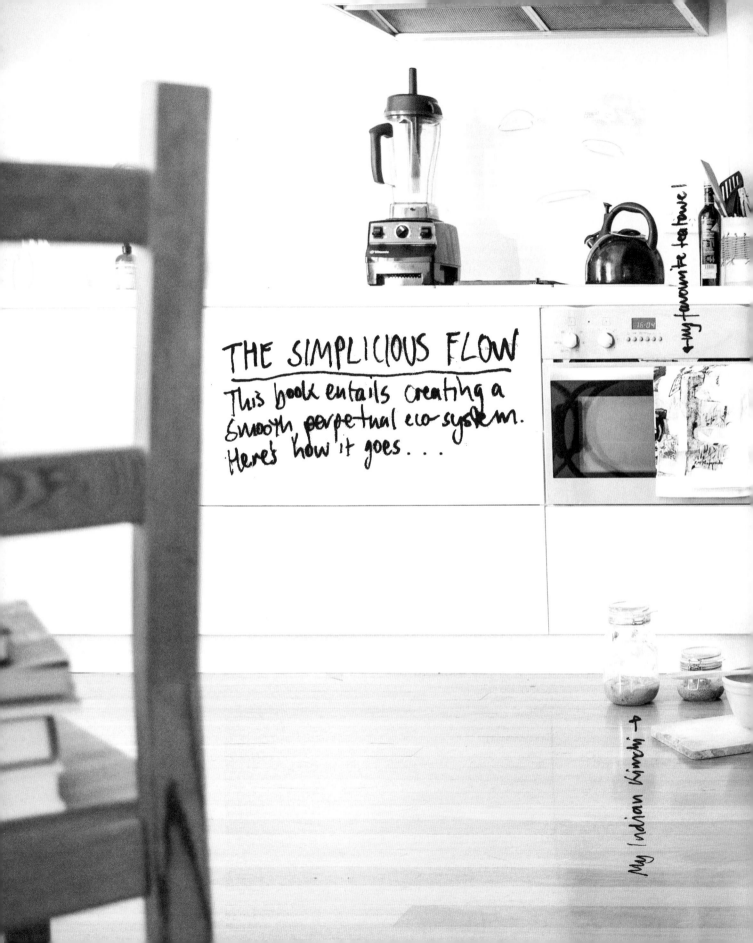

THE SIMPLICIOUS FLOW

This book entails creating a smooth perpetual eco-system. Here's how it goes . . .

my favourite feature!

My Indian kimchi →

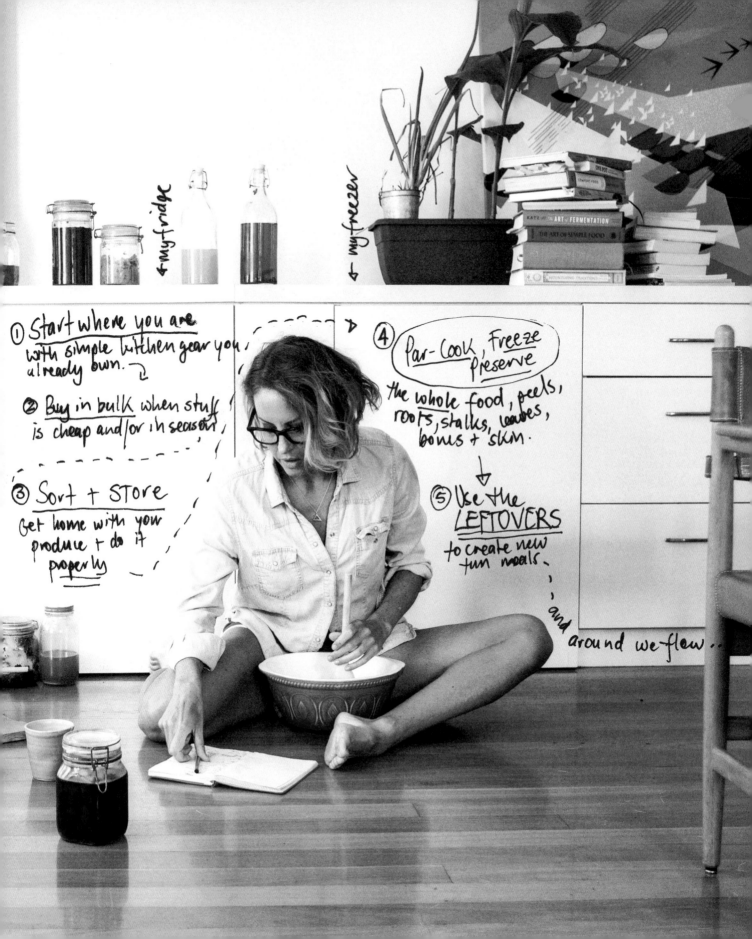

→ my fridge

→ my freezer

① Start where you are with simple kitchen gear you already own. ↵

② Buy in bulk when stuff is cheap and/or in season

③ Sort + STORE Get home with your produce + do it properly

④ Par-Cook, Freeze, Preserve the whole food, peels, roots, stalks, leaves, bones + skin.

⑤ Use the LEFTOVERS to create new fun meals.

...and around we flow...

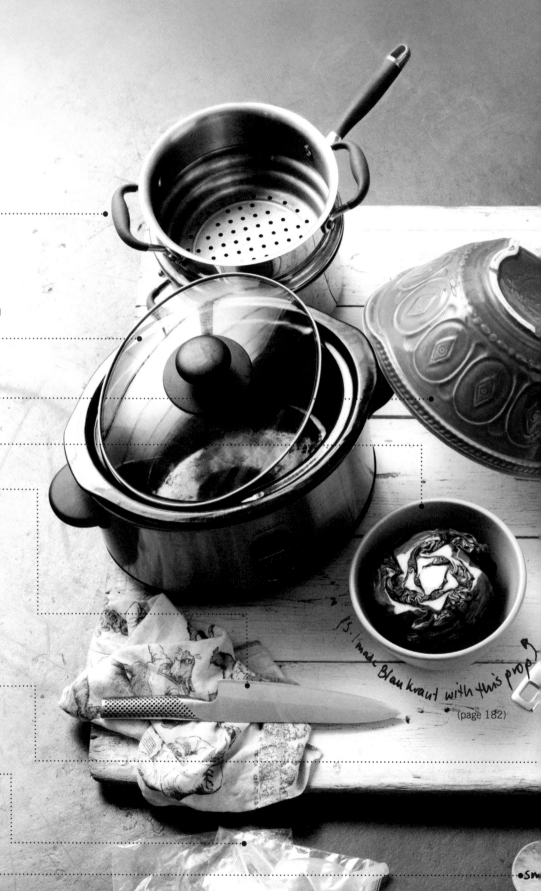

Double steamer – A 2–3 litre one is best. I boil my starchy veg down below, steam my greens up top.

4.5 litre slow cooker – These one-pot wonders cook your dinner while you're at work, are cheap, use less electricity than a light bulb, and cook slow and low, preserving minerals and enzymes thus making your food more digestible. There is really little discussion to be had here. PS An oval shape is best and if I had my time again, I'd get one with a timer.

Big mixing bowl – The old ones are best: nice lips! I got this for $4 at a garage sale after a bushwalk.

Little mixing bowl – Inherited from Grandma with this tea towel from the 1950s.

One big (chef's) knife – I've had mine for a decade. Go to a good knife shop and ask for their help.

Two paring knives for $5 – Knife blocks just take up too much room and I've never needed a bread knife in my life.

Stick blender – Also called an immersion blender, handheld blender or stab mixer. Again, cheap. Takes up no room. Allows you to blend stuff in the pot it was cooked in. Even better: you might like to buy yours as part of a multi-function processor kit (with grater, mincer etc). I did. I use most of the said kit, especially the grating and 'mandoline' blades.

Zip-lock bags – Worth the plastic investment if you wash and re-use. To dry, slap them to your kitchen window or splashback. When they're dry, they'll drop off. I use them daily but have only ever bought three packs in four years.

Wooden spoons – Generally inherited with character inbuilt.

P.S. I made Blaukraut with this prop (page 182)

START WHERE YOU ARE

The best cooks improvise. The worst kitchens are those with unused waffle-makers in the corner cupboard. The worst cookbooks are those with long lists at the front telling you what you should go and stock up on from scratch. This is not one of those lists. It's an illustration of what I use and why.

Large frying pan with lid – 32 cm should be large enough to serve 6. (This way I have a smallish skillet for meals to serve 1–3, and a bigger pan for dinner parties or cook-ups.)

Cast-iron skillet or frying pan – 25 cm is best for most things.

Cast-iron V non-stick V stainless steel frying pans

Cast-iron: This is my pick. It gives you even heat and a really anchored cooking experience, and will last a lifetime. Cast-iron pans are also best for one-pot simpliciousness (you can brown food on the stove then plonk in the oven or under a grill without transferring between pans). They're also naturally non-stick, if you care for them properly. Google 'How to season a cast-iron skillet'. If possible, buy one second-hand or nab Grandma's old one and Google 'How to bring cast iron back to life'.

Non-stick: Cheap and convenient, but only buy non-Teflon varieties. Drawbacks: You can't work up a hearty reduction or put them over super-high heat to get crusts and crispy bits. Also, they don't last long – they scratch and dint.

Stainless steel: Expensive but good for pots and bigger pans. Invest in triple-layers (aluminium between two layers of steel) and riveted handles.

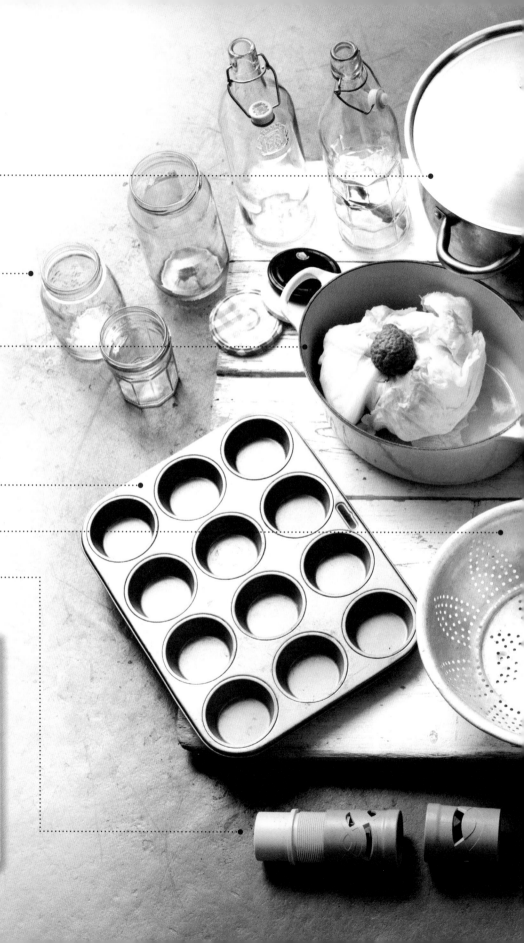

Big stockpot – About 8 litres is fine. I bought mine at St Vinnies for $3. No need to invest; no need for special features.

Glass jars and dishes – No need to buy fancy mason jars or plasticware. Most things can go in a jar instead. Added bonus – you can see what you've stored.

Enamelled cast-iron casserole – I got this 3.2 litre one for my birthday years ago from Mum and Dad. It's about perfect to serve 6.

Baking tins and dishes – My kit contains a 23 cm × 13 cm loaf tin, a 23 cm spring-form cake tin, and a couple of muffin trays. I've inherited most of these from people who had too many in their corner cupboard. A 23 cm × 20 cm glass, stoneware or enamel baking dish can be used not only for roasting veggies and baking pies and slices, but also for baking casseroles etc. One with a lid is great; it becomes a container after.

Old colander with no legs – From Grandma.

Spiraliser – Great for novelty noodles (I'd grab one if I had kids).

Microwave – Yes, I use one.

Are microwaves okay?

The science says they don't kill nutrients any more than boiling. Indeed, some studies show they retain more nutrients than other cooking methods. Nor do they radiate you. They use a form of non-ionising radiation (it can't directly break up atoms or molecules). Just stand back a little (1 metre) when it's in use to avoid the EMFs (electromagnetic fields) and don't put plastic in there. Use glass or ceramic containers instead.

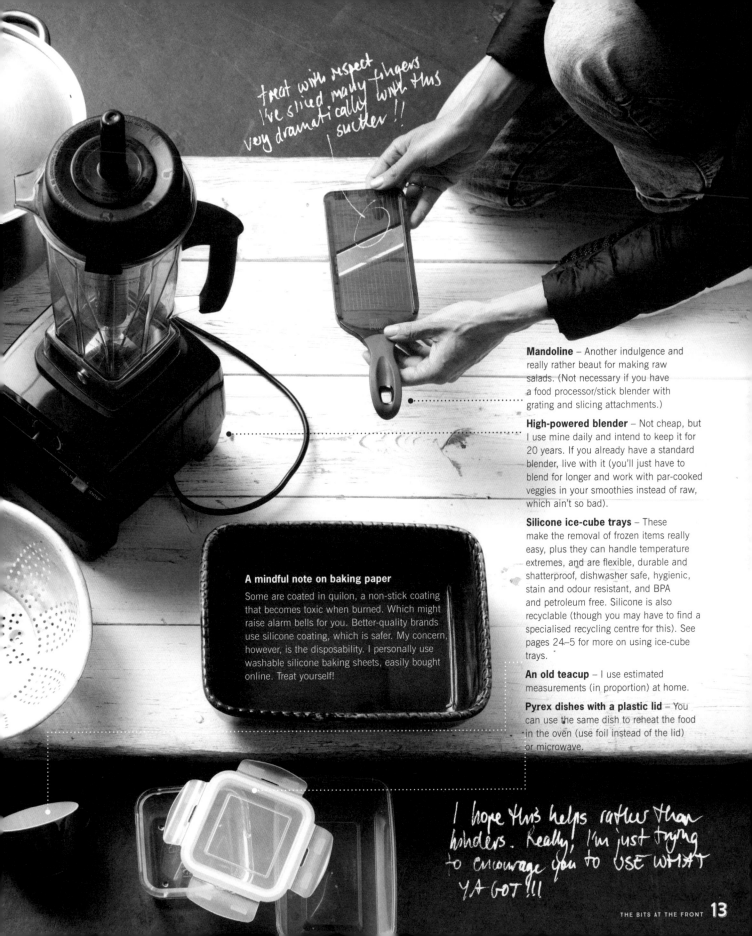

treat with respect I've sliced many fingers very dramatically with this sucker!!

Mandoline – Another indulgence and really rather beaut for making raw salads. (Not necessary if you have a food processor/stick blender with grating and slicing attachments.)

High-powered blender – Not cheap, but I use mine daily and intend to keep it for 20 years. If you already have a standard blender, live with it (you'll just have to blend for longer and work with par-cooked veggies in your smoothies instead of raw, which ain't so bad).

Silicone ice-cube trays – These make the removal of frozen items really easy, plus they can handle temperature extremes, and are flexible, durable and shatterproof, dishwasher safe, hygienic, stain and odour resistant, and BPA and petroleum free. Silicone is also recyclable (though you may have to find a specialised recycling centre for this). See pages 24–5 for more on using ice-cube trays.

An old teacup – I use estimated measurements (in proportion) at home.

Pyrex dishes with a plastic lid – You can use the same dish to reheat the food in the oven (use foil instead of the lid) or microwave.

A mindful note on baking paper

Some are coated in quilon, a non-stick coating that becomes toxic when burned. Which might raise alarm bells for you. Better-quality brands use silicone coating, which is safer. My concern, however, is the disposability. I personally use washable silicone baking sheets, easily bought online. Treat yourself!

I hope this helps rather than hinders. Really, I'm just trying to encourage you to USE WHAT YA GOT!!!

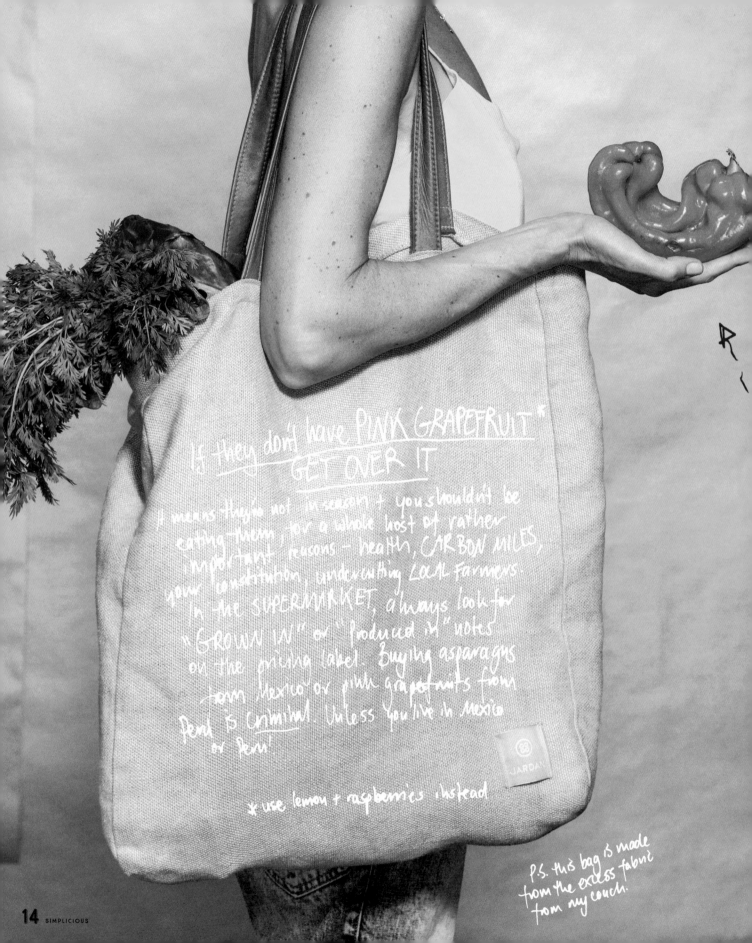

If they don't have PINK GRAPEFRUIT*
GET OVER IT

It means they're not in season + you shouldn't be eating them, for a whole host of rather important reasons – health, CARBON MILES, your constitution, undercutting LOCAL farmers. In the SUPERMARKET, always look for "GROWN IN" or "produced in" notes on the pricing label. Buying asparagus from Mexico or pink grapefruits from Peru is criminal. Unless you live in Mexico or Peru!

* use lemon + raspberries instead

P.S. this bag is made from the excess fabric from my couch.

BUY IN BULK

This really doesn't have to be complicated. And you don't have to be particularly organised – just fired up! Local produce markets are the best option. Not just for the free samples and overwhelming earnestness (and fewer carbon miles), but because you'll be buying stuff that's in season and therefore, the best food for your Ayurvedic constitution (see page 362). Yeah, we call it flow. (The greengrocer or supermarket is just fine, however.)

SAVE AT THE SUPERMARKET WITHOUT TRYING

This is how I cut corners, save coin and generally win.

Buy stuff in season: I'll say it again. This is the easiest way to save money (and the planet).

Buy discount meat, hard cheeses and smallgoods: Perishable items are often discounted a few days before their 'best before' date. If I'm going to eat something straight away or I can freeze it (or it's a food that improves with age anyway), I buy up. Mince is a great one to buy discounted. Turn it into meatballs (pages 144–5) and freeze immediately, thus rendering the use-by date redundant.

Buy secondary cuts of meat: These are the less popular and therefore cheaper cuts. They tend to be more muscly, leaner cuts, yet they have more flavour and nutrient density. Go for:

* **Chicken wings and legs** – not breasts (wings and legs are often half the price, plus dark meat contains more minerals than the white).
* **Lamb and pork shoulder, topside or leg cuts** – not loin chops, cutlets or tenderloin fillets.
* **Beef osso bucco, silverside, topside, chuck and brisket** – not fillet, rump or T-bone.
* **Fish offcuts** – if you're making soup or curry, why do you need a full fillet?

Look for imperfect veggies: Most supermarkets now stock these deformed 'rejects' at a portion of the price of the pretty picks. If you're not using your veg as props for an oil painting, always choose the rejects.

Grab some meat bones: My butcher gives them to me for free. Most will charge a few pounds for a big bag that will yield several litres of life-giving, joint-soothing, gut-calming bone broth/stock (see page 42).

Buy daggy roots 'n' shoots: Swedes, turnips, parsnips, sweet potato, cauliflower, cabbage . . . they're mostly available year-round and are generally cheaper than chips. Accordingly, I use them a lot in this book.

CHEAT, SOMETIMES WITH PACKET VERSIONS

I always prefer to buy fresh or make my own to avoid packaging. But sometimes the processed or packaged version is good (okay, better).

Frozen peas and corn: Freezing stops the starch in these little veggies from breaking down into sugars, helping them retain vitamins, fibre and minerals, and making the frozen versions 'fresher' than the, um, fresh ones.

Packets of slaw: They cost a few pounds and are dead nifty at times. Forgivable.

Roast chicken: If you can find a place that roasts organic chooks, then don't lose a second's sleep over buying a precooked one. It will probably be more energy-efficient this way anyway, seeing they roast stacks at once. Remember to boil up the bones to make stock afterwards (page 42).

Frozen berries: Just make sure they're organic and not from China (carbon miles). Even during berry season frozen berries are usually a fraction of the price of fresh ones. Plus, even the non-organic frozen berries contain less chemicals than fresh.

Curry paste: Yes, yes, yes. Grinding your own spices fresh is fab. And yes, yes, yes, most pastes use vegetable oil in the mix. But many don't contain sugar or other added nasties and can deliver a sound result, without having to keep 23,473,276 herbs and spices on hand. I tend to add Fermented Turmeric Paste (page 340) or kaffir lime leaves (which I keep in the freezer) to store-bought paste for some extra oomph.

'Use by' V 'best before'
The use-by date tells you when a food must be eaten for health and safety reasons. The best-before date gives a rough indication of when it's best to eat. Many countries have removed best-before dates. I personally ignore them. You should, too. If meat or fish is marked down because the 'use-by' date is approaching, buy it up and freeze it. The quality will be preserved instantly. Just ensure that you consume it within 2–3 months and that you don't refreeze it once thawed.

Ugly veggies made pretty

FOODS YOU SHOULD REALLY BUY ORGANIC

You might not be flush enough to buy your whole market haul from the organic section, but the following stuff is worth the investment. I've tried to keep this simple.

Almonds: Many toxic pesticides and herbicides are used on almond trees. Due to almonds' high fat content, the chemicals are easily retained.

Beef: Non-organic beef can be treated with growth-promoting hormones – regardless of whether it's grass-finished or not. Interestingly, Australia deems these hormones unfit for chooks but okay for cows.

USDA data shows 52 different pesticide residues on a fresh blueberry compared to 21 on a frozen blueberry.

Berries: These are more contaminated than any other fruit and have some of the highest levels of pesticide contamination recorded for any produce. If you can't find local, organic ones, it might be better to buy them frozen. Why? Berries farmed to be frozen are sprayed way less than those destined to be sold fresh since fresh ones need more chemicals to maintain shelf life.

Chicken and eggs: Organic is the ONLY way to eat chicken. Free-range birds might be able to move outside a cage but they can still be fed nasty chemical-laden feed and supplements. Most consumer authorities say it's worth investing in organic chook products. This is especially important if you're eating the whole chook (which we do in this book); you don't want chemicals leaching from bones. Or into the eggs.

Coffee: Not just a hipster affectation! Coffee can be a significant source of pesticides. Coffee beans are heavily sprayed (coffee from overseas is fumigated when entering Australia).

Dairy products: The high fat content in dairy retains any chemicals ingested by the cow.

Peanut butter: Peanut shells are super-porous and any chemical or pesticide is easily absorbed into the meat of the nut. The high fat content of peanuts also allows for easy absorption (and retention) of these chemicals. However, be careful with the organic stuff, too. Peanuts easily attract fungus and mould, the most problematic being aflatoxins, which have carcinogenic and liver-damaging effects. If you buy organic, be sure to refrigerate it.

Thin-skinned fruit: Soft fruits with fine skin (including stone fruit, apples and pears) absorb and retain more pesticides than fruits with thicker skin like bananas and melons. Scrubbing and even peeling doesn't eliminate the residue completely.

Veggies that can't be peeled: Especially thin-skinned veggies like peppers and celery. And leafy greens. With veggies that have no protective skin, it's almost impossible to wash off the chemicals. The leafiness of leafy greens and herbs means the chemicals permeate the plant's structure. Rosemary and spinach in particular have been shown to retain high levels of chemical residues.

SORT AND STORE

Once you get your shopping home, you need to sort it and store it. You might think, *Really!? I have to do annoying prep stuff after enduring the shops?* Yeah, you do. It doesn't take long and it will save you time down the track. PS I do my unpacking, storing, and the next bit – par-cooking, freezing and preserving (see page 22) – all in one hit.

HOW TO STORE YOUR FRESH STUFF

Most vegetables are best in the fridge. Onions and potatoes are outliers. Leave them in a cabinet or pantry, alone in the dark, away from the other vegetables and each other.

Cucumber, tomatoes, peppers, squash, aubergines and courgettes: Don't wash these until you need them. Leave at room temperature (if your house is cool i.e. 12–20°C, and you're eating them within 2–3 days) or in the fridge in paper bags (but off the bottom shelf, which is usually the coldest part).

Lemons: Keep in a *sealed* bag – they'll last up to a month this way. Yep.

Carrots: Trim off the green tops (they will draw nutrients and flavour from the roots) and store them as you would herbs (see opposite). Place the carrots in the fridge in a covered container filled with water.

If you've cut open an unripe avo, sprinkle the flesh with lemon juice, place back together, cover with cling film and return to the fridge. It'll soften up without browning.

Avocado: Store unripe avos in a paper bag on the worktop with a banana or apple – they'll ripen within 5 days.

Beetroot: Remove the leaves and store them as you would herbs (see opposite). Don't wash the beets – the dirt helps them hold moisture. Keep beetroot in the crisper, in a bag if you like.

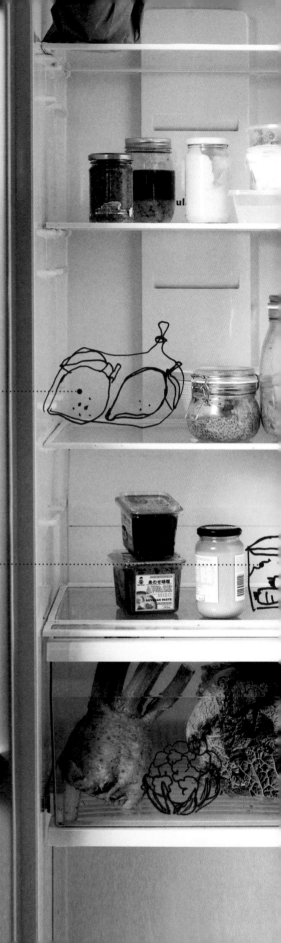

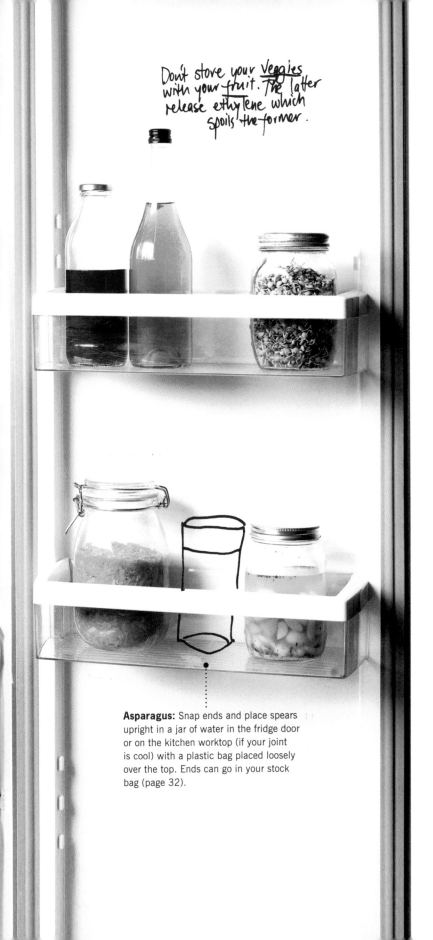

Don't store your veggies with your fruit. The latter release ethylene which spoils the former.

Spring onions: Plant the whole bunch in a pot of soil or in your garden, removing a whole stem as you need it. Or place in a jar, glass or clear vase of water on the windowsill and cut off the green tops as you need them.

Meat: Store in the meat compartment in your fridge if you're going to do a cook-up in the next 3 days; otherwise freeze in meal-sized batches.

Kale and other greens: To be honest, it's best to cook and eat these ASAP, but if you want to store them, do it the same way as you do lettuce (see below). Put the stalks in your stock bag (see page 32).

Or use the bath towel trick: lay the leaves on an old towel and roll up into a log. You then unroll as required, revealing a few leaves at a time!

Lettuce: Cut away the stalk, pull apart the leaves, wash in a sink of cold water, then dry and store as per the herbs, below.

Herbs: Wrap in tea towels or re-usable cloth (kitchen paper if you must), stacked together in a big container with a lid or in a large zip-lock bag. Or you can trim the roots and place in a jar or glass with water and stick a plastic bag loosely over the top. Both work well.

I use hospital bandage fabric you can get from the chemist.

Watercress: Wash immediately in a sink of water, dry really well (see below) and store as you would herbs.

How to dry watercress (and other leafy greens)
Place your washed greens inside a clean pillowcase or washing bag. Go outside and swing the bag around madly. Or place the bag in the washing machine on the spin cycle for 20 seconds. I'm serious. Cress will last more than a week this way.

Asparagus: Snap ends and place spears upright in a jar of water in the fridge door or on the kitchen worktop (if your joint is cool) with a plastic bag placed loosely over the top. Ends can go in your stock bag (page 32).

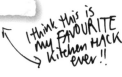

I think this is my FAVOURITE kitchen HACK ever !!

THINGS YOU CAN PUT STRAIGHT INTO THE FREEZER

As a general rule, proteins and fruit are best frozen raw, while most veggies are best frozen par-cooked. Freezing food that is as fresh as possible ensures the quality is maintained, as it slows the normal breakdown of foods by bacteria. Here are my tips for freezing your haul:

Always keep your freezer full.
It's more energy efficient than an empty one as solids freeze at a lower temperature than air.

Wash them in soapy water, rinse, turn inside out and stick to your splashback or window to dry.

If you use zip-lock bags:
Divide cooled veggies and meat into 'per serve' portions and line them up like books to save space and to generally be An Organised Person. (You can wash and re-use your bags.)

Avoid using plastic containers if you can.
But don't go out and buy new containers: use recycled jars as often as possible. Or invest in quality Pyrex baking dishes that can be used for cooking as well.

Always leave a good 2 cm free at the top.
Liquid expands when frozen, so this will ensure the container doesn't crack.

RAW BUCKWHEAT

PUMPKIN OR SWEET POTATO PURÉE
(see page 23)

PAR-COOKED 'N' FROZEN VEGGIES
(see page 22)

Other things people put in their freezer:
* credit cards (in a cup of water, frozen) — Ingrid
* ex-boyfriends' names written on a bit of paper
* jeans (instead of washing them; avoids fading)

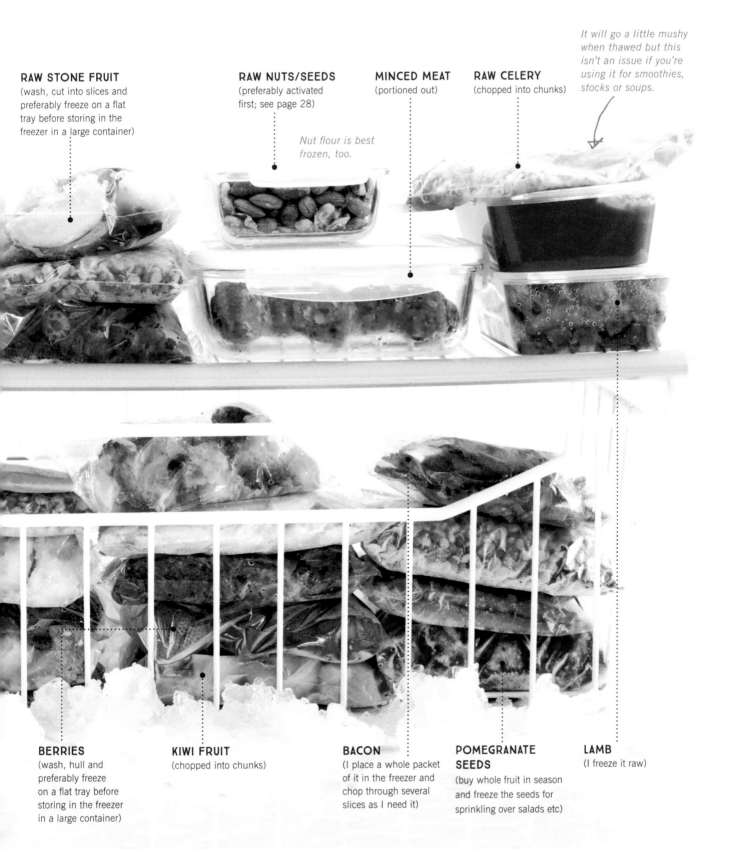

RAW STONE FRUIT
(wash, cut into slices and preferably freeze on a flat tray before storing in the freezer in a large container)

RAW NUTS/SEEDS
(preferably activated first; see page 28)

Nut flour is best frozen, too.

MINCED MEAT
(portioned out)

RAW CELERY
(chopped into chunks)

It will go a little mushy when thawed but this isn't an issue if you're using it for smoothies, stocks or soups.

BERRIES
(wash, hull and preferably freeze on a flat tray before storing in the freezer in a large container)

KIWI FRUIT
(chopped into chunks)

BACON
(I place a whole packet of it in the freezer and chop through several slices as I need it)

POMEGRANATE SEEDS
(buy whole fruit in season and freeze the seeds for sprinkling over salads etc)

LAMB
(I freeze it raw)

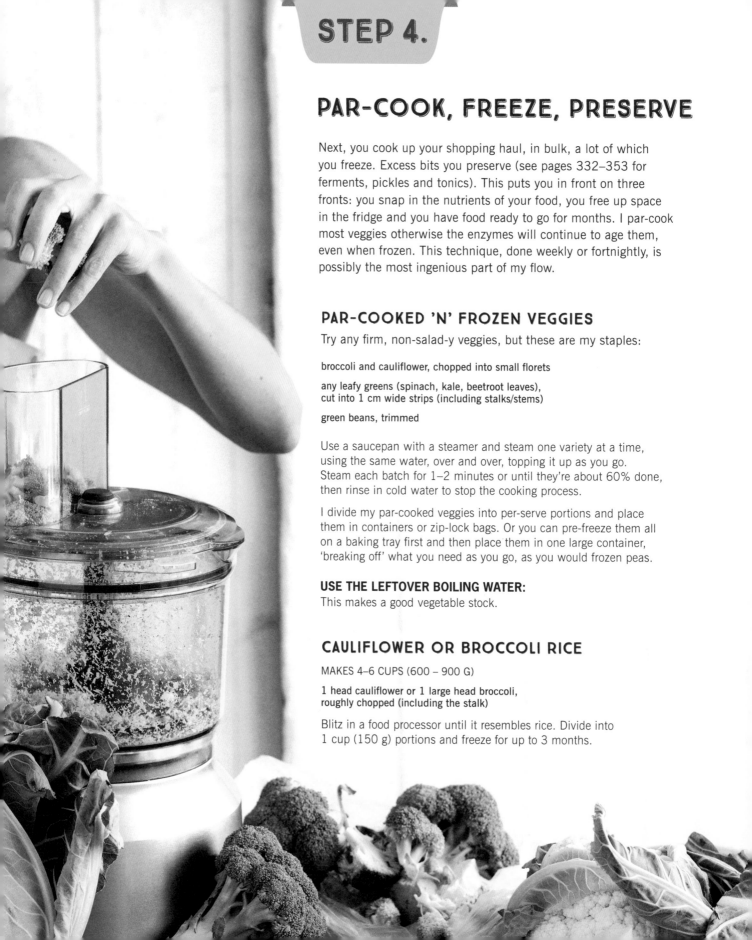

PAR-COOK, FREEZE, PRESERVE

Next, you cook up your shopping haul, in bulk, a lot of which you freeze. Excess bits you preserve (see pages 332–353 for ferments, pickles and tonics). This puts you in front on three fronts: you snap in the nutrients of your food, you free up space in the fridge and you have food ready to go for months. I par-cook most veggies otherwise the enzymes will continue to age them, even when frozen. This technique, done weekly or fortnightly, is possibly the most ingenious part of my flow.

PAR-COOKED 'N' FROZEN VEGGIES

Try any firm, non-salad-y veggies, but these are my staples:

broccoli and cauliflower, chopped into small florets

any leafy greens (spinach, kale, beetroot leaves),
cut into 1 cm wide strips (including stalks/stems)

green beans, trimmed

Use a saucepan with a steamer and steam one variety at a time, using the same water, over and over, topping it up as you go. Steam each batch for 1–2 minutes or until they're about 60% done, then rinse in cold water to stop the cooking process.

I divide my par-cooked veggies into per-serve portions and place them in containers or zip-lock bags. Or you can pre-freeze them all on a baking tray first and then place them in one large container, 'breaking off' what you need as you go, as you would frozen peas.

USE THE LEFTOVER BOILING WATER:
This makes a good vegetable stock.

CAULIFLOWER OR BROCCOLI RICE

MAKES 4–6 CUPS (600 – 900 G)

1 head cauliflower or 1 large head broccoli,
roughly chopped (including the stalk)

Blitz in a food processor until it resembles rice. Divide into
1 cup (150 g) portions and freeze for up to 3 months.

While you have the oven on ...
Make some Carrot 'Bacon' (page 115), Vegan 'Mince' (page 186), Celery Leaf Salt (page 265) or The Whole Brassicus Hummus (page 187).

COOKED 'N' FROZEN BEETROOT

4–5 beets (reserve the leaves for Leftovers Pesto; page 55), trimmed, scrubbed and pricked with a fork (don't peel them!)

Preheat the oven to 180°C (gas 4). Place the beets on a baking tray (no oil, no salt, no baking paper) and cook for 30 minutes until just tender. Cool and peel (I don't as I like the texture of the skin), then place in the freezer.

ROASTED ROOTS

Roasted vegetables taste better after a few days. Use them in Leftover Mishmashes (pages 246–65) and Abundance Bowls (pages 126–37). Depending on the season, you might choose from:

1 pumpkin or squash, peeled, seeded (use a big spoon to scrape them out) and chopped into 4 cm chunks

2–3 sweet potatoes, scrubbed and chopped into 4 cm chunks

4–5 parsnips, carrots and/or turnips, cut into 4 cm chunks

brussels sprouts, trimmed (halve them if they're particularly large)

a few sprigs rosemary

1–2 heads garlic, tops trimmed

butter, ghee or coconut oil, melted, for drizzling

sea salt

Preheat the oven to 180°C (gas 4).

Place the veggies on a large baking tray with the rosemary and garlic. Drizzle over the butter, ghee or oil and salt and toss with your hands. Place on the middle shelf in the oven and roast for 40–60 minutes. Squeeze out the garlic cloves and pull the rosemary leaves from the charred twig. Once cool, store the veg in the fridge for 3–4 days.

PUMPKIN OR SWEET POTATO PURÉE

MAKES 4–6 CUPS (1–1.5 LITRES) ← *Any pumpkin or squash is fine.*

1 pumpkin (about 2–3 kg), cut into 4 big wedges, or 4 large sweet potatoes, scrubbed and left whole

2 tablespoons butter, ghee or coconut oil

pinch of sea salt

Preheat the oven to 180°C (gas 4). Scoop out and discard the pumpkin seeds and pulp. Place the pumpkin or sweet potato on a baking tray and rub with the butter, ghee or oil and salt. Bake on the middle oven rack until tender – about 1 hour. (If you're pressed for time, cut the pumpkin or spuds into smaller chunks and bake for 30 minutes.) Scoop out the pumpkin flesh (or slip off the sweet potato skins when they've cooled) and purée using a stick blender or a potato masher. Once cool, freeze in 1 cup (250 ml) batches or ice-cube trays.

USE THE LEFTOVER SWEET POTATO SKINS:
Pan-fry in coconut oil or bacon fat over a high heat with a big sprinkle of salt to make chips.

MASSAGED KALE OR BEET GREENS

Don't laugh! There is seriously such a thing. Kale and beet greens are fibrous and, when eaten raw, hard on the guts and quite bitter. 'Kneading' or 'massaging' the stuff with some dressing with oil and acid softens it and pre-digests it for us. The leaves will darken, shrink in size and become silky in texture and sweeter in taste. Plus, a robustly massaged kale or beet salad will keep for up to a week in the fridge.

1 bunch kale, stems removed, leaves torn (or 1 bunch beetroot, leaves torn)

1/3 cup (75 ml) Powerhouse Dressing (page 53), or 2 tablespoons each of olive oil and lemon juice

1 teaspoon sea salt

In a bowl combine all the ingredients and massage the leaves – like, a deep-tissue one, squeezing and kneading – for 5 minutes or until soft and wilted. Eat as is or use in a salad.

TWO PAGES OF THINGS I LIKE TO DO WITH MY ICE-CUBE TRAY

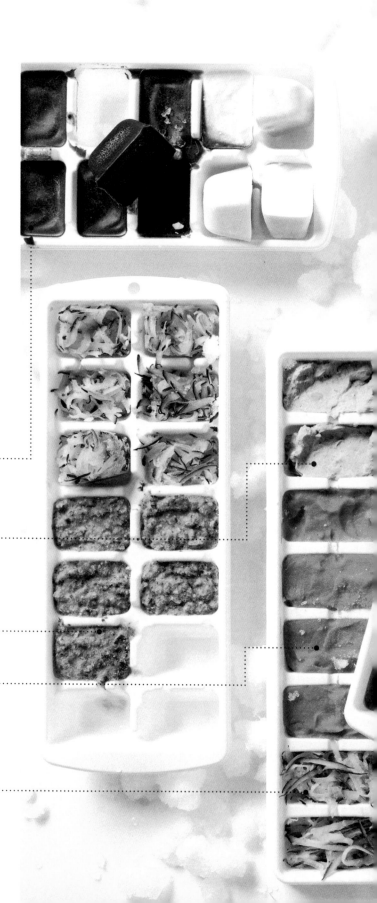

Here's how it works, for cooking flow:
1. Freeze leftover bits 'n' bobs in tray
2. Once frozen, pop your leftovers cube out + place in a freezer-proof container (thus freeing up your tray)
3. Label your bags
4. Use your cubes to deglaze, add liquid, bulk or flavour stuff.

Basic Raw Chocolate (page 56): Instant hot chocolate recipe: plonk a cube into a cup of simmering milk. Imbibe. Or for an instant treat, melt a cube and drizzle over ice cream.

Leftover avocado: Purée with coconut water or coconut cream and/or a little lime juice. Perfect for making Misomite (page 54), Green Minx Dressing (page 54), smoothies, and Leftovers Pesto (page 55).

Pesto and dressings: A cube is the perfect size for a single serve. Use with pasta, Abundance Bowls (pages 126–37), salad, fish, meat.

Pumpkin or Sweet Potato Purée (page 23): Add to casseroles, pasta and anything that needs a mock-tomato hit. Or toss into smoothies, hot chocolate, muffins or slices in place of sweetener (just add some chia seeds to soak up liquid if used in baking).

Grated raw courgettes: Smoothie fodder.

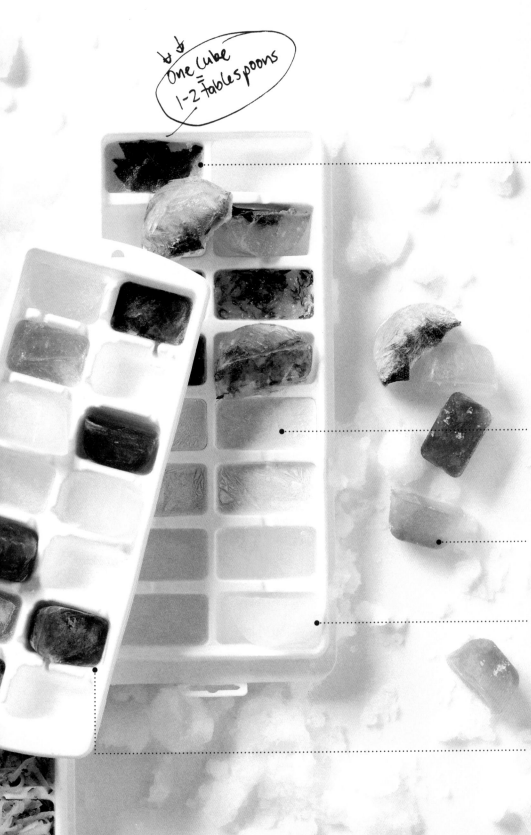

One Cube = 1–2 Tablespoons

Cooked greens: Purée and freeze – great to toss into smoothies, sauces or wherever you feel the need to up the nutrient ante.

Herbs in oil, wine or stock: One-third fill each cube with chopped fresh herbs (parsley, thyme, rosemary, sage and oregano work best) and top with the dregs of a wine bottle, stock or olive oil. Chuck into casseroles and soups, or use them to sweat your veggies instead of sautéing them in oil.

Egg whites: Transfer the cubes to a sealed freezer-proof container and use them within 12 months (really!). And make sure you thaw them completely before using – they'll beat better at room temperature.

Egg yolks: So that they don't turn to jelly, beat in ⅛ teaspoon salt for every 3 large yolks. When using in cooking, substitute 1 tablespoon thawed egg yolk for 1 fresh yolk.

Whole eggs: If you're worried you won't use the whole carton before they go off, whisk a few eggs and pour into a tray ready to add to omelettes.

Coconut milk, coconut cream, coconut water: Ready to toss into smoothies, or to use in recipes when you need small amounts.

Berries with coconut cream: Pop a few berries in and top with cream or yoghurt to eat as a sweet treat (or for smoothies).

Stock: Great for using up the stock that didn't fit into the bigger containers (see pages 42–3 for recipes). Use to deglaze your pan, or to sweat your veggies instead of sautéing in oil.

Lemon and lime juice: Citrus juice is a bugger to prepare a tablespoon at a time. Make in bulk in your blender (or juicer) and freeze in 1–2 tablespoon serves ready to go.

Lard and dripping: Use cubes to braise, deglaze or sauté your veggies. Or pour over herbs and freeze in cubes (see above).

Leftover sauces and stew liquid: A great way to keep the dregs of a delicious sauce (e.g. Watercress Sauce; page 176) or stew. Use for braising, deglazing and Leftover Mishmashes (pages 246–65).

BEANS, GRAINS, NUTS AND SEEDS

You might know the toxin drill surrounding BGNSs by now.
No? It goes like this:

* Most of the little buggers contain anti-nutrients – chiefly enzyme inhibitors that make them difficult to digest – and phytic acid, which binds to minerals and prevents their full absorption.

* This doesn't mean BGNSs should be banned from your diet. It just means choosing the least toxic varieties, preparing them right – soaking and fermenting (as our grandmothers did) – and eating them in moderation.

* Soaking and sprouting or fermenting BGNSs breaks down the phytic acid so you don't get the mineral-leaching thing going on; helps to release beneficial nutrients, making them more bioavailable (more easily digested); *and* creates enzymes that further assist digestion of the proteins and fibres. Triple boon!

COOKED QUINOA

Before cooking, quinoa must be rinsed well – twice – to remove the toxic but naturally occurring coating, saponin.

MAKES 4 CUPS (540 G)

1 cup (225 g) quinoa, rinsed
and drained twice

2 cups (500 ml) water

Place the quinoa in a saucepan and pour in the water. Cover and bring to the boil. Reduce the heat and simmer, covered, for 15 minutes or until all the water has been absorbed. Remove the pan from the heat and let it stand for 5 minutes, covered. Fluff the quinoa with a fork. Divide into 1 cup (135 g) portions and freeze for up to 6 months (or store in the fridge for 4–5 days).

MAKE IT EVEN MORE NUTRITIOUS:
Activate your quinoa first.
Cover 1 heaped cup (250 g) of well-rinsed quinoa with water and add 2 tablespoons of acid (apple cider vinegar, lemon juice or whey). Cover with a tea towel and leave for 12–24 hours before cooking.

ACTIVATED AND
COOKED QUINOA

RAW QUINOA

Buckwheat can get awfully confusing

Buckwheat 'groats' are the raw seeds that look like little light tan/green pyramids. You cook and eat these like you would quinoa or rice, and you can sprout them for salads. Activated groaties (also called buckinis) are soaked and then dried at a low temperature. They are ready to eat as is, as soup toppers or a crunchy cereal or in desserts. They can also be cooked as you would raw groats, but take less time. Kasha is the name for raw groats that have been toasted. Got it?

Buckwheat V quinoa

* Both are high in protein, containing all the essential amino acids. Buckwheat comes out slightly on top. (I'm not concerned about vitamin and mineral content – you'll get bigger doses from veggies and meat.)

* Both are gluten-free and relatively low in toxins, if prepared correctly.

* But buckwheat is much higher in antioxidants than quinoa.

* And buckwheat is more ethically sound. The popularity of quinoa in the West has left traditional South American communities starving as they can no longer afford the stuff.

* Also, buckwheat is often grown as a rotation crop to prime the soil for grains. It's a leftover before it even gets to the packet!

* Finally, buckwheat is faster to cook (less electricity!) and I personally love the toasty, caramel-y flavour and texture of activated groaties.

COOKED BUCKWHEAT

MAKES 8 CUPS (1.3 KG)

2 cups (350 g) raw buckwheat groats

3 cups (750 ml)) Homemade Stock (page 42) or water

½ teaspoon sea salt

I put mine on to soak just as I go to bed

Soak the buckwheat overnight in plenty of water (buckwheat is thirsty stuff). The next day, rinse well, drain and plonk in a saucepan with the stock or water, and the salt.

Bring to the boil, then reduce to a simmer and cook for about 8 minutes, until all the water is absorbed. When done, allow to sit for 5 minutes with the lid on and then fluff with a fork. Divide into ½ cup (80 g) serves and freeze for up to 3 months.

MAKE IT FASTER:

Instead of soaking, you can also reduce some of the phytic acid by toasting the groats in a dry frying pan (no oil) over a medium–low heat for 5 minutes before adding the water. Cook for 15 minutes.

Buckwheat is relatively high in phytase (the good enzyme that breaks down phytic acid), so keep the soak time to 7–8 hours max, or it will become too mushy. Bear in mind a bit of mushiness is normal, though.

ACTIVATED GROATIES

MAKES 4–6 CUPS (ABOUT 850 G)

2 cups (350 g) raw buckwheat groats, soaked overnight, rinsed and drained well

Spread the buckwheat on a large baking tray. Dry in the oven on the lowest temperature possible (no more than 50°C; for gas ovens, on the pilot light) for about 8 hours until crispy. Store in an airtight container in the pantry for 3 months.

MAKE THEM EVEN MORE NUTRITIOUS:

Sprout your buckwheat first by soaking the raw groats for 1–2 hours, then put them in a fine-meshed sieve over a bowl (or in a big jar with a muslin cloth secured over the top) and wash and drain twice a day for 1–2 days, until tiny little tails form (see page 352 for more info about sprouting). Then dry in the oven as above.

MAKE THEM SWEET SPICE GROATIES:

Combine soaked or sprouted buckwheat with 3 teaspoons of Pumpkin Spice Mix (page 45) or 2 teaspoons of ground cinnamon and 1 teaspoon of ground nutmeg.

MAKE THEM SALTED CARAMEL GROATIES:

Combine soaked or sprouted buckwheat with 2 teaspoons of maca, 1 teaspoon of sea salt and 1 teaspoon of ground cinnamon.

MAKE THEM MIDDLE EASTERN GROATIES:

Combine soaked or sprouted buckwheat with 1 tablespoon of Ras el Hanout Mix (page 45) and 1 teaspoon of sea salt.

SPROUTED BUCKWHEAT

ACTIVATED GROATIES

RAW BUCKWHEAT GROATS

COOKED BEANS AND LEGUMES

MAKES 3 CUPS (750 ML)

I'm not a paid-up fan of legumes (oh, the bloat), but when prepared and cooked properly they're a reasonably nutritious addition to the diet and an economical way to pad out a dish. Most books at this point feature a highly complex chart of different soaking and cooking times for the myriad beans and legumes out there. A waste of paper and your sweet time! I assure you it can be as flow-y as this:

I soak my lentils for 7 hours, even though most people don't.

1 cup (200 g) dried beans (any type, even lentils or mung beans)

3 cups (750 ml) hot water

1 tablespoon whey, apple cider vinegar or lemon juice

Optional, but it will break down the phytic acid even more.

Place all of the ingredients in a bowl and leave to soak overnight. The next morning, drain and transfer to a saucepan. Cover with water and bring to the boil over a medium heat. Boil for 10 minutes, then reduce the heat and simmer until the beans are soft (up to 1 hour).

Cool and divide into 1 cup (250 ml) portions (½ beans and ½ their cooking liquid). Beans and stock will keep in the fridge for 3–4 days like this. Or you can freeze for up to 6 months.

ACTIVATED NUTS AND SEEDS

Activating brings digestive benefits as well as producing a crunchier, slightly toasty version of the original nut or seed. Worth the stigma!

1 packet of raw nuts or seeds (e.g. almonds, pumpkin seeds, walnuts)

pinch of sea salt

Place the nuts or seeds in a bowl with plenty of water. Add the salt, cover and leave to soak overnight.

The next morning, drain the nuts/seeds. Spread them out on a baking tray (no oil, no baking paper) and dry in the oven for 12–24 hours at the lowest temperature possible (less than 65ºC; for gas ovens, on the pilot light). When cool, store in a sealed container in the freezer.

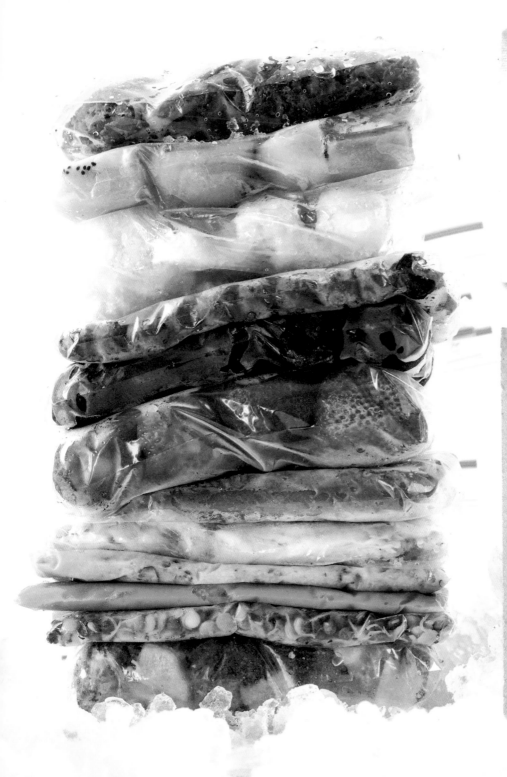

HOW LONG IN THE FREEZER?

You can actually freeze food indefinitely (from a safety POV) but for par-cooked and frozen veggies, a 3-month store is best for optimal texture and flavour. As for other foods, here are some recommended freezing times:

Fish (cooked) – 1 month

Meat soup – 2 months

Meat (cooked) – 2 months

Beans, grains, nuts and seeds (cooked) – 3 months

HOW TO FREEZE AND THAW STUFF PROPERLY

Always cool food first so it freezes fast; a slow freeze will cause the water cells to expand, which ruptures the food and denatures it.

Defrost food slowly in the fridge (over a day or two is best), though some ingredients can be tossed into your smoothie, stew, soup, pasta sauce etc frozen.

You can refreeze food that's been thawing in the fridge, if you realise you're not going to eat it . . . so long as it's still *very* cold or partially frozen.

Let meat, poultry and seafood thaw in the fridge (don't leave it out on the worktop for more than 2 hours). Stew meat, poultry and seafood should stay good for about 2 days, while red meat cuts (such as beef, pork or lamb roasts, chops and steaks) are good for 3–5 days after thawing.

USE YOUR LEFTOVERS

This is not really a separate step in my simplicious flow, but sort of happens along the way, both when I sort, store and pre-cook produce, and when I do cook-ups and make meals for mates. I've just put it in one spot so you can see how it fits in.

Please note that it would make me immensely happy if you were to regard this bit of the book and my Leftovers recipe chapter as the most important and interesting parts. Chuck on a Post-it, pull out a highlighter, if you must. I will hug you if I see evidence of this when you greet me at a book signing down the track. Promise!

FIRST, USE YOUR LEFTOVER SUGAR

Let's walk the leftovers talk from the get-go. Don't toss your sugar when you quit the stuff. Put it to good use.

1. MAKE AN AYURVEDIC FACE SCRUB

1 cup (225 g) sugar

1/3 cup (75 g) coconut oil, softened (or use 75 ml olive oil)

1 teaspoon pure vanilla extract (or make your own; page 45) and/or one of the oils or spices below

Combine all of the ingredients in a glass jar with a lid. It will keep in your bathroom for 2 months.

To use, take 1 tablespoon and apply to a very slightly moistened, clean face (you don't want it too wet, or the scrub will dissolve). Massage in circles. Rinse with warm water.

CHOOSE YOUR OWN SPICE ADVENTURE

For Kaphas (or during winter): Replace half the sugar with 1/2 cup (115 g) of salt and add some dried sage or rosemary and 5 drops of eucalyptus oil.

For Vatas (or when it's windy): Replace some of the sugar with honey and add 1 teaspoon of Pumpkin Spice Mix (page 45), or 1 teaspoon of ground nutmeg, cinnamon or cardamom, or 5–10 drops of lavender, rose, sandalwood or geranium oil.

For Pittas (or during summer): Add 1 teaspoon of ground turmeric or rosewater or 5–10 drops of jasmine or rose oil.

2. KEEP YOUR FLOWERS ALIVE

Dissolve 1 tablespoon of sugar in 2 tablespoons of white vinegar and add the syrup to a vase of water. The simple carbs in the sugar will help the flowers stay strong and the vinegar will kill bacteria and keep bugs away from the vase.

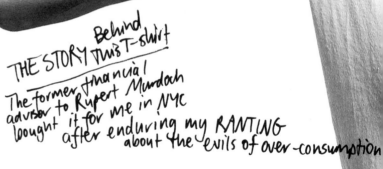

THE STORY Behind this T-shirt
The former financial advisor to Rupert Murdoch bought it for me in NYC after enduring my RANTING about the evils of over-consumption

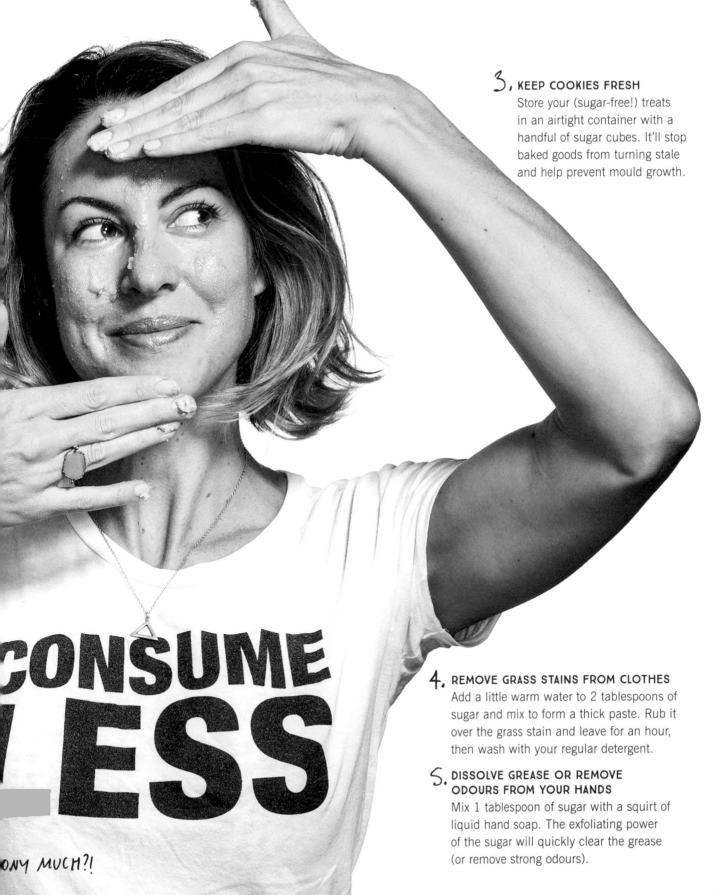

3. KEEP COOKIES FRESH
Store your (sugar-free!) treats in an airtight container with a handful of sugar cubes. It'll stop baked goods from turning stale and help prevent mould growth.

4. REMOVE GRASS STAINS FROM CLOTHES
Add a little warm water to 2 tablespoons of sugar and mix to form a thick paste. Rub it over the grass stain and leave for an hour, then wash with your regular detergent.

5. DISSOLVE GREASE OR REMOVE ODOURS FROM YOUR HANDS
Mix 1 tablespoon of sugar with a squirt of liquid hand soap. The exfoliating power of the sugar will quickly clear the grease (or remove strong odours).

CONSUME LESS

ONY MUCH?!

PACK UP YOUR SCRAPS AS YOU GO

I keep all the peels, leaves, stalks, offcuts, bones and other leftovers in bags or containers, ready to turn into stocks, smoothies and pestos. If I don't have time to make something straight away, I whack the bags in the freezer.

CREATE A VEGETABLE STOCK BAG

Place onion and carrot tops, celery bits, herb stalks, parmesan rinds etc in a freezer-proof bag in the freezer ready to make veggie stocks or to add to meat stocks or to cooked beans. Don't save the following for stocks (they're too overpowering): cabbage, brussels sprouts, broccoli, cauliflower, turnips or artichokes.

You'll need about 4 cups (600 g) of leftover veggies to make 2 litres of stock.

I keep a separate bag for asparagus stock (page 43).

CREATE A CHICKEN OR BEEF BONES STOCK BAG

Reserve raw bones or cooked bones from chicken or beef, literally off people's plates after they've eaten, until you have about 1–2 kg (see Homemade Stock; page 42).

CREATE A FISH STOCK BAG

You need a good couple of carcasses to make fish stock (see page 42). Collect them over time. Add leek and fennel offcuts to this bag.

CREATE A LEFTOVERS PESTO BAG

Put aside stems, stalks and excess leaves from your kale, beets, mint, parsley, coriander, leafy greens, carrot tops etc. The pesto works best if you use no more than 2–3 different herbs or greens in one batch (see page 55).

CREATE A SMOOTHIE BAG

Grated courgettes, celery offcuts, herbs, leftover cooked greens, and fruit offcuts go into this one.

HOW I USE CONDIMENT LEFTOVERS TO MAKE FLAVOUR BOMBS

* **THE BRINE OR OIL FROM OLIVES** goes into dressings.

* **THE OLIVE OIL FROM ANCHOVIES** goes into dressings.

* **THE OLIVE OIL AND HERBS FROM MARINATED FETA** go into dressings or are used for cooking.

* **THE BRINE OR SPRING WATER FROM TUNA** is used to sauté or deglaze.

* **THE SALT FROM CAPERS** seasons dishes.

* **THE JAR CONTAINING DRIED MUSTARD DREGS** becomes my salad-dressing shaking jar.

REGROW YOUR BUTT

Oh, the joy of taking a root and shooting it, watching it grow and eating it all over. Oh, and in the meantime, using the budding beauty as a room decoration. Here are my favourite regrowth projects:

Perpetual spring onions: Either plonk a bunch directly into a pot of soil, or sprout the white root ends in a glass jar filled with water, and leave in a sunny position. Within days it will shoot and you can use new shoots as required, leaving the white root in (fresh) water to keep growing.

Coriander and lemongrass: As above, using the 'white root in water method'.

Pak choi, celery and cos lettuce: As above, regrow the white root, but in a shallow bowl of water – enough to cover the roots but not the top of the cutting. Place in a sunny position, topping up the water as required. After a few days, roots and leaves will appear. After a week, transplant it into soil with just the leaves showing above the soil. The plant will continue to grow, and within a few weeks it will sprout a whole new head.

Ginger and turmeric: You know how they sprout if you leave them on the worktop too long? Simply place in a pot of soil with the newest buds facing upwards, leave in a filtered light position and water regularly. It will grow a big indoor-plant-like frond within days (rather handsome). After a few weeks, pull up the whole plant, roots and all. Remove a piece of the root (to eat), and re-plant it to repeat the process.

Pineapple: I don't actually eat the stuff (it's pretty high in fructose), but I inherited two recently and a) gave one to my parents; b) cut the fronds off the other to regrow a pineapple for fun and decorative purposes (it takes 2 years for the thing to reach edible stage); and c) froze the fruit, in pieces, to use sparingly in smoothies.

To regrow, grab the fronds and give them a hefty twist to remove them neatly from the fruit bit. Cut away any bits of fruit attached (if any). Pull off enough leaves to expose 2.5 cm of stalk. Then, carefully shave off small slices from the bottom of the stalk until you reveal root buds (small brown dots on the flat base of the stalk). Place in a jar of water in the sun for a week. Once roots shoot, pot in soil and enjoy its hipster, pot-planty effect for the next few years.

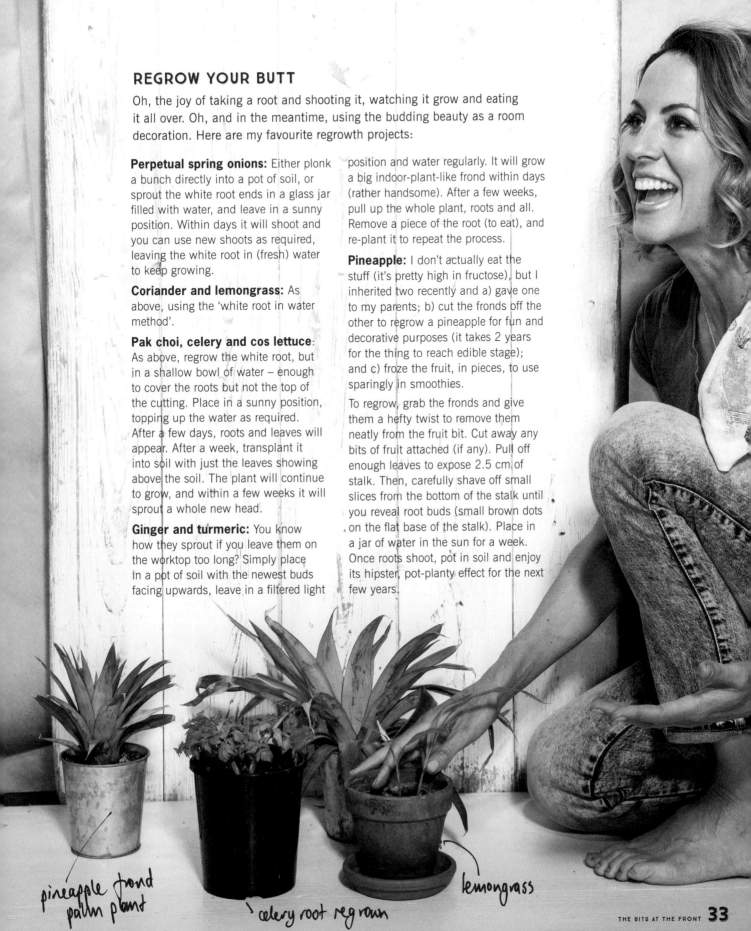

pineapple frond palm plant

celery root regrown

lemongrass

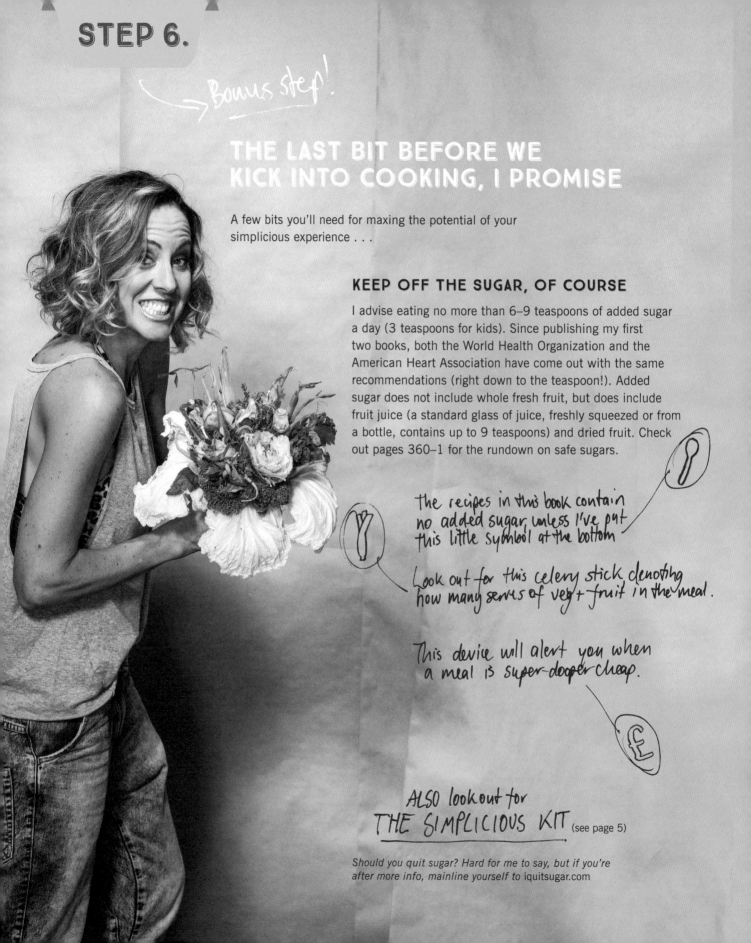

→ Bonus step!

THE LAST BIT BEFORE WE KICK INTO COOKING, I PROMISE

A few bits you'll need for maxing the potential of your simplicious experience . . .

KEEP OFF THE SUGAR, OF COURSE

I advise eating no more than 6–9 teaspoons of added sugar a day (3 teaspoons for kids). Since publishing my first two books, both the World Health Organization and the American Heart Association have come out with the same recommendations (right down to the teaspoon!). Added sugar does not include whole fresh fruit, but does include fruit juice (a standard glass of juice, freshly squeezed or from a bottle, contains up to 9 teaspoons) and dried fruit. Check out pages 360–1 for the rundown on safe sugars.

the recipes in this book contain no added sugar, unless I've put this little symbol at the bottom

Look out for this celery stick denoting how many serves of veg + fruit in the meal.

This device will alert you when a meal is super-dooper cheap.

ALSO lookout for
THE SIMPLICIOUS KIT (see page 5)

Should you quit sugar? Hard for me to say, but if you're after more info, mainline yourself to iquitsugar.com

This is also simplicious!

GET LOOSE AND BREAK THE RULES

This is an invitation, not an instruction. Don't peel your vegetables, don't bother browning meat to make stocks and slow-cooked casseroles. When making soup, toss the ingredients in without browning them in oil first. When you make a roast, shred or pull the meat rather than carve it. It generally tastes better and is more appropriate for a secondary cut. Use spice mixes that approximate the combo in a recipe. Go on! Use a microwave if it helps you get a nutritious meal on the table.

BUILD YOUR MEALS RIGHT

This is how I go about making my meals. Every meal should aim to work to these proportions.

1. **Start with 2–3 serves of vegetables.** Even at breakfast. 'Eat mostly plants' is a good way to operate.

2. **Add a bit of starch or bulk if you need it.** A starch/carb-free diet isn't sustainable for many. My preferred starches/carbs are sweet potato, buckwheat and frozen peas. Use these ingredients to provide sweetness, too.

3. **Toss on some protein.** I use meat to flavour and boost a meal, rather than focusing on it as the starting point.

4. **Add fat.** Generally about 1–2 tablespoons per person, in the form of oil, avocado, dressing, cheese or nuts, and even butter. This is partly for nutrient absorption, partly for flavour and partly for appetite control.

5. **Amp things with some ferment or bitters.** I try to do this at one meal a day. Two tablespoons of sauerkraut or kimchi or 100 ml of tonic or kombucha is enough.

There's a substitutions list on pages 358–9 if you want to be more certain about your creative licence.

What counts as '1 serve'?

Leafy greens (raw) = **1 cup (100 g)**

All other vegetables (raw) = **½ cup (75 g)**

Red meat and pork = **65 g cooked (90–100 g uncooked)**

Fish = **100 g cooked (115 g uncooked)**

Eggs = **2 large ones**

Beans = **1 cup (75 g)**

Nuts = **30 g**

Yoghurt = **100 g (½ cup)**

Milk = **1 cup (250 ml)**

Cheese = **40 g**

What are the daily requirements?

I work to standard dietary guidelines, but up the ante on the nutrients.

Vegetables: 6–8 serves per day; 5 for kids (Australian guidelines are 5–6 per day; 3 for kids)

Protein: 3 serves (Australian guidelines are 2–3)

Remember fat doesn't make us fat, sugar does. The most recent respected science shows there is no link between the consumption of saturated fat and cholesterol in food and cholesterol problems or heart disease.

Make a roster of weekend projects

Choose one or two of the following, set aside a quiet Sunday afternoon and start stocking up your pantry like a bona fide DIY enthusiast. Get the kids on board and work your way through a mix over the next 6 months. These are some fun items I have in my stash at all times:

* **Good for Your Guts Garlic** (takes 2½ minutes to make, but looks fully twee when displayed in your kitchen; page 340)

* **Kimchi** (fun, colourful, fast; page 337)

* **Sauerkraut** (the kids will enjoy the mushing into jars; page 337)

* **Mustard** (when it starts to puff after a few days, things get really exciting; page 336)

* **Sprouted buckwheat** (get the kids to spot when the little critters start to pop; page 27)

* **Cream cheese and whey** (because Miss Muffet liked to eat it; page 46)

Look out for this bit in my recipes, it's pivotal to the simplicious flow.

USE THE LEFTOVER EGG YOLKS: Make an omelette or frittata. Or freeze them.

EMBRACE THE SUNDAY COOK-UP

This concept is a big part of the I Quit Sugar programme. It entails bulk-cooking and freezing your veggies, but also bulk-cooking a dish that provides leftover serves that can be frozen for meals down the track – as well as fun projects that will stock your kitchen with clever condiments (and can be used as gifts, too).

CREATE YOUR OWN FLOWS

Feel free to devise or create your own flows, then share with me on social media. It's an art, a sport.

Create challenges for yourself. I do. Like:

* Making a meal from frozen bits and fridge-door condiments only.

* Just when you think you need to go to the shops, see if you can leave it one extra meal. And then another. And another. Until the fridge is truly bare.

* A meal needs something extra – will frozen peas, a handful of ferment, a portion of frozen sweet potato purée cut it?

* Collect your scraps from preparing a meal. Be deeply satisfied when they can fit into half a fistful. Social media it! I'll look out for your post.

SHARE, BRAG, CONNECT

I'm not just saying it; I do love to see your achievements and creations and flows and ideas on social media.

INSTAGRAM: @_sarahwilson_ and @iquitsugar

FACEBOOK: SarahWilson and IQuitSugar

TWITTER: @_sarahwilson_ and @iquitsugar

Hashtags: #simplicious (or #sarahwilsoneats for leftovers bragging and mishmash meals)

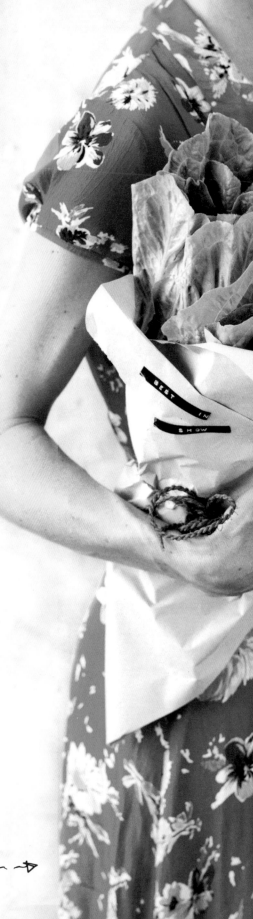

HERE'S ONE OF MY FLOWS

I set aside an hour or two (max) to bulk-cook and prepare a bunch of things. I keep the oven on and my steamer boiling away and off I go.

* Preheat the oven to 90°C (gas ¼). Roast 8 heads garlic.
* Meanwhile, fill the sink with water and dunk the watercress and lettuce. Remove and drain the greens (keep the sink water), then spin and store (page 19).
* Snap asparagus ends and place in stock bag (page 42); store the stems (page 19).
* Load up the slow cooker with veg and stewing steak for my Cheapest Stew Ever (page 212).
* Remove the garlic from the oven and set aside.
* Turn the oven up to 180°C (gas 4). Scrub a few roots in the sink water: 2 sweet potatoes; 1 bunch beets and 1 bunch baby carrots (on special for £1). Pop in the oven for 40–60 minutes. Meanwhile, wash and dry the beet greens and carrot tops, and 1 bunch Swiss chard.
* Boil water in the double steamer and cook a bunch of eggs, then use the same water to steam the beet greens followed by the chard. In the bottom, blanch the carrot tops.
* Use the sink water to cool the eggs and store (page 44).
* Make Leftovers Pesto (page 55) with carrot tops and parmesan. Add the rind to the asparagus stock bag.
* Make Sweet Potato Purée (page 23) with the sweet spud. Pop the carrots and beetroot into containers and leave in the fridge for salads during the week.
* Place all veggie scraps in a vegetable stock bag (page 32).
* Make Good for Your Guts Garlic (page 340) with the roasted cloves, using whey from last week's Homemade Cream Cheese.

And so on I flow . . .

> **Time taken:** 2¼ hours (including doing a load of washing)
> **Fridge/freezer items created:** 12
> **Meals created:** 6–8 (plus heaps more when the stew is cooked)

ENOUGH RUN-UP, LET'S GET TO IT!

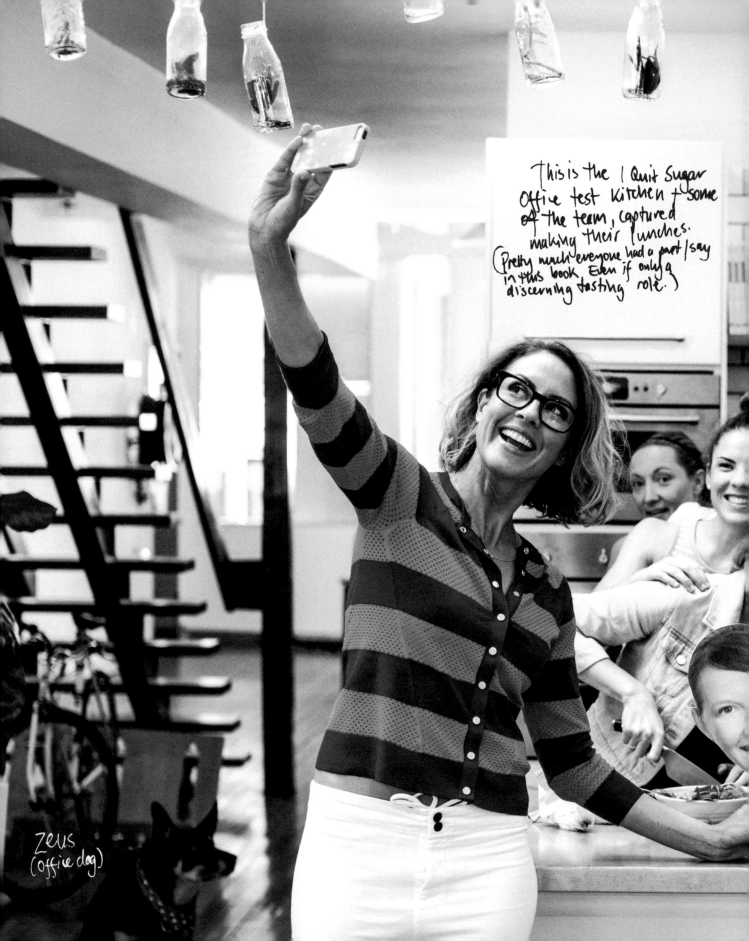

This is the I Quit Sugar Office test kitchen + some of the team, captured making their lunches. (Pretty much everyone had a part/say in this book. Even if only a discerning tasting role.)

Zeus (office dog)

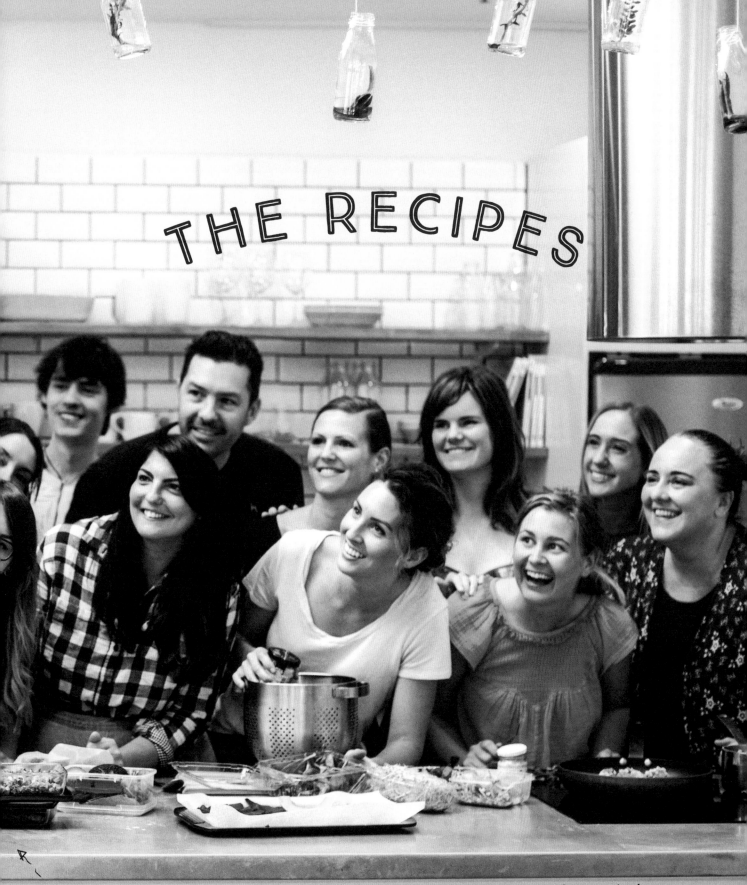

THE RECIPES

This, here, is Zoe my great mate + IQS general manager. On a stick.

THE
BASICS

really rather SIMPLE dressings.

'sauces'
JAMS'
fermented CHEESES
STOCKS

with which to fill
your pantry,
fridge and
FREEZER...

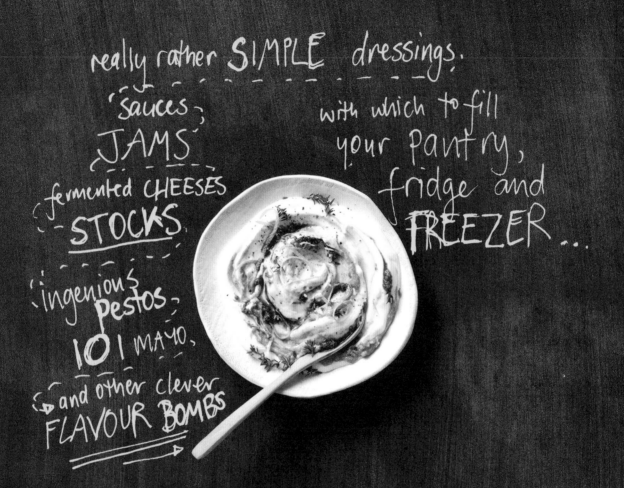

'ingenious Pestos'
101 MAYO,
and other clever
FLAVOUR BOMBS

... so you're 100% sorted + can just get on with cooking.....

HOMEMADE STOCK

Stock is the ultimate leftover foodstuff. I have jars of it in the fridge and freezer at all times. Later on I'll share how to make stock as you prepare meals, but here's how to make stock from scraps. Bone broth or stock is made with cheap bones or carcasses you can get from your butcher, and is simmered for a super-long time. Work to the amounts below, filling your pot with enough water to clear the contents by 5 cm but still leaving 2.5 cm of room at the top of the pot. Each batch you make will come out differently, so don't fret too much about getting it 'right'.

Be aware: food fad cynics hate it when stock is called "broth". Thus, I call it stock. It's the same stuff.

My butcher gives them to me.

FOR BEEF STOCK:

1–2 kg beef bones (marrow, knuckle, ribs, neck)

FOR CHICKEN STOCK:

1–2 leftover (cooked or uncooked) chicken carcasses plus extra bony chicken bits if you have them (wings, necks, feet)

FOR FISH STOCK:

1 kg fish carcasses (heads, tailbones or offcuts of white-fleshed fish – don't use oily fish!)

2 tablespoons apple cider vinegar (or just plain white will do)

1 onion, coarsely chopped

2 cups (300 g) veggie scraps, including peels, coarsely chopped

1 bay leaf or several sprigs of thyme

½ teaspoon dried green or black peppercorns

I include the skin, but some people don't because they reckon it makes the stock bitter.

Whatever you've got – carrot and celery are best. Avoid cabbage, turnips and bitter greens, as they'll make it bitter.

Sourcing fish carcasses
Next time you're at the fishmonger, ask for a bag of fish carcasses. Even better: when buying fillets for a dish, ask your fishmonger to fillet it fresh and keep the carcass. Then you know it's fresh and you have a longer chat with your fishmonger. Which I think is nice.

Place the bones in a very large stockpot with the vinegar and cover with cold water. (For beef stock, soak the bones for 30 minutes before cooking. You can also roast the meatier bones in a 200°C (gas 6) oven for 10 minutes first to make a browner broth. I rarely bother.) Add enough water to cover the bones, but the liquid should come no higher than within 2.5 cm of the rim of the pot, as the volume expands slightly during cooking. (The water should be cold – slow heating helps bring out the flavours.)

Bring to the boil. Reduce the heat and add the onion, veggie scraps, herbs and peppercorns, then simmer:

Beef: 12–72 hours
Chicken: 4–24 hours
Fish: 1–3 hours

When the stock is cool enough, remove the bones, then strain the liquid into a large bowl. (For beef bones, feel free to do a second batch with the same bones and new veggies. It won't be as 'gel-y' or flavoursome, but you'll get extra minerals from it.) Refrigerate the stock until cool and then, using tongs or large spoons, remove the layer of congealed fat on top – you can literally pick it up in chunks (like ice over a pond) – and toss it. (Not always pretty.) Divide the remaining liquid into 1 cup (250 ml) portions and freeze for up to 3 months (for fish stock, 1 month).

MAKE IT IN A SLOW COOKER:
Follow the method above, placing everything in your crock and cooking on low for 8–24 hours.

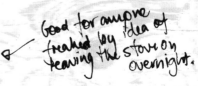

Good for anyone freaked by idea of leaving the stove on overnight.

Stock's healing qualities

* When cooked over a looooong time, minerals leach into the liquid. These minerals are easy to digest in this soupy form and boost the immune system.

* Also released from the bones: glucosamine and chondroitin, which have been shown to help arthritis and joint pain; gelatine, which is a boon for rebuilding the gut lining; and glycine, which is an 'inhibitory' neurotransmitter and promotes sleep and calmness.

* But wait, there's more! Bone broth is also said to be hydrophilic, which means that it facilitates digestion by attracting digestive juices to food, which helps break down tricky to digest foods. I drink the stuff, warmed, when I'm run-down and feel the benefits immediately. It courses through my very being and I'm instantly energised.

PROSCIUTTO–PARMESAN STOCK

Combine some prosciutto rinds or ends, a few pieces of parmesan rind, 2 crushed cloves garlic and a sprig of rosemary in a saucepan with 1–2 litres of water. Bring to the boil, reduce the heat and simmer for 1 hour. Strain.

ASPARAGUS STOCK

Boil the woody stems of 2–3 bunches of asparagus (preferably in leftover asparagus steaming water) for 45 minutes until super-soft. Remove the stems, purée in a blender or food processor then return the purée to the cooking water. Pass the lot through a sieve, pressing with the back of a spoon. You will be left with a purée-ish stock.

CORN COB STOCK

don't be scared of the slobber – all bacteria is boiled into oblivion!

Cover 6 corn cobs (pre-gnawed and stripped of kernels) with 1–2 litres of water. Add a couple of bay leaves and bring to the boil over a medium heat. Simmer for 1 hour. Strain.

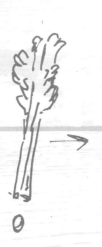

Why celery in stocks and sauces?

Have you noticed it features with carrots and onions in all the classic bases (soffrito, mirepoix)? There's a reason: Japanese scientists have found that when it's cooked slow and low, a bunch of volatile compounds are released that enhance the perception of sweetness and umami from the other ingredients.

PRECOOKED EGGS AND BACON — *true story!*

Eggs will keep for a while in the carton, but it's handy to cook a bunch at a time because they keep great when cooked, too. Ditto, bacon.

Eggs poach better when fresh and boil best when they've been sitting around a while – older eggs are easier to peel!

REALLY SIMPLE POACHED EGGS

I cook half a dozen poachies at a time and store them in a bowl of cold water in the fridge for several days.

white vinegar or rice vinegar (optional)

fresh eggs at room temperature

Fill a small shallow frying pan that has a lid with water (or pour water into a wide saucepan to a depth of 5 cm). Bring to the boil. Add a dash of vinegar if you like – this will help the egg whites to congeal neatly rather than spread out in the water. Break an egg into a teacup, then gently tip the egg from the cup into the water. (You can poach a few eggs at a time, if you like.) Turn off the heat immediately and cover the pan tightly. Leave for 3–4 minutes, then remove each egg with a slotted spoon.

PERFECT BOILED EGGS

I boil in bulk and store the eggs in their shells for up to a week. Place some older eggs (at room temperature) in a saucepan and cover with plenty of cold water. Bring to a gentle boil, uncovered. Remove from the heat, cover with a lid and set your timer.

Soft-boiled: leave in the pan for 4 minutes.

Medium: leave for 8 minutes.

Hard-boiled: leave for 12 minutes.

Drain, then plunge the eggs into cold water. Store in the fridge for up to a week.

How to perfectly peel a boiled egg
Half-fill a sturdy container with water, pop in your boiled egg, seal the lid tightly and shake. You'll have a very cracked egg, but the shell will fall off flawlessly, all done in less than 10 seconds. Rad.

BACON BITS

This entails one of my favourite kitchen hacks – it not only eliminates stinky splattering, but also renders the bacon perfectly.

Remove the rind only from 6–10 rashers of streaky bacon (keep all the fat on) and cut the bacon into 2 cm squares. Place in a frying pan or large saucepan and add just enough water to cover the bottom of the pan. Cook over a medium–high heat until the water has evaporated. Reduce the heat to medium and cook the bacon until crisp (about 10 minutes – no need to turn). This will take longer than frying but is more effective. Remove the bacon and allow to cool on a wire rack over the pan to catch all the juices.

To freeze bacon bits, lay them on a baking tray and place in the freezer. Once frozen, transfer to a freezer-proof container or zip-lock bag and return to the freezer (this will make it easier to snap off what you need).

USE THE LEFTOVER BACON FAT:
It's great for frying eggs and making popcorn. Just drain the rendered fat into a jar (or leave it in the pan ready to cook your next meal). It will keep for a month in the fridge.

PANTRY
FLAVOUR BOMBS

I'll be using these time-saving, entirely useful mixes throughout this book. So feel free to make up a batch of each.

RAS EL HANOUT MIX

MAKES ABOUT 8 TABLESPOONS

2½ tablespoons ground coriander seeds

2½ tablespoons ground cinnamon

2½ tablespoons ground cumin

1 tablespoon cayenne pepper

Put all the ingredients in an airtight jar, seal with the lid and shake. Will keep for 6 months.

SEAWEED DUKKAH

MAKES ABOUT 1½ CUPS

1 cup (225 g) macadamias

2 teaspoons cumin seeds

1 teaspoon coriander seeds

3 tablespoons white sesame seeds

4 tablespoons dulse flakes or 4 nori sheets

2 teaspoons dried Greek oregano

sea salt and freshly ground black pepper

Toast the macadamias in a skillet or frying pan over a medium heat until golden (about 4 minutes). Remove from the pan and leave to cool, then finely chop.

Grind the seeds (and nori if using) finely in a blender (or use a mortar and pestle). Add to the pan and toast until fragrant (about 2 minutes). Cool, then stir in the macadamias, oregano and dulse flakes (if using). Season to taste with salt and pepper. Will keep for 1 month in an airtight container.

PUMPKIN SPICE MIX

MAKES ABOUT 8 TABLESPOONS

5 tablespoons ground cinnamon

1 tablespoon ground ginger

1 tablespoon ground nutmeg

1 tablespoon ground allspice

Put all the ingredients in an airtight jar, seal with the lid and shake. Will keep for 6 months.

NEVER-ENDING VANILLA EXTRACT

I use this stuff a lot so I figured it was time to share a recipe for it. Try to use a long, narrow bottle or jar (an old capers jar – well washed or sterilised – is perfect).

3 vanilla pods

½ cup (125 ml) vodka (or bourbon, brandy or rum)

Split the vanilla pods lengthways. Place in your bottle or jar (cut them in half to fit if need be) and cover with vodka or whatever booze you're using. Seal, shake and store in the dark. Whenever you see it in your cupboard, give it a shake (a few times a week); it will be ready to use in 4 weeks.

Note: it will get stronger the longer you keep it.

MAKE IT BOTTOMLESS:

Simply add more booze as you drain the bottle. Also add another pod or two as the flavour wanes (a great way to use up pods when you've used the seeds for something else).

See also Celery Leaf Salt (page 265) and Kale Flakes (page 179).

A FEW DAIRY THINGS

Which yoghurt?
Go for plain (unflavoured), organic and full-fat (most low-fat varieties have added sugar). I find the Greek styles are often best. BUT look at the nutrition label. It should contain no more than 4.7 g of sugar per 100 g serve. This is the natural lactose contained in dairy foods and is perfectly fine (unless you're lactose intolerant). Anything more than 4.7 g per 100 g is added sugar.

HOMEMADE CREAM CHEESE AND WHEY

It's so simple to make your own cream cheese and whey.

1 kg full-fat organic plain yoghurt

Pour the whole tub of yoghurt onto a large handkerchief-sized square of clean cheesecloth or muslin (or use a new J-cloth). Bunch the ends together like you're tying a sack and secure with an elastic band or string. Suspend the bag over a large bowl – I attach mine to a wooden spoon placed across the bowl, while others hang theirs from a cupboard doorknob, or even a chandelier! You're going to be straining out the whey, leaving a beautifully creamy curd in the sack. Drain for 12–24 hours. Store the cream cheese in the fridge for up to 1 month, and use it as you would the commercial stuff (see the Cream Cheese Frosting recipe on page 56).

Transfer the whey into an ice-cube tray. When frozen, store the cubes in a freezer-proof container in the freezer. Use for fermenting or making pesto or mayonnaise.

Be sure to use full-fat organic yoghurt – I've found that this recipe doesn't work well if you use the commercial stuff.

MARINATED GOAT'S CHEESE

Buy the feta-type goat's cheese in bulk (feel free to double the quantities below) and make it last 3 months by preserving it in oil.

200 g organic soft feta-type goat's cheese, chilled

½ cup (125 ml) good-quality extra-virgin olive oil

1 clove garlic, peeled

3 sprigs thyme or 2 bay leaves

1 teaspoon fennel seeds, peppercorns or allspice berries

pinch of sea salt

Cut the cheese into 1.5 cm cubes. Place a little olive oil in the bottom of a smallish, squat jar. Add half the cheese, the garlic clove and half of your chosen herbs and spices. Sprinkle with salt. Add some more oil and the remaining cheese, herbs and spices until you've filled the jar. Pour over the rest of the oil, adding more, if necessary, to ensure the cheese is completely covered. Seal the jar and refrigerate for 2–3 days to allow the flavours to infuse before eating.

USE THE LEFTOVER HERB-INFUSED OIL:
Combine it with apple cider vinegar or lemon juice in a 2:1 ratio (oil to acid) and use as a dressing.

The above cost me £3.79 to make. The equivalent store-bought stuff is £6.08

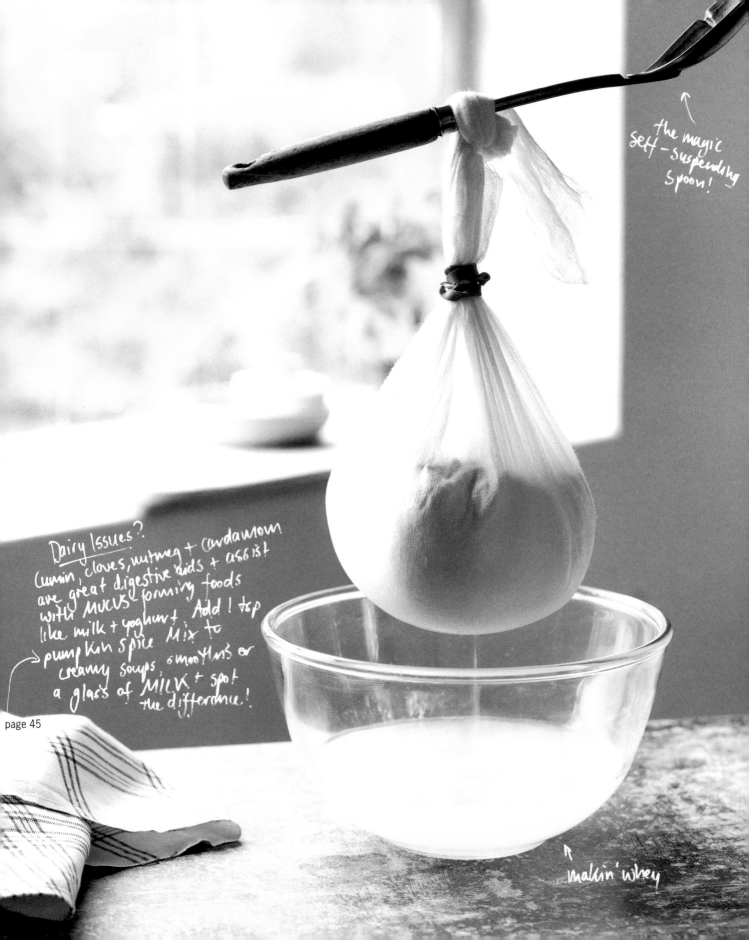

the magic
self-suspending
spoon!

Dairy Issues?
Cumin, cloves, nutmeg + cardamom
are great digestive aids + assist
with MUCUS forming foods
like milk + yoghurt. Add 1 tsp
pumpkin spice Mix to
creamy soups, smoothies or
a glass of MILK + spot
the difference!

page 45

makin' whey

HOMEMADE PANEER

This Indian version of the IQS community's much-loved haloumi is one of the easiest cheeses to make at home. Plus it's also one of the easiest to digest, which I guess is why it features a bit in Ayurvedic recipes (it's chiefly recommended for nourishing and calming Vata and increasing Kapha). It's also often recommended as an Ayurvedic cure for female infertility. There you go!

2 litres full-fat milk

juice of 4 lemons

1 teaspoon sea salt

Warm the milk in a large saucepan over a medium heat until it reaches 'almost boiling' point (around 90°C). If it looks like it might boil over, take it off the heat and blow directly across the rising foam (taking it off the heat won't be enough). Your breath is much cooler than the boiling milk and should get it back down in the pot quickly. When ready, the milk should be foamy and steamy.

Stir in the lemon juice really quickly for no more than 5 seconds until the milk curdles. If it doesn't separate properly, then VERY carefully stir through a little more lemon juice, again without disturbing the curd too much, then simmer for a few seconds until the milk curdles.

I.

I Quit Sugar's Marly, also a cheese maker, told me that excessive stirring can break up the curd too much.

Remove from the heat and allow to sit, uncovered and undisturbed for 20 minutes while the curd separates from the whey (which will be yellow and milky).

Line a colander with a piece of cheesecloth or muslin (or a new J-cloth) and place over a bowl. Pour in the curdled milk. Tie the corners of the cloth together and squeeze out the excess liquid. Open the 'sack', sprinkle over the salt and massage it gently through the cheese. Form the cheese into a square, then re-wrap the cloth around it as you would a book you're giving as a present. Place it on a plate or tray. Place another plate or tray on top with a weight (e.g. a bowl of water or a can of tomatoes) and allow it to flatten for at least 1 hour (3–4 hours is best). Refrigerate before use. It will keep in the fridge for about a week.

2.

3.

4. cut into cubes.

USE THE LEFTOVER WHEY:
Add it to smoothies for a protein hit or use it in place of water in baking recipes. Note: This whey doesn't have fermentable properties as it's been heated.

Cold paneer is less likely to crumble.

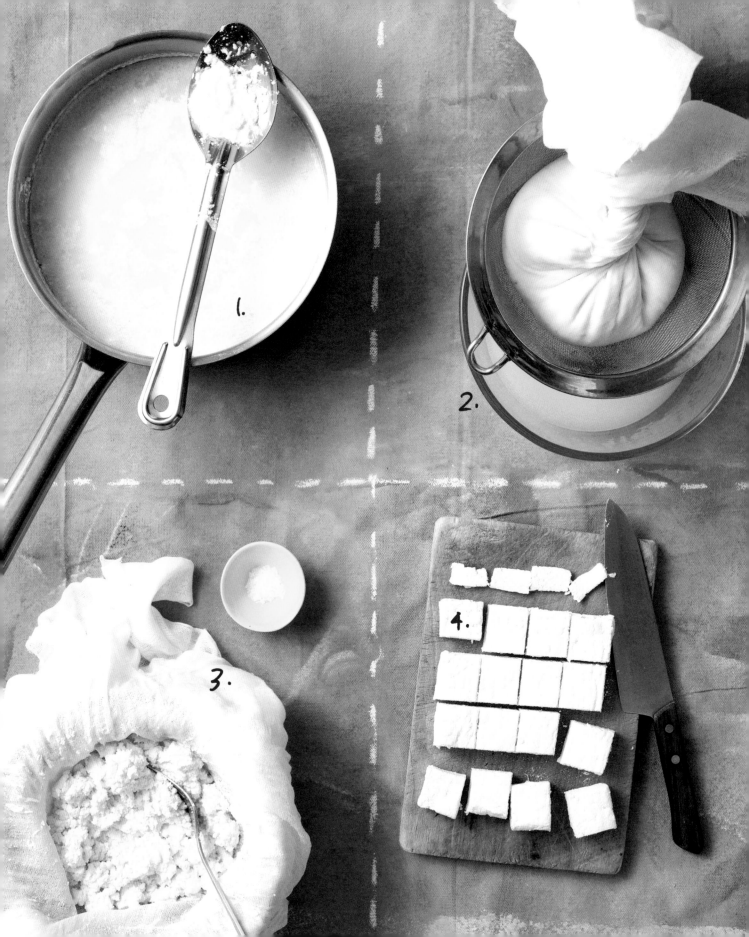

A WHOLE BUNCH OF SAUCES, DRESSINGS AND PESTOS

This is how I do dressings. I make one based on the ingredients I have lying around, then I put it in a jar in the fridge and use it on Abundance Bowls (pages 126–37), Leftover Mishmashes (pages 246–65), pizzas, dosas etc. As it starts to run low, I make up another sauce or dressing and do the same. This way I have two at a time to choose from and I don't get bored.

The following recipes are designed to last as long as possible. If you're worried they might not keep for the prescribed distance, please do this: pour a portion into an ice-cube tray, freeze, then pop the blocks into a freezer-proof container or zip-lock bag so you can thaw and use one cube at a time.

WHEY-GOOD MAYO

MAKES ABOUT 1½ CUPS (350 ML)

1 egg

1 teaspoon Dijon mustard

1 tablespoon lemon juice

1 tablespoon Homemade Whey (page 46)

big pinch of sea salt

1 cup (250 ml) good-quality extra-virgin olive oil

Whizz all the ingredients except the oil in a food processer on a low speed for 30 seconds. With the motor running (still on low), very slowly drizzle in the oil until the mayo is thick and smooth. (Did I mention drizzling it very slowly? You want it to pour in a very, very fine stream, otherwise it won't form an emulsion.) Cover the mayonnaise and let it sit at room temperature for 8 hours before refrigerating. This activates the enzymes in the whey and means it will last for 3 months in the fridge.

MAKE IT A QUICK MAYO:
To make a mayo you can use straight away, omit the whey, and prepare as above without the fermenting stage. Refrigerate the mayo immediately and use within a week or two.

MAKE IT A HOMEMADE AIOLI:
Make the mayo, then simply stir through 2 cloves garlic, crushed to a paste, at the end. (You might like to divide your batch in half to make one portion of mayo and one portion of aioli; though if you do this, use 1 clove garlic instead.)

NOMATO SAUCE

MAKES ABOUT 1 LITRE

Tomato passata with no 'matoes? No mata … this concoction is infinitely better than any tomato sauce or passata you've tasted. As someone in the office said: 'It's liquid pizza!' Make it in big robust batches (I triple the mixture) and freeze as cubes, ½ cup (125 ml) and 1 cup (250 ml) batches.

2 tablespoons extra-virgin olive oil

4 shallots (or 2 onions),
finely chopped

6 cloves garlic, finely chopped

1 large beetroot (400 g), trimmed, scrubbed
and coarsely grated

2 celery stalks, coarsely grated

3 carrots, coarsely grated

1 teaspoon sea salt

1 tablespoon finely chopped oregano

2 cups (500 ml) Homemade Stock (page 42), or water

¼ cup (40 g) pitted black olives, such as kalamata
(for the umami flavour)

2 tablespoons lemon juice

Heat the oil in a saucepan over a medium–low heat. Cook the shallots, garlic, beetroot, celery and carrot for 10 minutes or until the shallot is translucent. Add the salt, then the oregano and stock or water and bring to the boil. Reduce the heat to a simmer and cook for 15 minutes or until the vegetables are tender. Transfer the mixture to a blender with the olives and lemon juice and process until smooth. Store in a sealed container in the fridge for 1 week or in the freezer for up to 6 months.

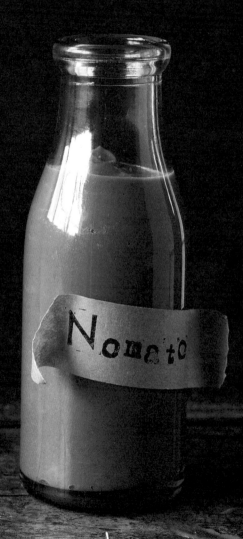

when used instead of tomato sauce, it counts as 1–2 serves of veggies!

2 SERVES VEG + FRUIT PER SERVE

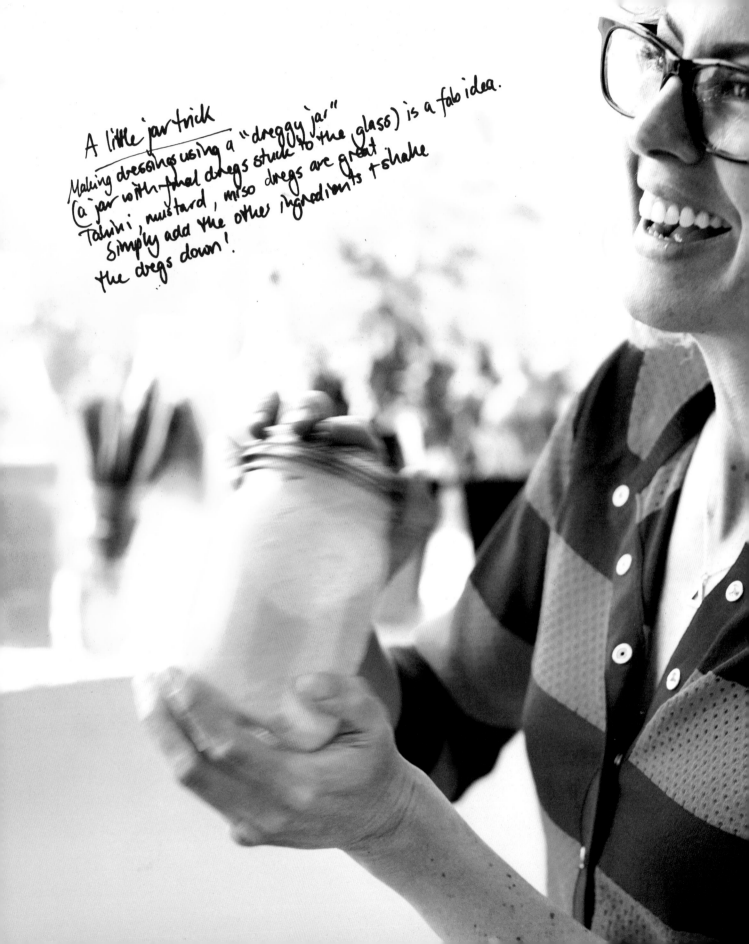

A little jar trick
Making dressings using a "dreggy jar"
(a jar with final dregs stuck to the glass) is a fab idea.
Tahini, mustard, miso dregs are great.
Simply add the other ingredients + shake
the dregs down!

TMT DRESSING
(TAHINI MISO TURMERIC)

MAKES 1½ CUPS (350 ML)

¾ cup (210 g) tahini

½ cup (125 ml) hot water

4 tablespoons red miso paste
(or 8 tablespoons white miso paste)

1 tablespoon Fermented Turmeric Paste
(page 340) or a 3 cm piece of turmeric,
chopped (or 1 teaspoon ground turmeric)

1 tablespoon finely chopped Good for Your
Guts Garlic (page 340), or 2 cloves garlic

4 tablespoons lemon juice, apple cider vinegar
or ferment brine (page 334)

If you're using fresh turmeric and garlic, throw them in the blender whole.

Place all the ingredients in a blender and blitz until
lovely and smooth. Transfer to an airtight container or
jar and keep in the fridge for up to 1 week, adding a
little extra water and shaking before each use.

Tahini V peanut butter

In this book I play with the
former quite a bit, in part
because so many are allergic
to the latter, but also …

* Tahini is an excellent
  source of calcium and
  is higher in protein than
  most nuts.
* It's high in vitamin E and
  B vitamins (B1, B2, B3,
  B5 and B15) that promote
  healthy cell growth and
  function.
* It's rich in magnesium,
  lecithin, potassium and
  iron.
* It's also a great source
  of methionine, which
  aids liver detoxification.
* It's easier to digest than
  peanut butter due to
  its high alkaline mineral
  content.
* And it is high in good
  (unsaturated) fat.

POWERHOUSE DRESSING

MAKES ABOUT 1½ CUPS (350 ML)

Choose your own adventure with this one and
create your family or group-house special flavour.

¹/₃ cup (75 ml) good acid (kombucha,
apple cider vinegar, lemon juice,
or some excess brine from one
of your ferments)

1 cup (250 ml) oil
(olive, avocado or walnut)

1 teaspoon sea salt

1 clove garlic, finely chopped

1 tablespoon finely chopped soft herbs
such as basil, tarragon or chives and/or
1 teaspoon Dijon mustard, ground allspice
or ground cloves

I make mine with Kombucha dregs (the stuff at the end of a batch thats gone sour).

Place all the ingredients in a large jar, seal with a tight-fitting
lid and shake until well combined. Keep in the fridge for
1–3 weeks.

If you use a brine or kombucha it will last longer.

GREEN MINX DRESSING

MAKES ABOUT 2 CUPS (500 ML)

There are 101 Green Goddess dressings out there these days. They're based on a dressing created in the 1920s as a nod to the play by the same name (and here I was thinking it was Just Another Instagram Fad). With my version, I undress things with a little saucy thrift and voluptuous nutrition.

1 large avocado or 1 cup (250 ml) Whey-Good Mayo (page 50)

1 large handful of coriander, including stalks (or you can use parsley, chives or basil, or a combo)

1 large handful of chopped lettuce

1 small courgette (or ½ cup/75 g Par-Cooked 'n' Frozen courgettes; page 22)

2 cloves garlic (preferably fermented; page 340)

3 tablespoons apple cider vinegar, ferment brine (page 334) or lemon juice

¼ teaspoon each of sea salt and freshly ground black pepper

Blend all the ingredients in a blender or use a stick blender and a large mixing bowl. Thin, if required, with a little water.

If you use avocado, this will keep for 3–4 days in the fridge, or it can be frozen for 1–2 months in a freezer-proof airtight container, as long as the dressing is totally puréed (lumps make the dressing icy). To use, simply thaw in your refrigerator or in a bowl of cold water. Whisk to bring everything back together and serve cold!

MAKE IT LAST LONGER:
If you use Whey-Good Mayo instead of avo, it will last for up to a month in the fridge.

MISOMITE

MAKES ABOUT 1 CUP (250 ML)

Yep, a yeast-free, sugar-free salty fermented spread in, like, two ingredients flat.

1 avocado

½–1 tablespoon red miso

Blend together with a fork. Done. Will keep in the fridge for 1–3 days. Use as a dip or spread.

See also 'Bucha Mustard (page 336) and my other ferments (pages 337–40)

1 SERVE VEG + FRUIT PER SERVE

Leftovers Pesto.

MAKES ABOUT 1½ CUPS (350 ML)

I wanted to find a way to use up stalks and leaves you'd normally throw out. I figured fermenting them could be the way to go. I contacted ferment maestro Sandor Katz to get his take. He hadn't tried it himself but reckoned it might just work. I can report back from the mouldy frontline: it does! Kale stalks become edible after a bit of lacto-breakdown. Plus you get the digestive benefits. There's also this: frankly, I'm sick of my homemade pesto going off. Fermenting increases pesto's fridge shelf life from a few days to 6 weeks. Bam!

mine = £1.66
bought = £4.13

Parsley, basil and/or coriander leaves and stalks; celery leaves; kale stalks (blanch in boiling water for 2–3 minutes first); carrot tops (blanch in boiling water for 1–2 minutes first); beetroot leaves; broccoli or cauliflower stalks (blanch first, if you like).

3–4 cups leftover leaves and/or stalks, roughly chopped

½ cup (70 g) cashews, pumpkin seeds or almonds or ½ cup (50 g) grated parmesan

4 cloves garlic, finely chopped

½ cup (125 ml) extra-virgin olive oil

1 tablespoon lemon juice

½ teaspoon sea salt

2 tablespoons Homemade Whey (page 46), ferment brine (page 334) or ¼ teaspoon salt dissolved in 2–3 tablespoons water

Time on the worktop will depend on the temperature at your place. Once you start to see a few little bubbles rise, it's time to whack it in the fridge. In summer in Sydney this happens overnight.

Process all the ingredients in a food processor until finely chopped. Spoon into a jar and press down with the back of the spoon so that the liquid rises to cover the greens but leaves 3 cm of space at the top of the jar. Seal and leave on the worktop for 1–3 days. Once fermented, keep it in the fridge for up to 6 weeks.

MAKE IT UNFERMENTED:

If you know you're going to use it quickly, simply omit the whey and place in the fridge after you've processed the mixture.

1 SERVE VEG + FRUIT PER SERVE

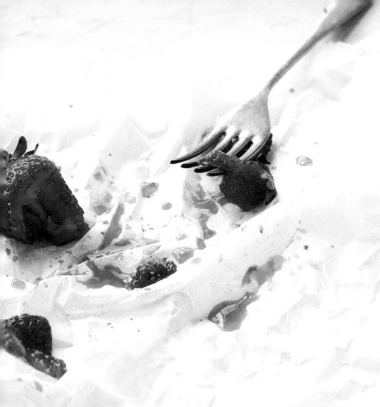

WHIPPED COCONUT FROSTING

MAKES ABOUT 1½ CUPS (350 ML)

400 ml can full-fat coconut cream, refrigerated upside down

2 tablespoons rice malt syrup or ½–1 teaspoon granulated stevia

Open the can the right way up without shaking it. Spoon out the top layer of liquid and freeze it for smoothies or other recipes requiring coconut milk or coconut water.

dish-saving trick →

Leave the rest of the firm cream in the can, add the syrup or stevia and then blend with a stick blender until creamy. (If you don't have a stick blender, remove the cream from the can and place in a blender.)

MAKE IT SUPERCHARGED COCONUT FROSTING:

Make as above, but blend in a small bowl, adding 3 tablespoons of powdered gelatine in a thin, steady stream before you add the sweetener. Continue mixing until soft peaks form. Use immediately or store in the fridge and use within 4–5 days.

½ TSP ADDED SUGAR PER SERVE

A FEW FROSTINGS, TOPPINGS AND JAMS

These can be frozen in ice-cube trays and stored in the freezer ready for making or decorating muffins or cakes as required.

CREAM CHEESE FROSTING

MAKES ABOUT 1½ CUPS (375 G)

250 g Homemade Cream Cheese (page 46)

1–2 tablespoons rice malt syrup or ½–1 teaspoon granulated stevia

zest of 1 lemon (optional)

4 tablespoons coconut cream or unsalted butter

Blend the cheese in a high-speed blender along with the syrup and zest (if using). Slowly add the coconut cream or butter until the mixture is nice and thick. If needed, add more coconut cream or butter. This will last for up to 1 month in the fridge.

½ TSP ADDED SUGAR PER SERVE

BASIC RAW CHOCOLATE

MAKES ABOUT 1⅓ CUPS (325 ML)

1 cup (225 g) coconut oil, softened

⅓ cup (40 g) raw cacao powder

1 tablespoon rice malt syrup or 1 teaspoon granulated stevia, to taste

2 pinches of sea salt

Blend all the ingredients in a blender until smooth (or mix by hand). Use immediately in recipes, or pour into small silicone moulds or ice-cube trays and keep in the freezer for up to 3 months.

Snack trick: pop out a cube to eat as a choc treat. Or melt + use as a chocolate drizzle on fruit etc.

½ TSP ADDED SUGAR PER SERVE

STRAWBERRY CHIA JAM

MAKES ABOUT 1¼ CUPS (300 ML)

1 cup (150 g) hulled strawberries, fresh or frozen

2 tablespoons rice malt syrup
or ½–1 teaspoon granulated stevia

3 tablespoons chia seeds

Throw all the ingredients into a saucepan with 2 tablespoons of water and use a stick blender to combine (or whizz in a blender first). Heat the pan over a medium heat until the mixture begins to bubble. Reduce the heat and whisk constantly until thickened (about 3–5 minutes). Store in an airtight container in the fridge for 1 week or freeze in an ice-cube tray and store the cubes in a container in the freezer for up to 3 months.

MAKE IT RASPBERRY CHIA JAM:
Um, use raspberries instead.

½ TSP ADDED SUGAR PER SERVE

mine = £1.82
bought = £4.13

AGAINST-THE-GRAIN
BREAKFASTS

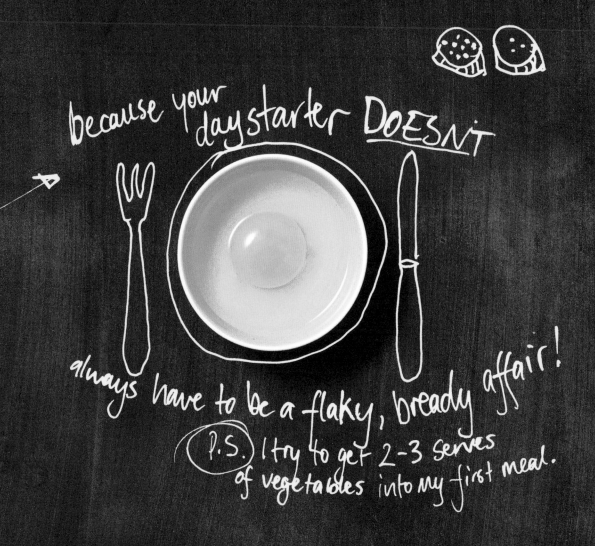

because your daystarter DOESN'T

always have to be a flaky, breacly affair!
(P.S.) I try to get 2-3 serves
of vegetables into my first meal.

'PIZZA' MUGGINS

Kids are naturally 'simplicious'. They totally get the hands-in, cut-the-guff, intuitive approach. The ingredients in these mini-muffins-in-a-mug are just to give you some ideas – use leftovers and whatever you have to hand.

olive oil, coconut oil or butter, for greasing

some red things: cherry tomatoes, halved; diced red pepper

some green things: Par-Cooked 'n' Frozen broccoli (page 22) or tiny florets of raw broccoli

some sweetness: frozen peas, 1–2 cubes frozen Pumpkin or Sweet Potato Purée (page 23)

some pizza flavour: 1–2 olives, pitted and chopped

some meat: Bacon Bits (page 44) or a small portion of chopped Pulled Beef (page 223) or Shredded Chicken (page 214)

2 eggs

grated cheese or crumbled feta

Rub the insides of two mugs with a little oil or butter. Now hand them over to the kids and invite them to add whatever ingredients they like until the mug is half-full. Cover the mug (I use a saucer or small plate) and heat in the microwave for about 45 seconds.

Now get the kids to crack an egg into their cup(s) and sprinkle over the cheese. They can then stir the lot with a fork. Microwave again for another 30–60 seconds.

MAKE IT WITHOUT A MICROWAVE:
The kids can assemble all the ingredients in a ramekin and then crack an egg over the top and sprinkle over some cheese. Bake in an oven preheated to 180°C (gas 4) for 15 minutes.

MAKE IT FOR THE LUNCHBOX:
Make the muggins in a microwave-safe container and, once cooled, top with the lid.

½ SERVE VEG + FRUIT PER SERVE

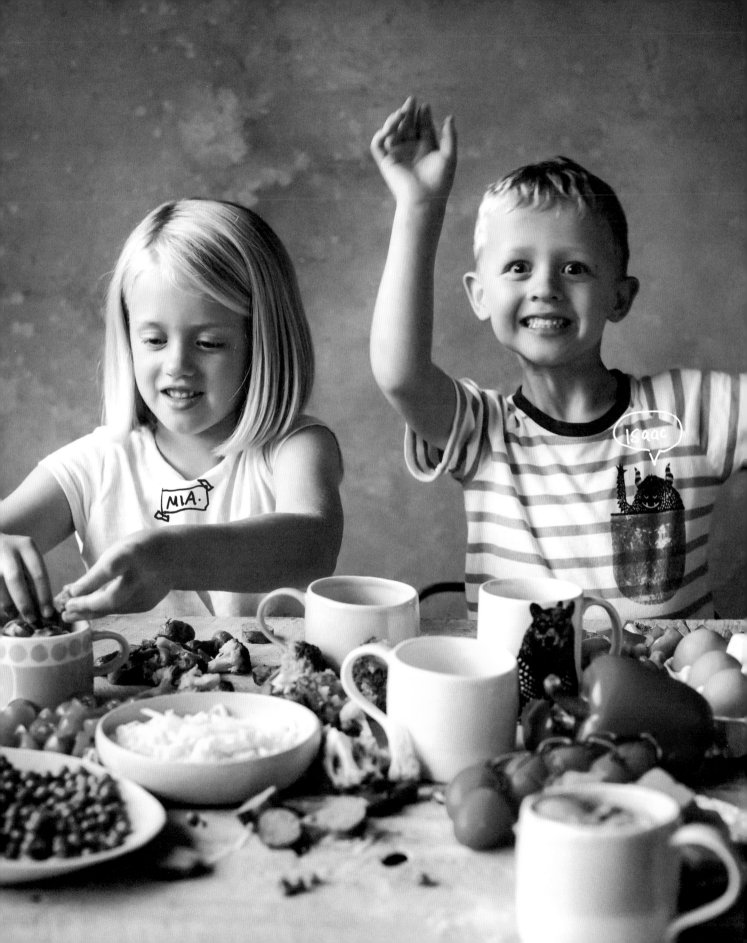

SLOW-COOKER COURGETTE AND PUMPKIN SPICE BREAKFAST PUDDING

SERVES 6

If you have a slow cooker with a timer, work things so the pudding greets you with a warm cinnamon vibe as you rise. Equally, this works really well made in advance, divvied up into lunch containers to be heated in the office microwave and served with a big splodge of yoghurt.

coconut oil, butter or ghee, for greasing

½ cup (115 g) butter, softened

4 tablespoons rice malt syrup

2 eggs

1 cup (250 ml) Pumpkin or Sweet Potato Purée (page 23) or 2 cups (400 g) grated raw pumpkin or sweet potato

1½ cups (250 g) grated courgettes

3 tablespoons milk (any kind)

2 teaspoons pure vanilla extract (or make your own; page 45)

2 cups (200 g) almond meal

1 cup (125 g) plain flour (gluten-free if you prefer)

1 teaspoon bicarbonate of soda

1 teaspoon sea salt

2½ teaspoons Pumpkin Spice Mix (page 45) or 2 teaspoons ground cinnamon and ½ teaspoon ground nutmeg

4 tablespoons chia seeds

½ cup (55 g) pecans, lightly toasted and roughly chopped

Lightly grease the slow-cooker insert with coconut oil, butter or ghee and line with baking paper so that it reaches quite high up the inside of the pot.

Using a stick blender, beat the butter and rice malt syrup together in a large bowl. Add the eggs, one at a time, beating after each addition. On low speed, beat in the pumpkin or sweet potato, courgettes, milk and vanilla. Using a wooden spoon, stir in the almond meal, flour, bicarbonate of soda, salt, spices and chia seeds and mix until well combined.

Pour the batter into the slow-cooker insert and sprinkle the pecans over the top. Cover and cook on low for 4–5 hours, or on high for 2–3 hours. Check the pudding by inserting a skewer in the centre – it should come out clean. If not, continue cooking on high with the lid off.

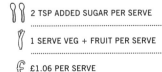 2 TSP ADDED SUGAR PER SERVE

1 SERVE VEG + FRUIT PER SERVE

£1.06 PER SERVE

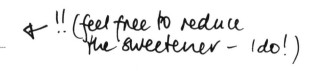 ← !! (feel free to reduce the sweetener – I do!)

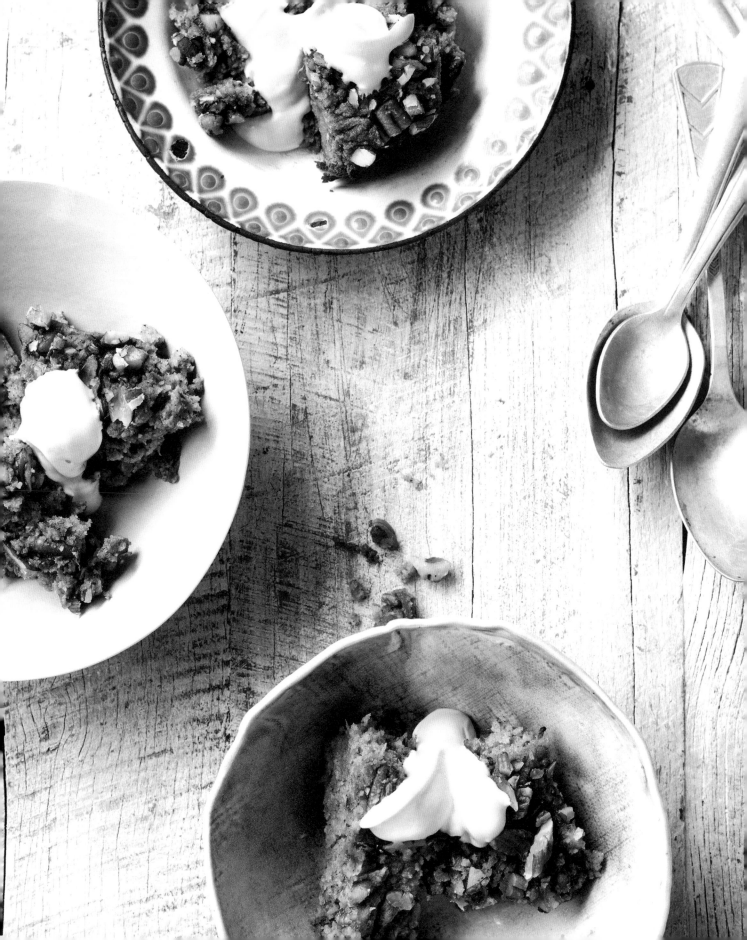

MUSHROOM, THYME AND HAZELNUT PORRIDGE

Savoury porridge. For real. And it will probably change your life.

1 teaspoon butter or olive oil

1 small onion, chopped

1 cup (75 g) sliced button mushrooms

1 teaspoon dried thyme or 1 tablespoon thyme leaves, plus extra to serve

1 cup (100 g) whole rolled oats, or 135 g Cooked Quinoa (page 26) or 170 g Cooked Buckwheat (page 27)

¾ cup Homemade Stock (a veggie variation; page 43) mixed with ½ cup (125 ml) water

50 g feta-type goat's cheese

4 tablespoons hazelnuts, toasted and chopped

Heat the butter or olive oil in a saucepan over a medium heat and sauté the onion until translucent (about 3 minutes). Add the mushrooms and thyme and cook until soft. Add your chosen 'grain', the stock and water and, if using oats, also add an extra 1¼ cups (300 ml) water. Stir and cook for 6–8 minutes or until the liquid has been absorbed. Remove from the heat and stir in half of the cheese and half of the hazelnuts.

Divide the porridge between two bowls and serve topped with the remaining cheese and hazelnuts and a sprinkle of thyme.

2 SERVES VEG + FRUIT PER SERVE

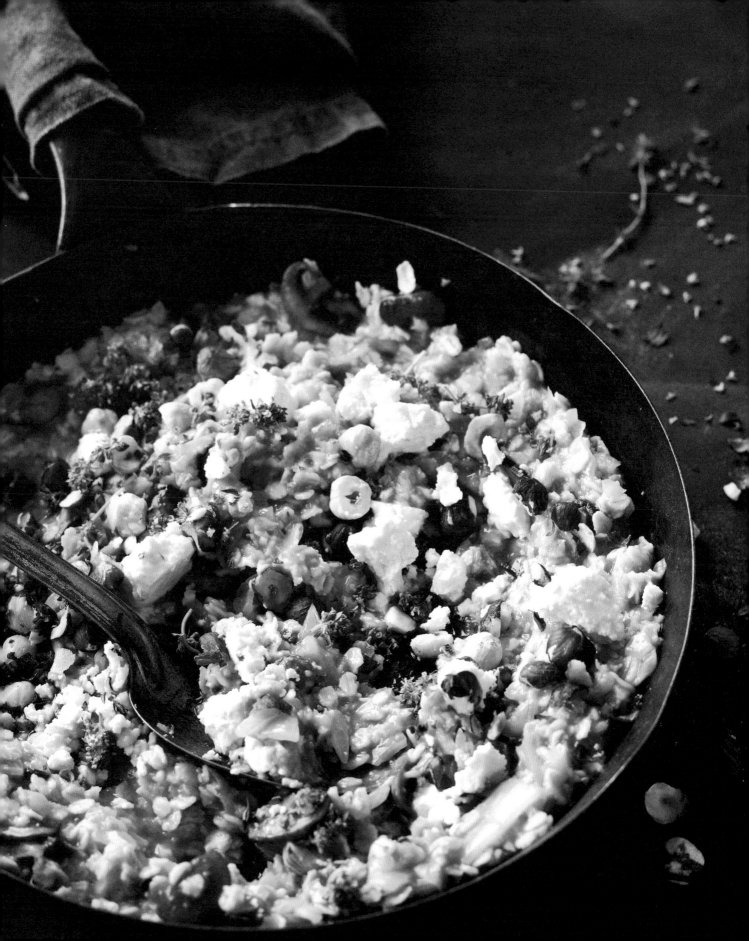

BACON 'N' EGG PORRIDGE

Another talking-point savoury porridge for you.

2 teaspoons coconut oil, olive oil, butter or ghee

1 small onion, chopped

1 cup (100 g) whole rolled oats, or 150 g Cooked Quinoa (page 26) or Cooked Buckwheat (page 27)

¾ cup (175 ml) Homemade Chicken Stock (page 42) or any stock

8 tablespoons Bacon Bits (page 44), or 4 rashers bacon, chopped and fried

3 tablespoons grated cheddar

2 soft-boiled eggs, halved

sea salt and freshly ground black pepper

fennel fronds, to serve (optional)

Heat the oil, butter or ghee in a saucepan over a medium heat and sauté the onion until translucent (about 3 minutes). Add your chosen 'grain', stock, and if using oats also add 1¼ cups (300 ml) water. Stir and cook for 6–8 minutes until the liquid has been absorbed.

Take the porridge off the heat. Stir through half of the bacon and all of the cheese. Divide the porridge between two bowls, top with the egg halves and remaining bacon, and season to taste with salt and pepper. Garnish with fennel fronds if you like.

You can also toss in 1 tablespoon of chia seeds and an extra 4 tablespoons of water or stock to the soaking bowl, if you like, to really bulk things out.

MAKE IT ACTIVATED OVERNIGHT PORRIDGE:
Soak ¾ cup (75 g) of whole rolled oats (or raw quinoa or buckwheat groats) in 1½ cups (350 ml) of stock overnight. Add this to the sautéed onions to heat through, along with a little stock or water to stop the 'grains' from catching, then continue with the rest of the recipe.

½ SERVE VEG + FRUIT PER SERVE

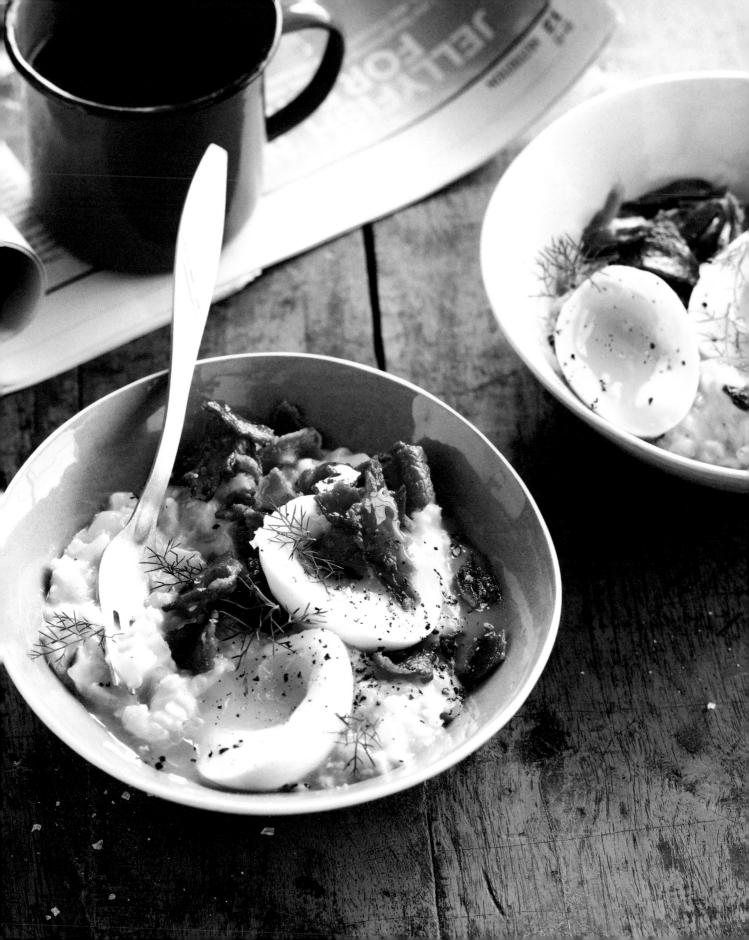

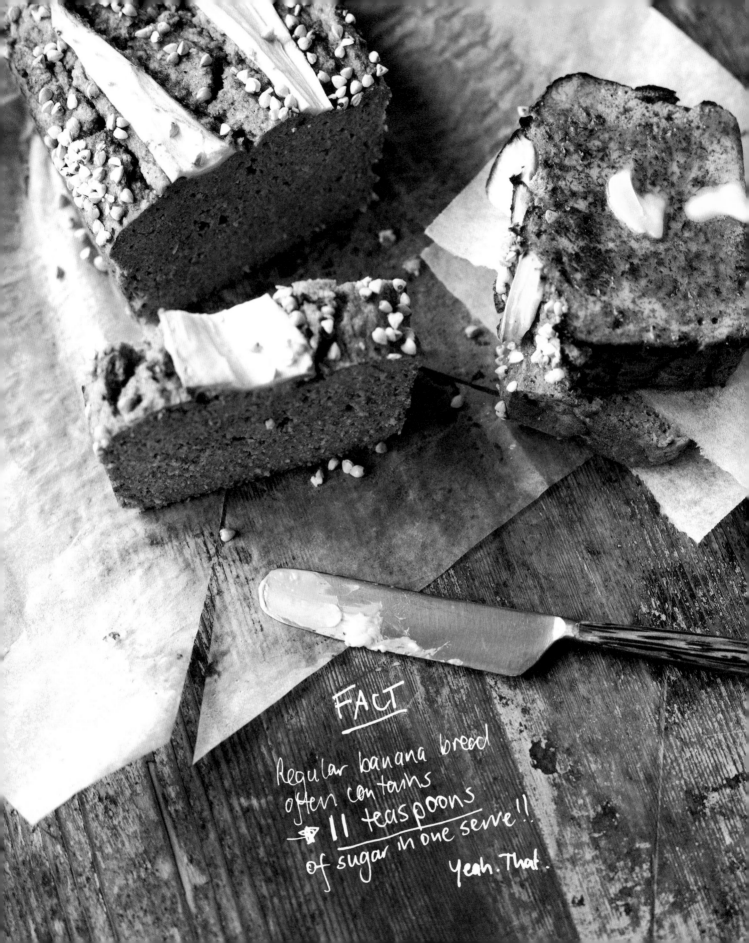

FACT

Regular banana bread
often contains
11 teaspoons
of sugar in one serve!!

Yeah. That.

NOT QUITE
BANANA BREAD

This fake banana trick is a really good one for anyone wanting to up the nutritional count of their breakfast and cut back on fructose. It's great as is. Better toasted under a grill, in a sandwich press or in a frying pan with a dash of coconut oil (or butter if you don't mind dairy).

A bit of history for you
During World War II, bananas were scarce. So housewives of the era used parsnips – boiled and mashed with spices – as mock bananas. Ha!

2 large, very ripe bananas

1 cup grated parsnip
(about 150 g or 2 parsnips)

4 eggs

1/3 cup (75 g) coconut oil

3 tablespoons (or 1–2 frozen cubes) full-fat coconut milk

2 teaspoons Pumpkin Spice Mix (page 45) or 1½ teaspoons ground cinnamon and ½ teaspoon ground nutmeg

½ teaspoon ground cardamom

1 teaspoon pure vanilla extract (or make your own; page 45)

3 tablespoons chia seeds stirred into 1 cup (250 ml) water and soaked for 10 minutes

½ cup (55 g) coconut flour, sifted

4 tablespoons buckwheat or quinoa flour, sifted

1½ teaspoons baking powder

pinch of sea salt

TO GARNISH (OPTIONAL)

1 small, thin parsnip, halved lengthways

Activated Groaties (page 27) or shredded coconut

Preheat the oven to 180°C (gas 4). Grease and line a 23 cm × 13 cm loaf tin with baking paper.

Place the bananas, grated parsnip, eggs, coconut oil, coconut milk, spices and vanilla in a food processor and process until smooth. Add the chia seed 'goo' and pulse to combine. Transfer the mixture to a large bowl and fold through the flours, baking powder and salt until just combined. Transfer to the prepared tin and top with garnishes that float your boat. Bake for 1 hour or until cooked – a skewer inserted in the middle should come out clean. Check after 45 minutes, and if the top is browning too quickly, cover with foil.

Let the loaf sit for 5 minutes then transfer to a wire rack to cool. Slice and serve.

Store the cooled bread in the fridge for up to 5 days, or freeze (place individual slices between baking paper) for up to 3 months.

MAKE IT BLUEBERRY BANANA BREAD (BBB):
Add an extra 4 tablespoons of chia seeds to the chia seed 'goo', and 1 cup (115 g) of blueberries to the main mixture.

THREE SMOOTHIE BOWLS: something between a smoothie, a sou and a porridge.

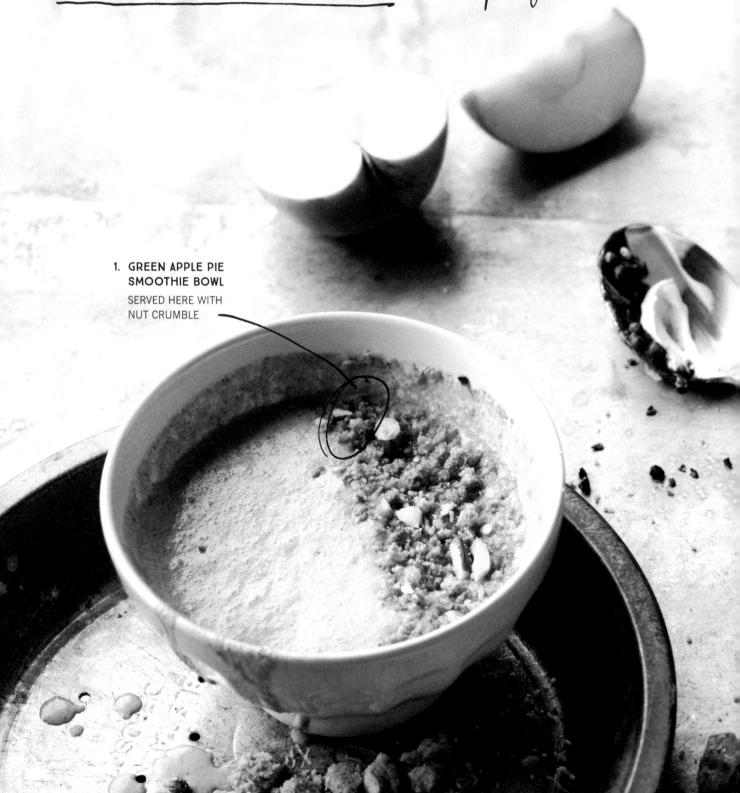

1. GREEN APPLE PIE SMOOTHIE BOWL

SERVED HERE WITH NUT CRUMBLE

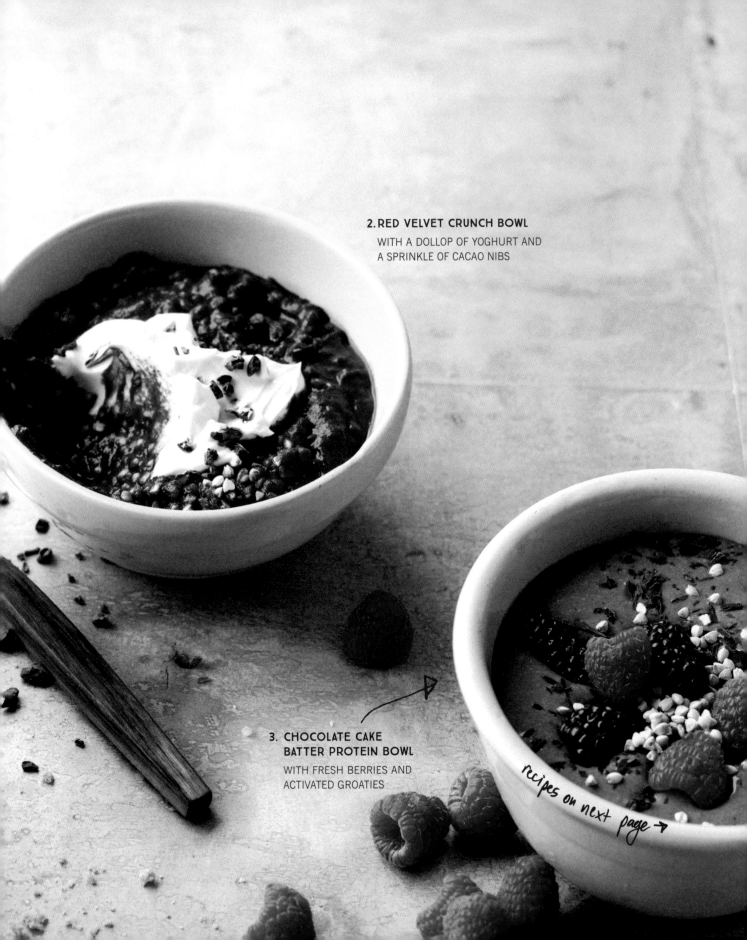

2. RED VELVET CRUNCH BOWL
WITH A DOLLOP OF YOGHURT AND
A SPRINKLE OF CACAO NIBS

**3. CHOCOLATE CAKE
BATTER PROTEIN BOWL**
WITH FRESH BERRIES AND
ACTIVATED GROATIES

recipes on next page →

1. GREEN APPLE PIE SMOOTHIE BOWL

SERVES 2

1 green apple, roughly chopped

1½ cups (350 ml) full-fat coconut milk

1½ cups (75 g) baby spinach leaves

4 tablespoons vanilla protein powder (optional)

3 teaspoons Pumpkin Spice Mix (page 45) or 2¼ teaspoons ground cinnamon and ¾ teaspoon ground nutmeg

3 tablespoons nut butter (any kind; almond is probably best)

½ cup (125 ml) ice cubes

Nut Crumble (see below), to serve

Chuck all the ingredients in a blender and blitz until smooth. Pour into two bowls and top with some nut crumble.

 1½ SERVES VEG + FRUIT PER SERVE

NUT CRUMBLE

4 tablespoons roughly chopped activated almonds (page 28)

2 tablespoons desiccated coconut

1 teaspoon rice malt syrup

2 teaspoons coconut oil, melted

Combine the lot in a small bowl, spread out on a lined baking tray and cook for 5 minutes at 180°C (gas 4) until golden. Feel free to make in bulk and store in an airtight container in the fridge for 2 weeks.

 ½ TSP ADDED SUGAR PER SERVE

2. RED VELVET CRUNCH BOWL

SERVES 2

1 frozen (or fresh) banana

1 cup (150 g) Cooked 'n' Frozen beetroot (page 23) or 2 small beetroots, trimmed, scrubbed and grated

1 cup (250 ml) unsweetened almond milk (or regular milk if you prefer)

²/₃ cup (75 g) frozen raspberries

4 tablespoons raw cacao powder

1 cup (170 g) Activated Groaties (page 27) or coconut flakes

Whipped Coconut Frosting (page 56) or full-fat organic plain yoghurt, to serve

raw cacao nibs, to serve

Place the banana, beetroot, milk, raspberries and cacao powder in a blender and blitz until smooth. Add the groaties to the blender jug and stir through (or if you use coconut, blitz briefly). Pour into two bowls. Serve with a dollop of coconut frosting or yoghurt and a sprinkle of cacao nibs.

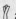 2 SERVES VEG + FRUIT PER SERVE

MAKE IT A BIT FANCY:
Swap the cacao nibs for a few basil and mint leaves.

3. CHOCOLATE CAKE BATTER PROTEIN BOWL

SERVES 2

½ cup (125 ml) coconut cream or full-fat organic plain yoghurt

4 tablespoons vanilla protein powder

1 frozen (or fresh) banana

1½ cups (350 ml) unsweetened almond milk (or any milk)

4 tablespoons raw cacao powder

4 tablespoons chopped activated almonds (page 28) or almond meal

½ cup (80 g) buckwheat groats or whole rolled oats (or a combo)

Activated Groaties (page 27), berries, nuts, coconut flakes or raw cacao nibs, to serve

Dump all the ingredients except the buckwheat and/or oats in a blender and blitz until smooth. Add the buckwheat and/or oats, stir and pour into two bowls. Cover and place in the fridge overnight.

The next morning, scatter over your chosen toppings and serve.

 1 SERVE VEG + FRUIT PER SERVE

SALTED CARAMEL CARDAMOM COFFEE

FOR THOSE OF US WHO 'SHOULDN'T REALLY BE DRINKING COFFEE'

SERVES 1

This is actually a recipe for folk trying to cut back on coffee, or who love the coffee but not the adrenaline spike. How so? Coconut oil lengthens and softens out the caffeine hit and cardamom neutralises the over-stimulating effects.

2 cardamom pods, crushed

1 serve of ground coffee

1 tablespoon coconut oil

pinch of sea salt

¼ teaspoon pure vanilla extract (or make your own; page 45) or pinch of pure vanilla powder

pinch of granulated stevia

Add the cardamom to the ground coffee in your plunger, filter or stovetop coffee maker and make 1 cup.

Place all the ingredients in a blender and blitz until well combined and frothy. (Or use a stick blender in a beaker.)

I have a mate who takes a shaker of ground cardamom to cafés and sprinkles it over her coffee at the table.

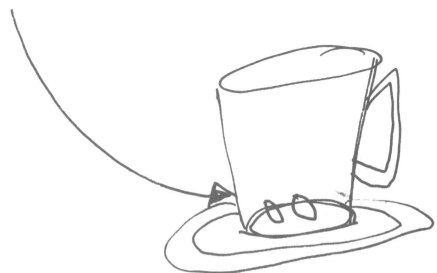

THREE SAVOURY YOGHURTS

yep, it's a thing!

I came across this concept – yoghurt as a meal with savoury toppings – in New York at the Chelsea Market.

1. THE REAL GREEK YOGHURT

SERVES 2

300 g Greek-style full-fat organic plain yoghurt

8 cherry tomatoes, halved

1 small cucumber, cubed

8 pitted kalamata olives, halved

¼ red onion, thinly sliced

small handful of basil leaves and/or mint leaves

3 tablespoons pine nuts, lightly toasted

3 tablespoons extra-virgin olive oil

1 tablespoon lemon juice

sea salt and freshly ground black pepper

Divide the yoghurt between two bowls and top each with half of the tomatoes, cucumber, olives, onion, herbs and pine nuts. Drizzle over the olive oil and lemon juice. Season to taste.

1 SERVE VEG + FRUIT PER SERVE

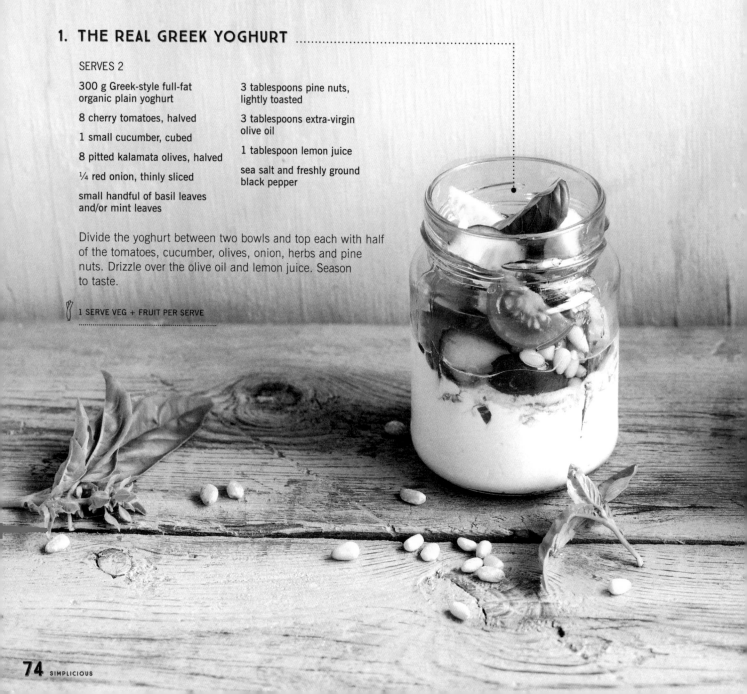

2. WALDORF SMASH-UP

SERVES 2

300 g Greek-style full-fat organic plain yoghurt

1 celery stalk, finely chopped

80 g vintage cheddar, crumbled

4 tablespoons walnuts, chopped and toasted

½ pear, thinly sliced

sea salt and freshly ground black pepper

Divide the yoghurt between two bowls and top each with half of the celery, cheddar, walnuts and pear. Season to taste.

Combining cheese and yoghurt might seem odd. But then so is beetroot on a burger. Give this a crack. You'll get it.

3. THE BLAT (Bacon, Leaves, Avocado, Tomato)

SERVES 2

300 g Greek-style full-fat organic plain yoghurt

small handful of watercress (or rocket or basil leaves)

1 avocado, cubed

8 cherry tomatoes, halved

2 rashers streaky bacon, chopped and fried (or 4 tablespoons Bacon Bits; page 44)

2 tablespoons extra-virgin olive oil

sea salt and freshly ground black pepper

Divide the yoghurt between two bowls and top each with half of the leaves, avocado, tomatoes and bacon. Finish with a drizzle of olive oil and season to taste.

3 SERVES VEG + FRUIT PER SERVE

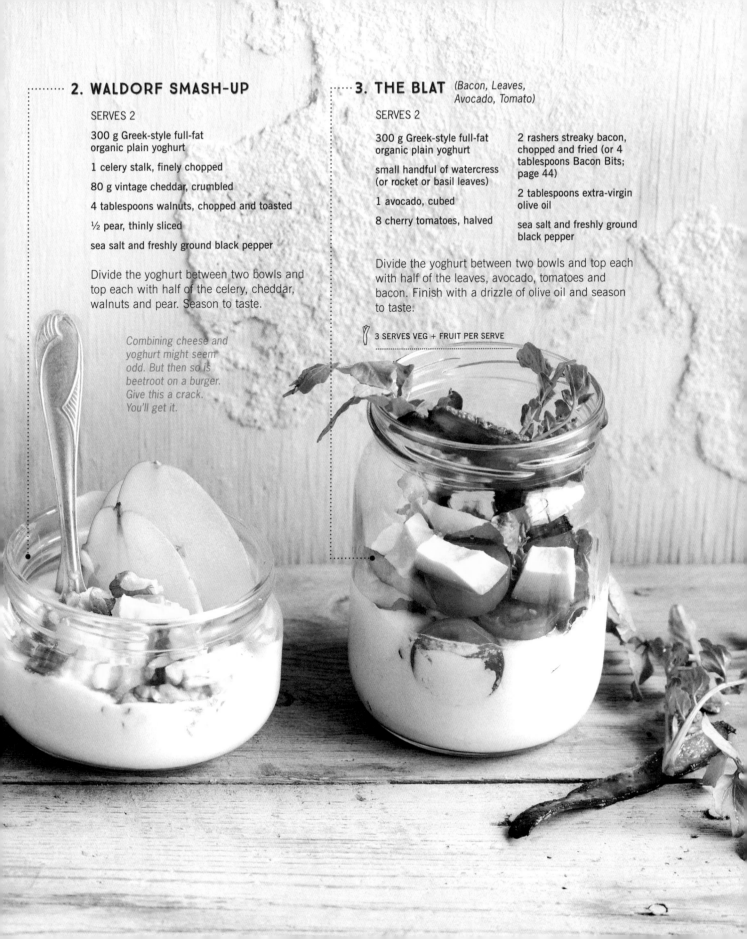

SPROUTED CACAO POPS

MAKES 6 CUPS

If you've already made up some Activated Groaties (page 27), feel free to use those instead of sprouting from scratch. Here, I'm going the full witchy distance – soaking *and* sprouting the buckwheat before I roast it.

3 cups (500 g) buckwheat groats

1/3 cup (75 g) coconut oil

4 tablespoons rice malt syrup

1/3 cup (40 g) raw cacao powder

Rinse the buckwheat and place in a large bowl. Add plenty of water (more than enough to cover) and leave to soak overnight.

The next day, rinse the groats really well (they can sometimes get a little slimy), transfer to a large sieve over a bowl and cover with a cloth (or put them in a sprouting jar or tray). Leave the buckwheat for 1–3 days until it starts to sprout, rinsing a few times a day.

Once you see small sprouts appear, preheat the oven to 120°C (gas 1/4) (or lower if possible) and line a baking tray with baking paper.

Melt the coconut oil and rice malt syrup in a large bowl. Mix in the cacao powder, then add the sprouted groats and stir gently to coat.

Make it just like a chocolate milkshake only crunchy: add 4 tablespoons tahini or natural peanut butter (melted) to the coconut oil mixture.

Plonk the lot onto the lined baking tray, spreading it out to a thin layer (you may need to use two trays). Bake for 1–2 hours, depending on how low you get your oven to go. Stir frequently (every 20 minutes or so) and make sure they don't burn.

Cool, then serve with milk.

MAKE IT QUICKER:
Use 3 cups (500 g) of Activated Groaties (page 27) instead of soaking and sprouting raw buckwheat. Halve the ingredients for the cacao mixture then coat as above. Bake for 10–15 minutes in a preheated 180°C (gas 4) oven, stirring a couple of times to break up any clusters.

1/2 TSP ADDED SUGAR PER SERVE

Sarah

Robbie

Robbie + Sarah have been sugar free
since reading my first book, I Quit Sugar

Three WINTER SPICE breakfast ideas

To make these rippers you'll need to make
up a batch of Pumpkin Spice Mix (page 45)

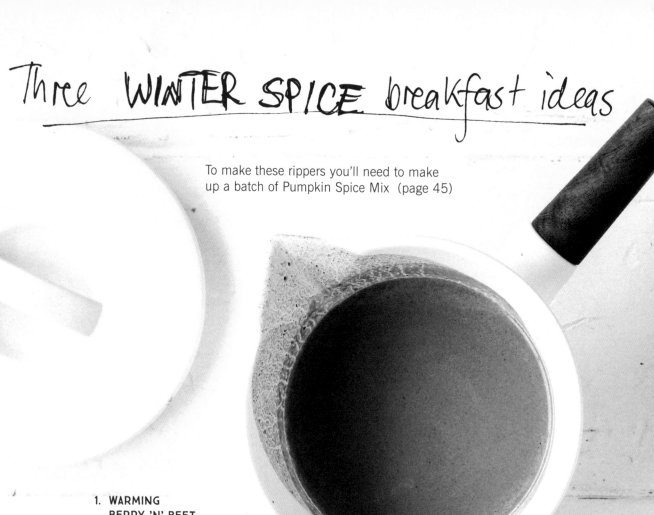

**1. WARMING
BERRY 'N' BEET
SMOOTHIE**

Forgive me!
This is indeed a
MASON JAR

pumpkin spice

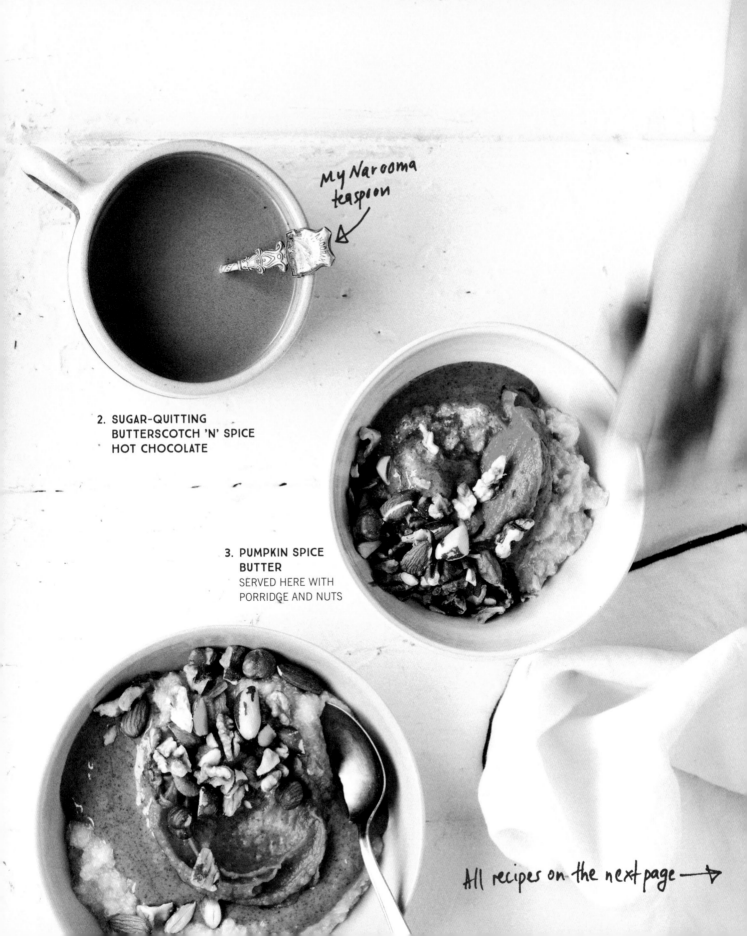

My Narooma teaspoon

2. **SUGAR-QUITTING BUTTERSCOTCH 'N' SPICE HOT CHOCOLATE**

3. **PUMPKIN SPICE BUTTER**
   SERVED HERE WITH PORRIDGE AND NUTS

All recipes on the next page →

1. WARMING BERRY 'N' BEET SMOOTHIE

SERVES 2

I have a real issue with folk drinking cold smoothies outside of summer. It ain't good for our anxious little souls to be cooled when we need some cosy comfort. The antidote is this nutrient-rich concoction.

2 cups (500 ml) full-fat milk

1 tablespoon chia seeds

2 teaspoons Pumpkin Spice Mix (page 45), plus extra to serve

1 cup (120 g) fresh or thawed frozen mixed berries (raspberries, blueberries and blackberries work best)

1 beetroot, trimmed, scrubbed and grated (or ½–1 cup/75–150 g) Cooked 'n' Frozen beetroot, thawed; page 23)

½ banana

1 tablespoon coconut oil

1 tablespoon aloe vera (optional)

Activated Groaties (page 27), to serve

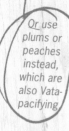

Or use plums or peaches instead, which are also Vata-pacifying

Combine all of the ingredients in a blender and blitz until smooth. Pour into a small saucepan and heat gently. Serve with groaties and a sprinkling of spice mix.

1½ SERVES VEG + FRUIT PER SERVE

Don't have Pumpkin Spice? Combine cinnamon + nutmeg in a 3:1 ratio.

2. SUGAR-QUITTING BUTTERSCOTCH 'N' SPICE HOT CHOCOLATE

SERVES 2

400 ml can full-fat coconut milk (or milk of your choice)

3 tablespoons raw cacao powder

1 tablespoon coconut oil

2 teaspoons maca powder (optional, but great)

Maca helps with cravings, increases metabolism, balances thyroid and improves glucose tolerance.

1½ teaspoons Pumpkin Spice Mix (page 45)

½ teaspoon ground white pepper

pinch of sea salt

pinch of granulated stevia, to taste

Place all the ingredients in a saucepan and bring to the boil. Reduce the heat to low and simmer for several minutes while whisking to remove any lumps. Pour into two mugs and sip away.

White pepper helps lower blood sugar levels and has antibacterial, antioxidant and antispasmodic properties.

3. PUMPKIN SPICE BUTTER

MAKES ABOUT 2½ CUPS (600 ML)

3 cups (750 ml) Pumpkin Purée (page 23)

1 tablespoon Pumpkin Spice Mix (page 45)

4 tablespoons apple cider vinegar or lemon juice

1 teaspoon granulated stevia

Place all the ingredients in a medium-sized saucepan, stir well and bring to the boil over a medium heat. Reduce the heat and simmer for 15 minutes, uncovered, stirring often, until the mixture thickens. Cool, then store in an airtight container in the fridge for up to 3 weeks, or freeze for up to 6 months.

MAKE IT IN A SLOW COOKER:
Simply cook on low for 5–6 hours until it's thickened.

2 SERVES VEG + FRUIT PER SERVE

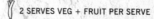

WARMING GOLDEN MILK

SERVES 1

A cup of Vata-calming goodness for your cockles. You can add a little stevia or rice malt syrup to taste, if you like.

1 cup (250 ml) milk (coconut or almond milk is best)

¼–½ teaspoon Fermented Turmeric Paste (page 340)

1 teaspoon coconut oil

generous sprinkle each of pure vanilla powder and ground cinnamon

Heat all the ingredients in a saucepan over a medium heat, stirring constantly. Serve warm.

MAKE IT A GOLDEN MILKSHAKE:
Place all the ingredients in a blender and whizz until foamy.

FIVE WAYS TO USE PUMPKIN SPICE BUTTER:

1. Spread over pancakes, dosas and toast.

2. Swirl into yoghurt, ice cream, porridge and smoothie bowls.

3. Make a Pumpkin Spice Butter, Walnut and Sauerkraut Toastie (page 84).

4. Try an Apple and Peanut Butter with Pumpkin Spice Butter Snack (page 120).

5. Make Socettes with Nomato Sauce and Pumpkin Spice Butter (page 106).

'BUT THE KITCHEN SINK' BREAKFAST MINCE

SERVES 6

I've been waiting for this moment for years. Yep, I'm finally including a recipe from Jo, my right-hand mate who's supported me in the writing of all my books. Not a massive fan of a pan and a set of hotplates, she arrived in the I Quit Sugar office one day with what she calls 'My Chop Suey'. Mercifully it doesn't contain packet chicken noodle soup or pineapple. She eats it naked (the meal, that is!), but you could serve it with a fried egg or poachie.

Which bread is best?

Mass-produced bread generally uses a high-gluten flour (gluten makes bread fluffy) and can contain a lot of sugar. Gluten-free versions generally contain even more sugar. The best options are:

* My Allergy-Free Bread (page 113).
* A sprouted bread – sprouting breaks down the gluten.
* Sourdough – the cultures in the sourdough partially break down gluten and slow our absorption of the sugars in white flour, plus they activate the enzymes required to break down the phytic acid. Even commercial sourdoughs contain less sugar than most other breads.

1 tablespoon coconut oil, olive oil, butter or ghee

1 large onion, finely chopped

3 cloves garlic, crushed

800 g beef mince

3 tablespoons curry powder

3 tablespoons tamari

2 cups (300 g) grated or finely chopped vegetables (cabbage and courgettes are best, but use whatever you have in the fridge – celery, beans, sweet potato, carrot)

1 cup (150 g) frozen peas

Heat the oil, butter or ghee in a large frying pan over a medium–high heat. Add the onion and garlic and sauté until the onion softens (about 5 minutes). Add the mince, breaking it up with a wooden spoon. Cook until browned (about 5 minutes). Stir in the curry powder and tamari and cook for 1 minute. Add the grated or chopped vegetables and peas, stirring until cooked through. Serve as is or with toast or a fried or poached egg.

 This dish keeps in the fridge for a week and is a great base for creating Leftover Mishmashes (see pages 246–65).

1 SERVE VEG + FRUIT PER SERVE

£0.72 PER SERVE

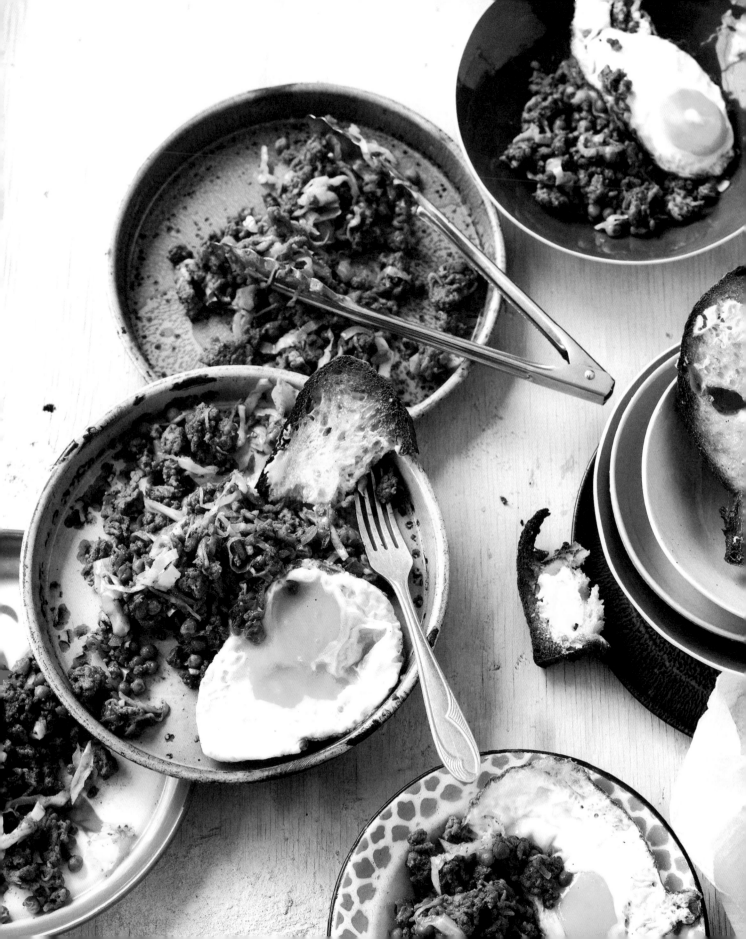

FOUR-INGREDIENT (or less) TOASTIES : If you're going to eat toast, you should really make it count

Layer up your ingredients between two slices of bread (see pages 113–14 for my homemade bread recipes), scrape with a bit of butter, and toast in a sandwich press, under a grill or in a skillet.

PUMPKIN SPICE BUTTER, WALNUT AND SAUERKRAUT

- Pumpkin Spice Butter (page 80)
- chopped walnuts
- Simplicious Sauerkraut (page 337), drained

even better with a smear of tahini

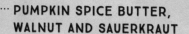

PINK BEET AND GOAT'S CHEESE

- Cooked 'n' Frozen Beetroot (page 23), thawed and sliced
- crumbled goat's cheese or sliced brie
- watercress, basil or spinach

1 SERVE VEG + FRUIT PER SERVE

KIMCHEESE

- 'But the Kitchen Sink' Kimchi (page 337) or Simplicious Sauerkraut (page 337), drained
- sliced gruyère or emmental
- thinly sliced apple or pear

½ SERVE VEG + FRUIT PER SERVE

which bread is best?

THE GREEN GODDESS

- Leftovers Pesto (page 55) or Green Minx Dressing (page 54)
- sliced avocado
- sliced cheddar, emmental or mozzarella
- spinach or watercress

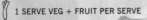 1 SERVE VEG + FRUIT PER SERVE

BROCCOLI AND CHEESE MELTS

- steamed or roasted broccoli, chopped
- sliced cheddar
- sprinkle of Seaweed Dukkah (page 45) or dob of mustard

1 SERVE VEG + FRUIT PER SERVE

BLUEBERRY, BASIL AND MOZZARELLA

- frozen blueberries, thawed
- sliced mozzarella or feta
- basil (or watercress or baby spinach)

½ SERVE VEG + FRUIT PER SERVE

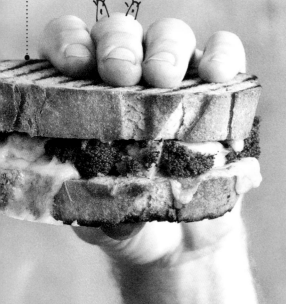

THE NEW GREEN "ZMOOTHIE"

Green smoothies are the new Starbucks-coffee-cup-as-accessory (worn with yoga mat slung over shoulder). Yawnful Instagram clichés aside, I tend to have a few issues with them: they can be mighty expensive, not particularly sustainable (um, carting coconuts across the globe?) and too complex and cold. Worry not. I've applied a few simplicious fixes to the formula, starting with my favourite vegetable, the courgette (that's zucchini for us Aussies), used in place of the less nutrient-dense cucumber, the more expensive avocado and the too-sweet banana. Blend on . . .

The courgette is creamier and 200–300% denser in nutrients than the cucumber.

Smoothies V juices
Liquefying your breakfast or lunch has some health benefits – it can jam in a bunch of greenery, while giving your digestion a bit of a break. But puréeing instead of juicing fruit and veggies is a far better way to go. It not only retains the fibre and extra nutrients from the skin but also helps you metabolise any sugar content. Oh, and it involves no wastage.

CHOCOLATE CHERRY BLITZ

SERVES 2

½ cup (115 g) frozen pitted cherries
(or any frozen berries)

1 cup (150 g) grated or chopped fresh or frozen courgettes

2 handfuls of baby spinach leaves
(or just add extra courgettes)

4 tablespoons raw cacao powder

3 tablespoons vanilla protein powder
or 1 tablespoon chia seeds and a pinch
of powdered stevia (optional)

1 cup (250 ml) milk (any kind)

Place all the ingredients in a blender with ½ cup (125 ml) of water and blend until smooth. Add a little more water or milk if you need to.

1½ SERVES VEG + FRUIT PER SERVE

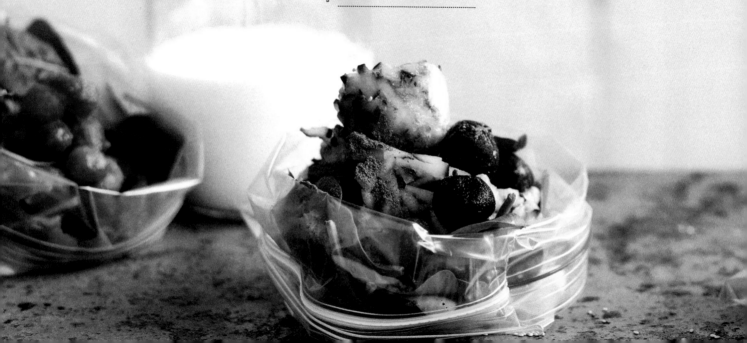

COURGETTE BREAD THICKIE

SERVES 2

Meet the thickie: a smoothie made over into a full meal. This thickie will keep you going 'til late lunch.

2 cups (300 g) grated or chopped fresh or frozen courgettes

½ frozen banana (or add extra courgettes and a big pinch of powdered stevia)

1 cup (250 ml) milk (any kind)

½ cup (70 g) Cooked Quinoa (page 26) or 50 g whole rolled oats (raw, soaked or cooked)

3 tablespoons nut butter (pecan or almond is best)

1 tablespoon chia seeds

1 teaspoon Pumpkin Spice Mix (page 45) or ¾ teaspoon ground cinnamon and ¼ teaspoon ground nutmeg

Place all the ingredients in a blender with ½ cup (125 ml) water and blend until smooth. Add a little more water if you need to.

2 SERVES VEG + FRUIT PER SERVE

MY GUT-HEALING BREW

SERVES 2

When I pitched the idea of a smoothie made with bone broth/stock to the I Quit Sugar office they thought I was mad. But then they tasted it. Makes a great lunch or light dinner, too.

1–2 cups (150–300 g) grated or chopped fresh or frozen courgettes

½ cup (75 g) frozen peas

½ avocado

2 cups (500 ml) Homemade Stock (page 42; beef or chicken is best)

juice of 1 lemon

1 clove Good for Your Guts Garlic (page 340), finely chopped

sea salt and freshly ground black pepper

1 teaspoon Fermented Turmeric Paste (page 340)

2 cups (100 g) watercress leaves (optional)

full-fat organic plain yoghurt (optional)

Place all the ingredients in a blender and process until smooth. Add extra stock or water to achieve your desired consistency. Try not to serve this *too* cold as warm foods are more settling. In fact, feel free to heat it a little. Serve with a little yoghurt if you like.

3 SERVES VEG + FRUIT PER SERVE

Smoothie bags:
Freeze ingredients together in zip-lock bags and have them ready to plonk into your blender.

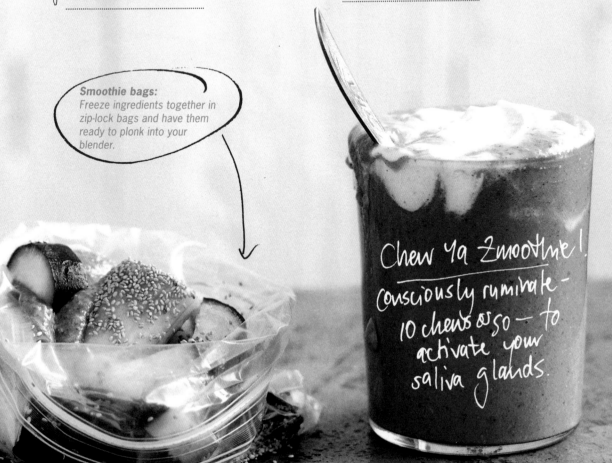

Chew Ya Zmoothie!
Consciously ruminate - 10 chews or so - to activate your saliva glands.

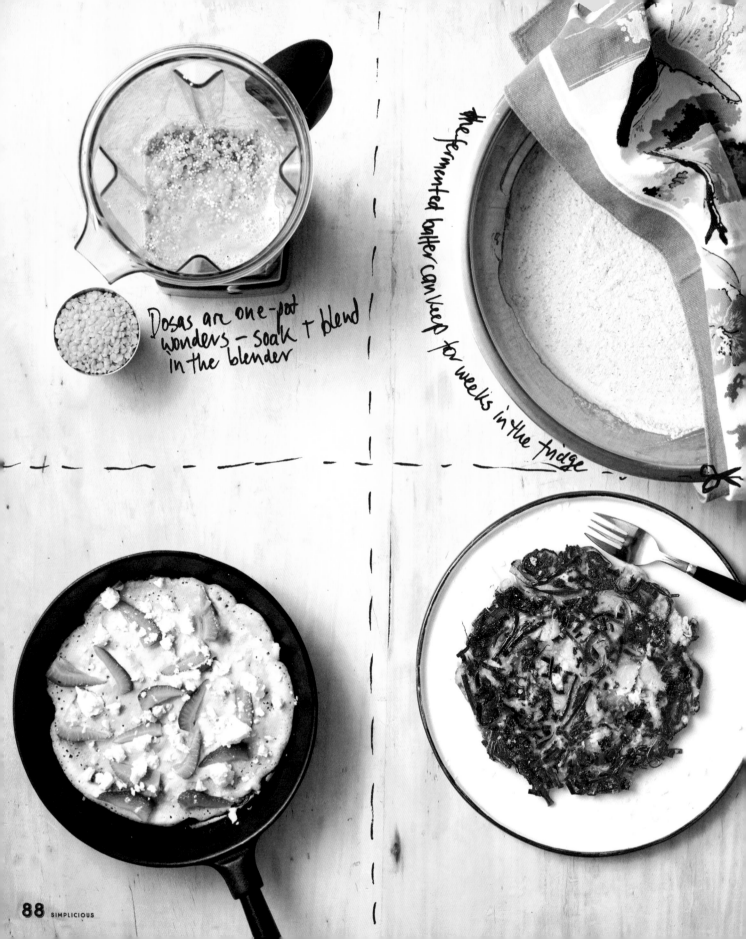

Dosas are one-pot wonders — soak + blend in the blender

the fermented batter can keep for weeks in the fridge

FERMENTED DOSAS

Does a dosa do things for you like it does for me? Not tried one? Well, let's get you dosed up. These traditional Indian pancakes tick a buncha boxes for me.

Dosas are:

* **Fermented.** Flick back to page 26 to read why fermenting grains is a win-win-win and kind of non-negotiable.

* **Low-toxin.** Especially mine. Traditional dosas are made with lentils and rice. I make mine with red lentils – the least toxic legume on the planet – and quinoa, which is gluten-free.

* **Brimful of protein.** Especially mine. Quinoa has both more and better protein than any other grain and one serve deals up 28% of your daily protein intake. But wait! Lentils contain double the amount of protein of quinoa. A protein punch right there.

1 cup (225 g) quinoa

1 cup (200 g) red lentils

1 tablespoon ground fenugreek

1 teaspoon sea salt

olive oil, coconut oil or ghee, for frying

Place all the ingredients in a blender. Add 2 cups (500 ml) water and let it sit for 4–6 hours or overnight. The next day, blend until smooth. Pour the batter into a large bowl and leave it to sit for 1–2 days, covering the bowl with a tea towel to prevent bugs taking their fill. Bubbles will form and the batter will puff up a lot, so ensure the bowl is big enough for this. If it's cold or wintry, add 2 teaspoons of apple cider vinegar, lemon juice or whey (see page 46) to oomph the fermenting process.

When ready to cook, heat a skillet or small frying pan with 1 teaspoon oil or ghee. Stir the batter a little (adding extra water if necessary to ensure a pouring consistency) and pour in 4 tablespoons or so. Swirl or use a spatula to spread the mixture to the pan's edge. Feel free to make a thicker pancake (called an igli), covering with a lid when you cook it.

Once the batter has big bubbles on top, flip it over and cook for another minute or two. Make as many as you need, then put the rest of the batter in the fridge. Before using again, stir it (and add a little water if necessary) each time.

MAKE IT AN ONION CURRY DOSA:
Add a sprinkle of ground turmeric or cumin to the batter before cooking. Slice half a red onion and sauté in the hot pan before adding the batter. Serve with Watercress Sauce (page 176) or Green Minx Dressing (page 54) and a dollop of yoghurt.

I keep a batch in the office fridge and the team dip in when they need a quick snack or lunch accompaniment.

SNACKALICIOUS

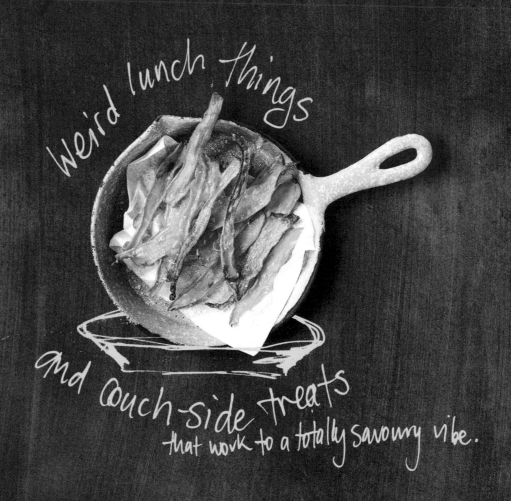

Weird lunch things and couch-side treats that work to a totally savoury vibe.

BROC BITES

MAKES ABOUT 20

These are like lovely little scones and are delicious served warm or cold.
Make up a big batch and freeze them – they make great health-bombs for
the lunchbox.

coconut oil, olive oil, butter or ghee,
for greasing

2–3 cups (300–450 g) Par-Cooked 'n'
Frozen broccoli (page 22), thawed and
chopped

1½ cups (150 g) grated cheese (cheddar,
parmesan or whatever you have)

3 eggs

1 cup (125 g) flour (plain, gluten-free
or almond)

1 teaspoon dried oregano
or 1 tablespoon chopped
oregano

sea salt

Preheat the oven to 190°C (gas 5). Line two baking trays with baking paper and
lightly grease the paper.

Combine all the ingredients in a large bowl and mix well. Roll the mixture into
bite-sized balls and place on the prepared trays. Bake for 25 minutes or until
golden. Store in an airtight container in the fridge for 4–5 days, or freeze for up
to 1 month.

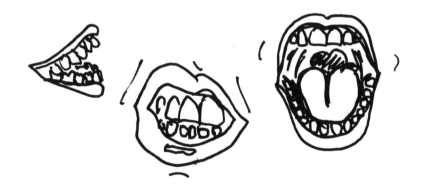

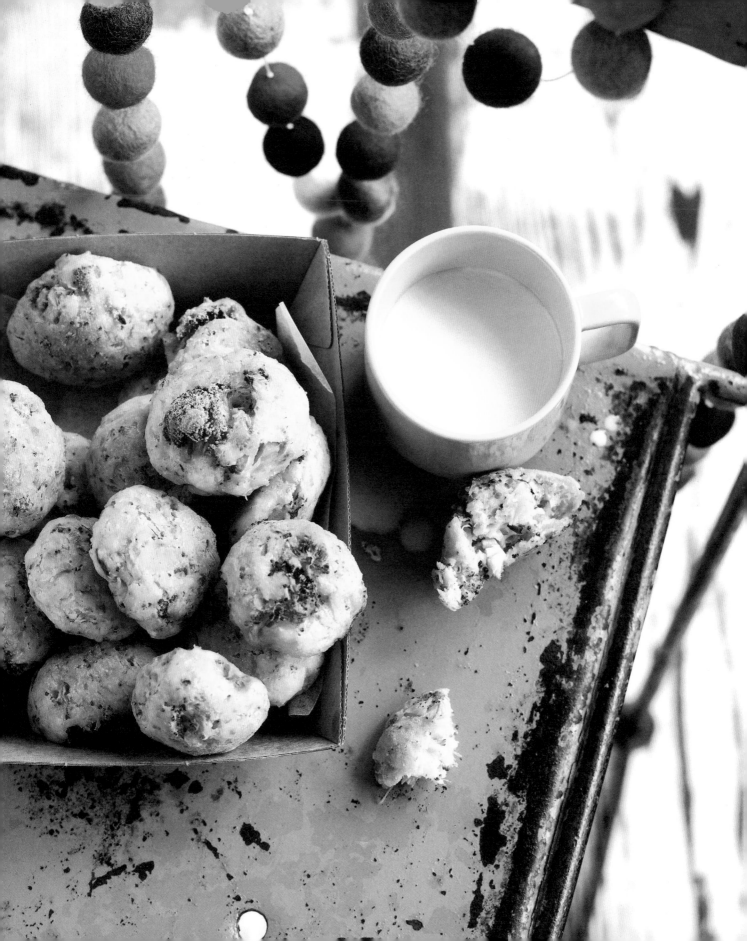

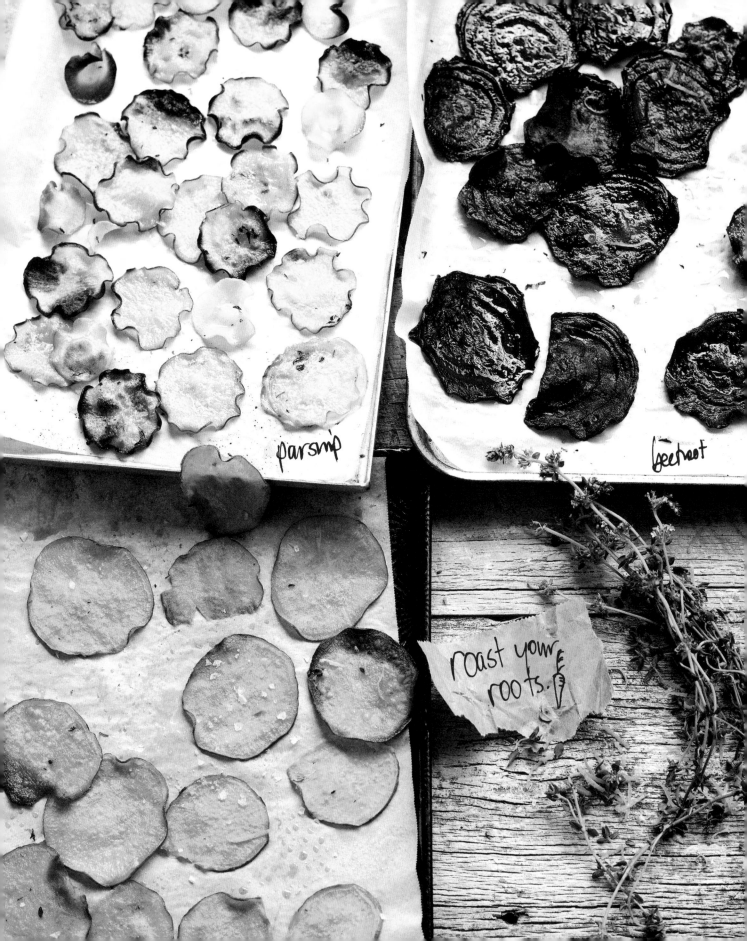

parsnip

beetroot

roast your roots.

ORANGE AND THYME RAINBOW CHIPS

SERVES 12

Make these rippers when you do your Sunday cook-up. Try to buy even-sized roots for this recipe, so your chips match nicely.

1 parsnip

1 swede, peeled

1 beetroot, peeled

1 sweet potato

1/3 cup (75 g) coconut oil,
butter or ghee, melted

zest of 1 orange

½ cup (125 ml) orange juice

1 tablespoon finely chopped thyme

1 teaspoon sea salt

Preheat the oven to 200°C (gas 6) and line two baking trays with baking paper.

Using a sharp knife or a mandoline, slice all of the vegetables into even, thin rounds (2 mm thick). Mix the oil, butter or ghee, orange zest and juice, thyme and salt in a large bowl. Add the parsnip and swede and toss to coat. Transfer the rounds to the first baking tray in a single layer (no overlapping). Repeat the process with the beetroot and sweet potato placing them on the other tray.

Bake the parsnip and swede chips for around 15 minutes and the beetroot and sweet potato chips for 25 minutes, or until golden. Remove from the oven and transfer to wire racks to cool. You can store them in an airtight container for 2–3 days, though they'll lose a bit of their crunch.

½ SERVE VEG + FRUIT PER SERVE

SLICE 'N' BAKE MISO BUTTER BISCUITS

The beauty of these is twofold: four ingredients only, and you can portion out what you need to bake a fresh batch.

1¼ cups (150 g) buckwheat flour

3 tablespoons sesame seeds, plus extra for sprinkling

5 tablespoons red miso paste   *You can use black, white or a combo.*

125 g butter, cubed

3 tablespoons iced water

coconut oil, butter or ghee, for greasing

Place the flour, sesame seeds and miso in a food processor and whizz for a few seconds until combined and crumbly. Add the butter cubes and iced water and process, turning the processor off and on frequently, until the mixture starts to ball around the blade.

Turn the dough out onto a floured surface and knead very lightly. Halve the dough and place each portion on a piece of cling film. Roll each half, with the help of the film, into a log 3 cm in diameter. Wrap the log up completely and place in the fridge to chill for 30 minutes. You can keep these in the fridge for up to a week before baking, or in the freezer for 2 months before thawing and baking.

When ready to bake, preheat the oven to 200°C (gas 6) and lightly grease two baking trays. Cut the dough into 5 mm slices and arrange on the prepared trays. Sprinkle each with a pinch of extra sesame seeds. Bake for 12–15 minutes, or until light golden and crisp. Transfer to a wire rack to cool. These biscuits are best eaten fresh though you can store them in an airtight container for 3–4 days.

Cut + bake what you need as you need

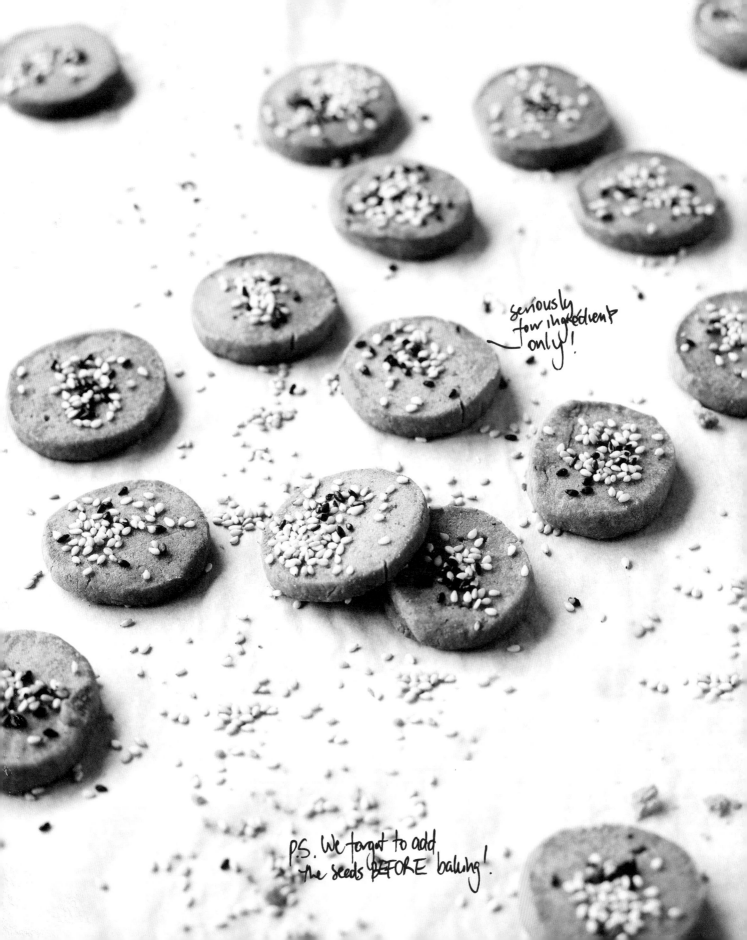

seriously
two ingredient
only!

P.S. We forgot to add
the seeds BEFORE baking!

ROAST CHOOK 'MEFFINS'

Meffins are meat muffins. Eat two for lunch. Meffins that make a meal
out of a deconstructed roast dinner are the money.

2 teaspoons coconut oil, olive oil, butter
or ghee, plus extra for greasing

1 small onion, chopped

500 g chicken mince

2 eggs

1½ cups (350 ml) Sweet Potato Purée
(page 23)

¾ cup (115 g) frozen peas, thawed

3 sprigs thyme, leaves chopped

1 sprig rosemary, leaves chopped

juice of ½ lemon

1 clove garlic, finely chopped

sea salt and freshly ground black pepper

Preheat the oven to 180°C (gas 4) and grease an 8-hole muffin tray.

Heat the oil, butter or ghee in a frying pan over a medium heat. Add the onion
and sauté until soft (about 3 minutes). Transfer the onion to a bowl and toss in
the mince, eggs, 1 cup (240 ml) of the Sweet Potato Purée, ½ cup (75 g) of
the peas, half the thyme, the rosemary, lemon juice and garlic, then season with
a good pinch each of salt and pepper. Using your hands, mix the ingredients
together until well combined. Divide the mixture into eight portions and press
firmly into the prepared muffin holes. Bake for 25 minutes, or until the meat is
cooked through and the tops are lightly browned. Remove from the oven and cool
before serving.

To serve, place 1 tablespoon of Sweet Potato Purée on each of the meffins and
sprinkle with the remaining peas and thyme. These will keep in the fridge for
2–3 days. Or you can freeze them (without the purée or peas) for 2–3 months.

½ SERVE VEG + FRUIT PER SERVE

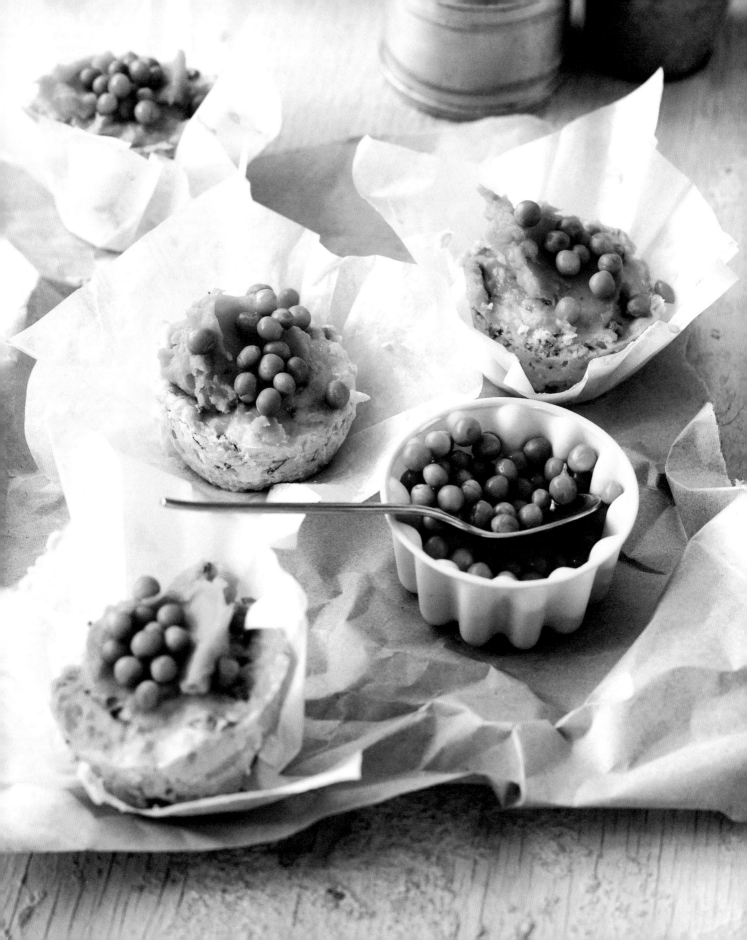

CAULI POPCORN

¼ cup (50 g) coconut oil, melted
½ teaspoon paprika (smoked or sweet) or ground turmeric
¼ teaspoon ground cinnamon

1 teaspoon sea salt
1 large head cauliflower, cut into bite-sized florets

Preheat the oven to 200°C (gas 6). Place the oil, spices and salt in a large bowl. Toss in the cauliflower and coat well. Transfer the cauli to a baking tray and bake, tossing once, for 30 minutes or until golden brown and popcorny.

MAKE IT CHEESY CAULI POPCORN:
Add 3 tablespoons of nutritional yeast powder or grated parmesan and omit the cinnamon.

1 SERVE VEG + FRUIT PER SERVE

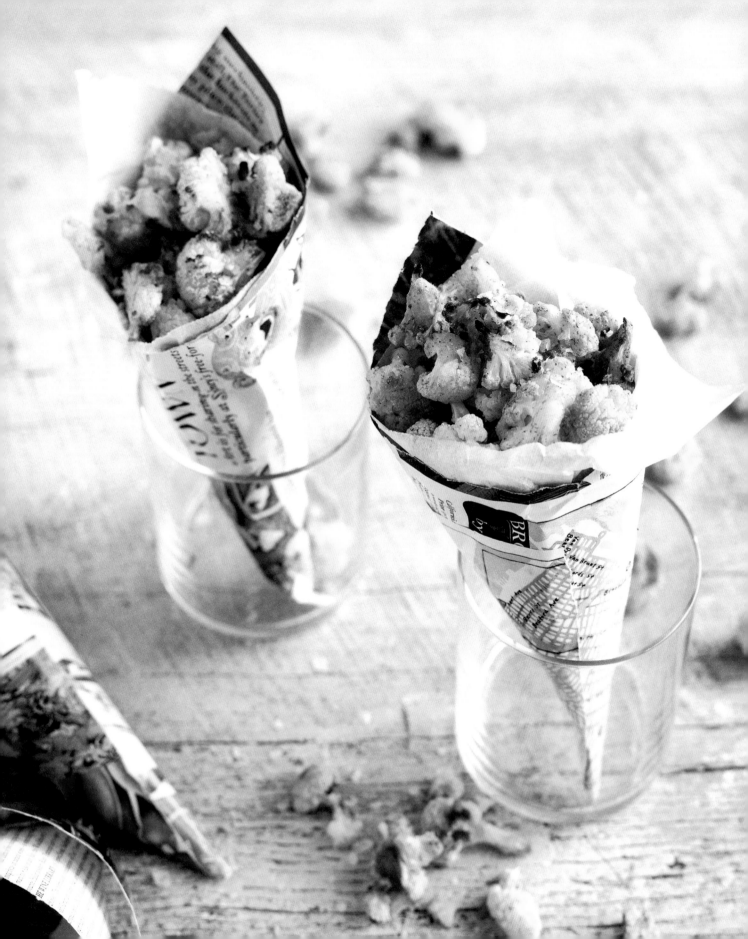

CHEESEBURGER DIM SIMS

Yep, seriously!

So much potential wrongness, right? But, I tell you,
this is close to my favourite recipe in this book.

2 teaspoons coconut oil, olive oil,
butter or ghee

1 small onion, finely diced

250 g beef mince

4 tablespoons buckwheat flour
or plain flour

½ cup (75 g) grated beetroot

8 small pickles (preferably no sugar added),
finely diced (or 1 tablespoon capers, finely
chopped)

75 g cheddar, grated

sea salt and freshly ground black pepper

15 rice paper sheets (22 cm diameter)

Nomato Sauce (page 51), to serve

Preheat the oven to 180°C (gas 4) and line a large baking tray with baking paper.

Heat the oil, butter or ghee in a frying pan over a medium heat. Add the onion
and cook until translucent (about 3 minutes). Transfer to a mixing bowl along
with the mince, flour, beetroot, pickles or capers, and cheese. Season to taste
with salt and pepper and use your hands to combine.

Fill a shallow dish (large enough to fit a rice paper sheet) with warm water.
Submerge a sheet in the water for 15 seconds, or until soft. Transfer to a clean
chopping board and use a sharp knife to slice it in half.

Place 1 tablespoon of the mince mixture in the centre of each half, fold to form
a parcel and place on the prepared tray. Repeat with the remaining rice paper
sheets and mixture. Bake for 10–15 minutes or until the meat has cooked
through. Serve with Nomato Sauce.

These were done with whole pickles. It's much easier to chop & mix it with the mince.

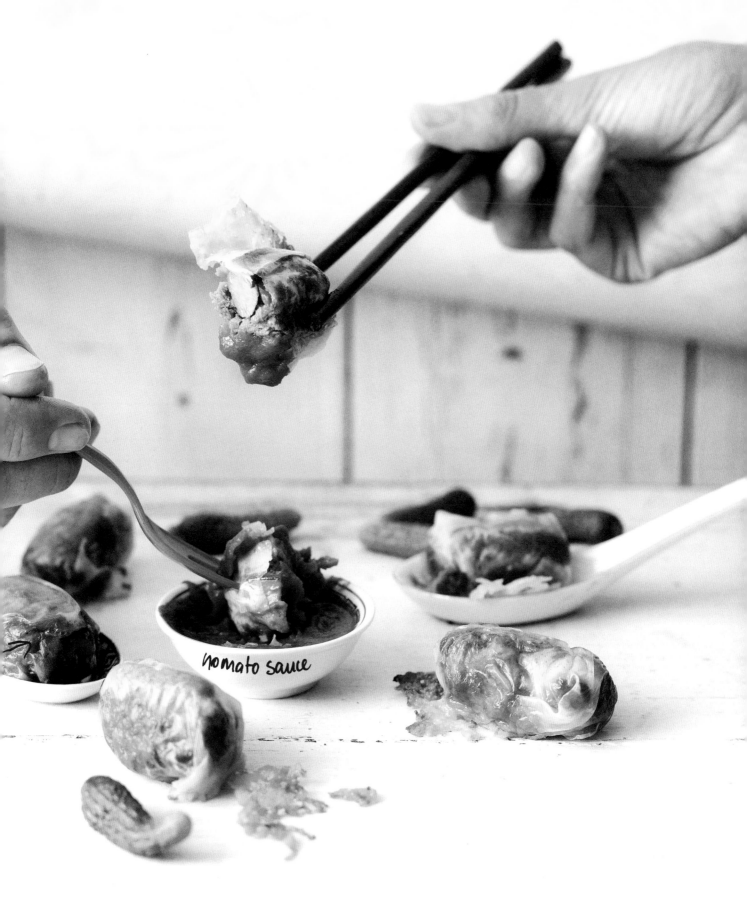

tomato sauce

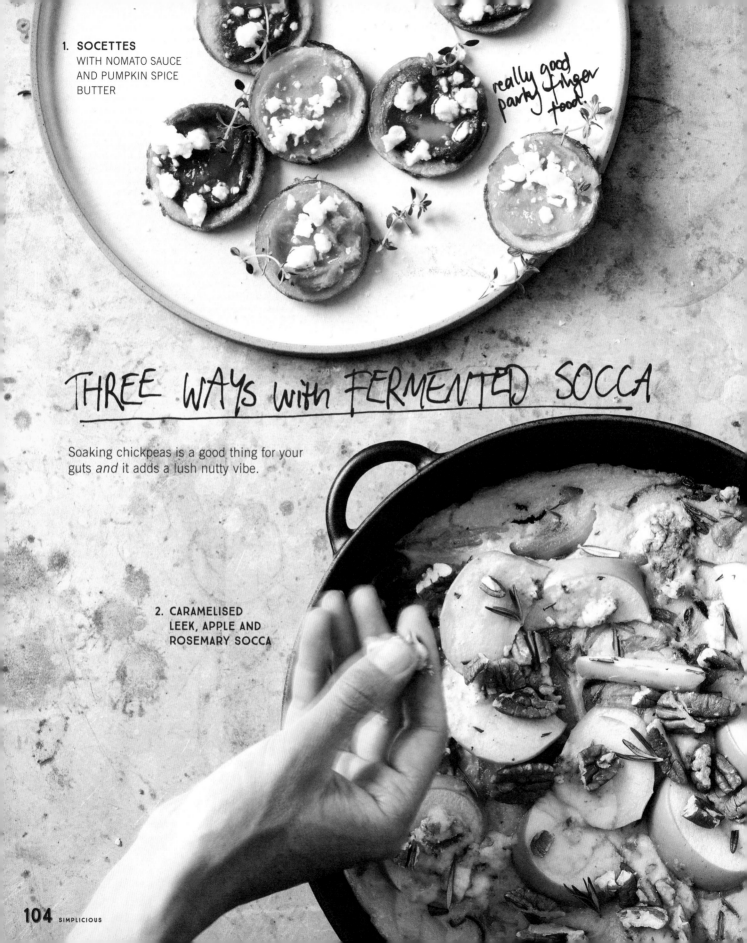

1. **SOCETTES**
   WITH NOMATO SAUCE
   AND PUMPKIN SPICE
   BUTTER

really good party finger food.

THREE WAYS with FERMENTED SOCCA

Soaking chickpeas is a good thing for your guts *and* it adds a lush nutty vibe.

2. **CARAMELISED
   LEEK, APPLE AND
   ROSEMARY SOCCA**

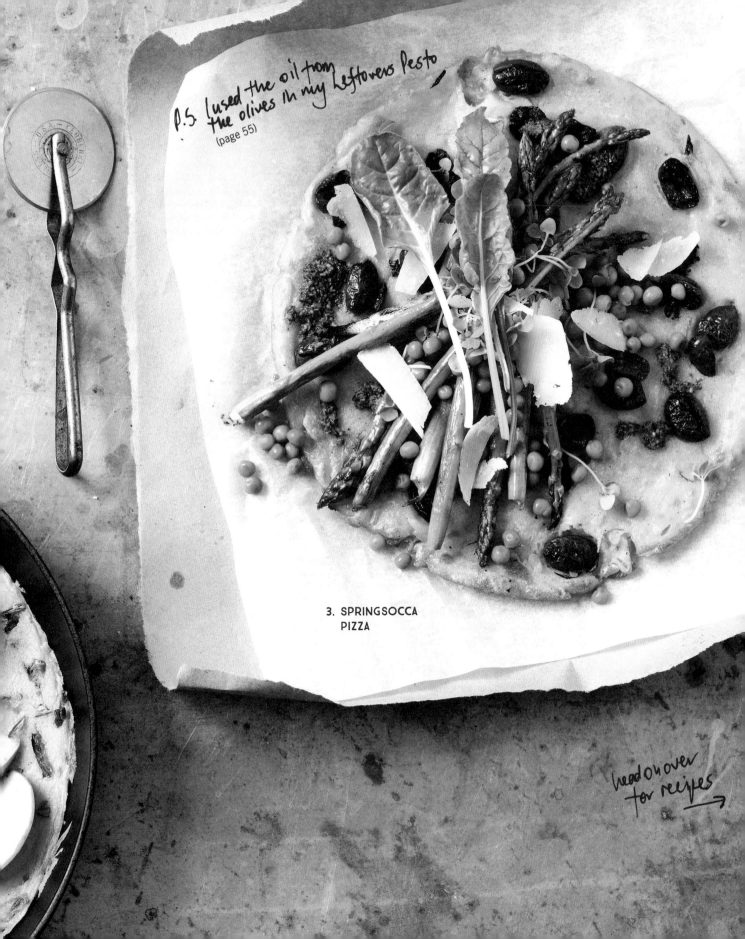

P.S I used the oil from
the olives in my Leftovers Pesto
(page 55)

3. SPRING SOCCA
PIZZA

head on over
for recipes →

First make... your...

BASIC SOCCA

SERVES 6 AS A SIDE

1 cup (100 g) chickpea flour

1 teaspoon apple cider vinegar, Homemade Whey (page 46) or lemon juice

2 tablespoons coconut oil, butter or ghee, plus extra for greasing

½ teaspoon sea salt

Place the flour and vinegar, whey or lemon juice in a bowl with 1¼ cups (300 ml) water. Whisk until combined. Cover with a tea towel and allow to rest at room temperature overnight (24 hours is even better). It should bubble slightly and become lighter and airier. Whisk in the oil, butter or ghee and the salt until the mixture forms a thin, smooth batter.

Preheat the grill to high and place the rack about 15 cm below the element. Place a dob of oil, butter or ghee in a cast-iron skillet and heat under the grill for a few minutes, until hot. Pour half to one-third of the batter into the skillet, swirling to create a thin layer. Grill for 5–10 minutes, or until the edges crisp. Remove from the pan and repeat with the remaining batter. Cut into wedges and serve with soups, dips, stews etc. Freeze any unused wedges to reheat and serve.

MAKE IT ON YOUR STOVETOP:
Heat a little oil, butter or ghee in a non-stick frying pan over a medium–high heat. Pour in the batter and swirl to evenly coat the pan. Cook, flipping once the batter comes away from the side (about 2–3 minutes). Cook for an extra 2 minutes on the other side.

then mix things up

1. SOCETTES

MAKES 24

Generously grease two 12-hole muffin trays with coconut oil and heat them in a 180°C (gas 4) oven for 2–3 minutes. Spoon 1 heaped tablespoon of Basic Socca batter into each muffin hole and return the tray to the oven for 8 minutes – the batter will pull away from the sides of the holes a little. Remove the socettes gently (using a spatula) and cool on a wire rack. Turn the oven up to 200°C (gas 6). Top each socette with Pumpkin Spice Butter (page 86), Nomato Sauce (page 51) or Courgette Butter (page 189); a crumble of feta or Homemade Cream Cheese (page 46) and a sprinkle of thyme. Return to the oven for a few minutes or until the cheese melts.

2. CARAMELISED LEEK, APPLE AND ROSEMARY SOCCA

SERVES 2 AS A LIGHT LUNCH

Preheat the grill to high and place the rack about 15 cm below the element. Caramelise a sliced leek in butter or oil in a cast-iron skillet for a good 10 minutes, adding 1 tablespoon of chopped rosemary after 5 minutes. Add ⅓ cup (75 ml) Basic Socca batter to the leek and place under the grill for 5–10 minutes or until the edge crisps. (Or you can do all of this on the stovetop as per the variation above.) Once cooked, layer with sliced apple, crumbled blue cheese and smashed pecans and place back under the grill to melt the cheese a little (about 3 minutes).

3. SPRING SOCCA PIZZA

SERVES 2

Make as per the main recipe, but toss in ½ cup (75 g) pitted kalamata olives, halved, once you've poured the batter into the hot pan and cook as above. While the grill is on (and if there is enough room), cook a bunch of asparagus spears cut into shards and coated in a little oil. Once everything is cooked, smear your pizza with Leftovers Pesto (page 55) and layer with the asparagus as well as some mint, peas, watercress . . . whatever takes your fancy. Sprinkle with parmesan gratings and a raining of lemon juice.

PEACH AND PEANUT BUTTER FROZEN YOGHURT

SERVES 2

3 tablespoons natural peanut butter
or other nut butter, softened

1 teaspoon rice malt syrup (optional)

½ cup (100 g) full-fat organic plain yoghurt
(Greek-style is best)

pinch of sea salt

pinch of ground cinnamon (optional)

2 peaches, roughly chopped

Basic Raw Chocolate (page 56), to serve

crushed peanuts, to serve (optional)

In a bowl (or your stick-blender beaker), combine the peanut or nut butter and
the rice malt syrup if using (you might need to heat them in the microwave for
a few seconds so they combine properly). Add the yoghurt, salt and cinnamon
(if using) and stir. Place in the freezer for 45 minutes. Transfer to a blender with
the peaches. Pulse a few times to mix but not purée. Return to the freezer for
1–2 hours. To serve, melt the chocolate in a cup in the microwave (do it gradually
on low). Divide the frozen yoghurt between two bowls and top with a swirl of
melted chocolate and a sprinkle of crushed peanuts (if using).

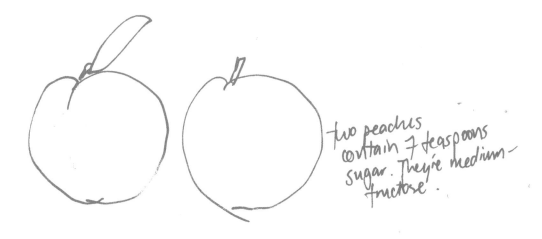

two peaches
contain 7 teaspoons
sugar. They're medium-
fructose.

½ TSP ADDED SUGAR PER SERVE

½ SERVE VEG + FRUIT PER SERVE

BACON GRANOLA

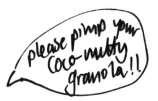

I was asked by precisely 23 of you to pimp my original granola recipe (the one featured in my first book, *I Quit Sugar*). In my second book we have chocolate granola. However, I think this bacon version is the tastiest and most versatile of the cousins. Use as a soup topper, on savoury yoghurt or as a trail mix ('scroggin' for my Kiwi mates).

10 rashers streaky bacon, rind removed (keep all the fat on)

3 (175 g) cups coconut flakes

2 cups (250 g) mixed nuts or seeds (use whatever you have – almonds, cashews, pecans, walnuts, pumpkin seeds), activated if possible (page 28) and roughly chopped

3 tablespoons chia seeds

2 tablespoons Pumpkin Spice Mix (page 45) or 1½ tablespoons ground cinnamon and 2 teaspoons ground nutmeg

I don't sweeten mine at all.

4 tablespoons rice malt syrup (optional)

Preheat the oven to 120°C (gas ½) and line a baking tray with baking paper.

Place the bacon in a large, heavy-based saucepan and add just enough water to completely coat the bottom of the pan. Cook over a medium–high heat until the water has evaporated. Reduce the heat to medium and cook until the bacon is crisp (about 10 minutes – no need to turn). Remove the bacon and place in a strainer over the pan to drain all the fat. When cool, break the bacon into bits and retain the fat.

Combine the remaining ingredients in a big bowl. Add the bacon bits and stir in 4 tablespoons of the bacon fat (if you don't have enough, top it up with coconut oil). Spread the mixture over the tray and bake for 20–25 minutes, until golden, stirring after 10 minutes.

Store any leftover bacon fat in a sealed glass jar in the fridge and use it instead of cooking oil. It will keep for up to 1 month.

MAKE IT FASTER:
Use ¼ cup (50 g) coconut oil instead of the bacon fat and add 5 tablespoons of frozen Bacon Bits (page 44) in the last 5 minutes of baking.

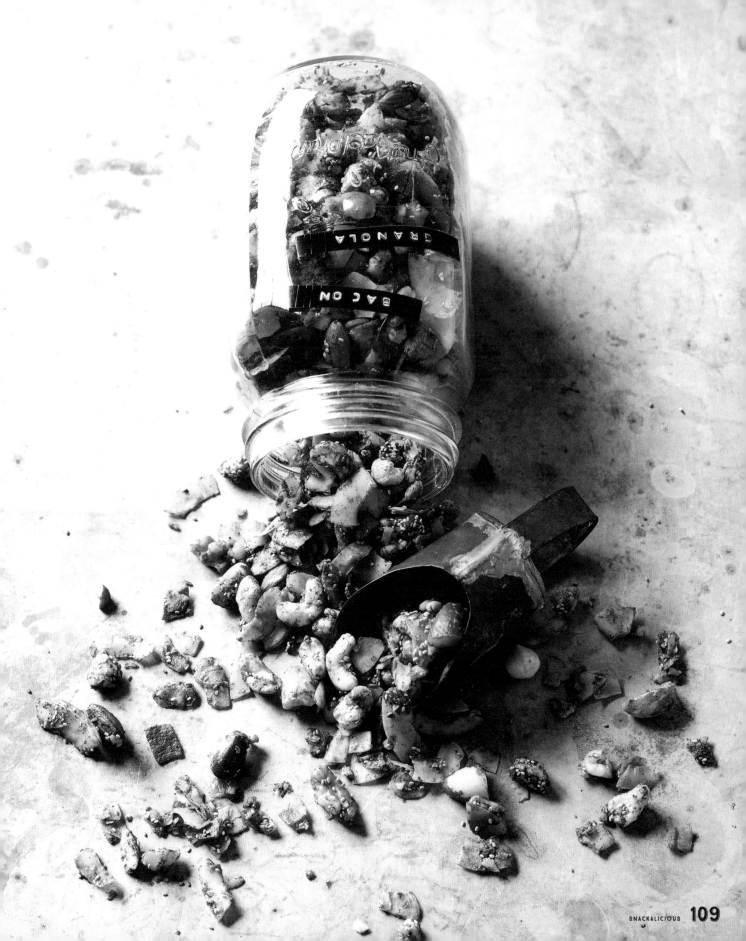

SPICED PANEER 'N' PEAS

IN WHICH I 'PIMP' ANOTHER OF MY CLASSICS

SERVES 2

I was also asked by you guys to overhaul the 'Salted Caramel' Haloumi and Apple recipe from my first book, which all of us got a bit obsessed about. Rather than go another sweet route I thought I'd just share my latest cultured cheese obsession.

1 teaspoon ghee or coconut oil

½ cup (120 g) Homemade Paneer (page 48), cubed

¼ red onion, finely diced

½ teaspoon garam masala or Ras el Hanout Mix (page 45)

½ teaspoon ground cinnamon

1 bay leaf (optional)

½ cup (75 g) frozen peas, thawed

Powerhouse Dressing (page 53), to serve

Heat the ghee or coconut oil in a small frying pan over a medium heat. Add the paneer and cook for 1–2 minutes. Add the onion, spices and bay leaf, if using. Cook until the paneer is golden and the onion is soft. Add the peas and a dash of water and cook briefly to combine and reduce the liquid.

Serve with a drizzle of Powerhouse Dressing.

½ SERVE VEG + FRUIT PER SERVE

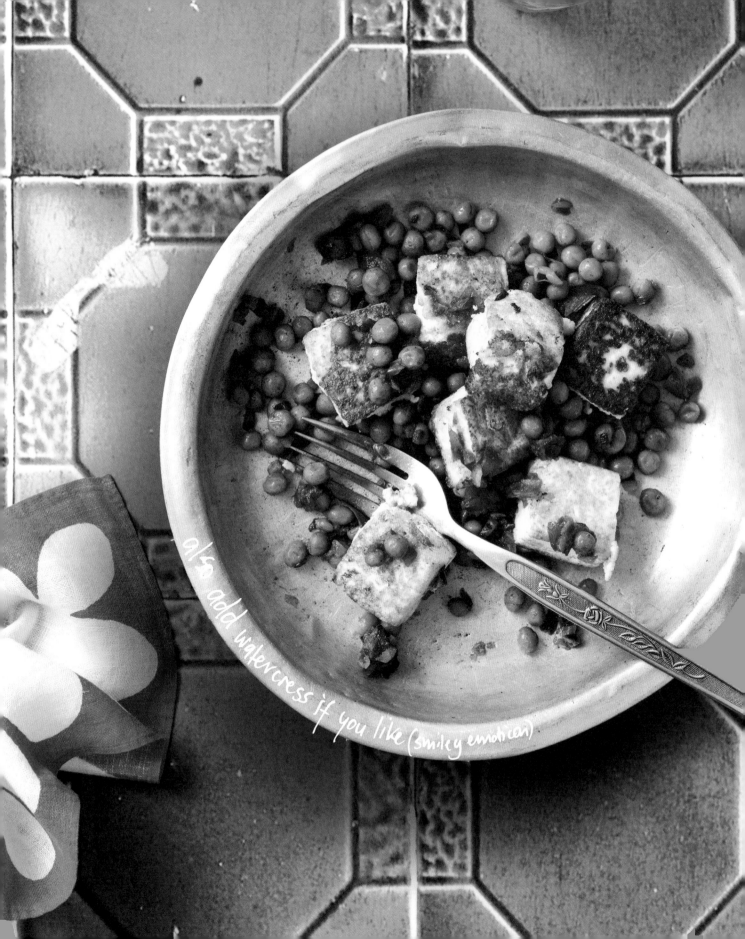

also add watercress if you like (smiley emoticon)

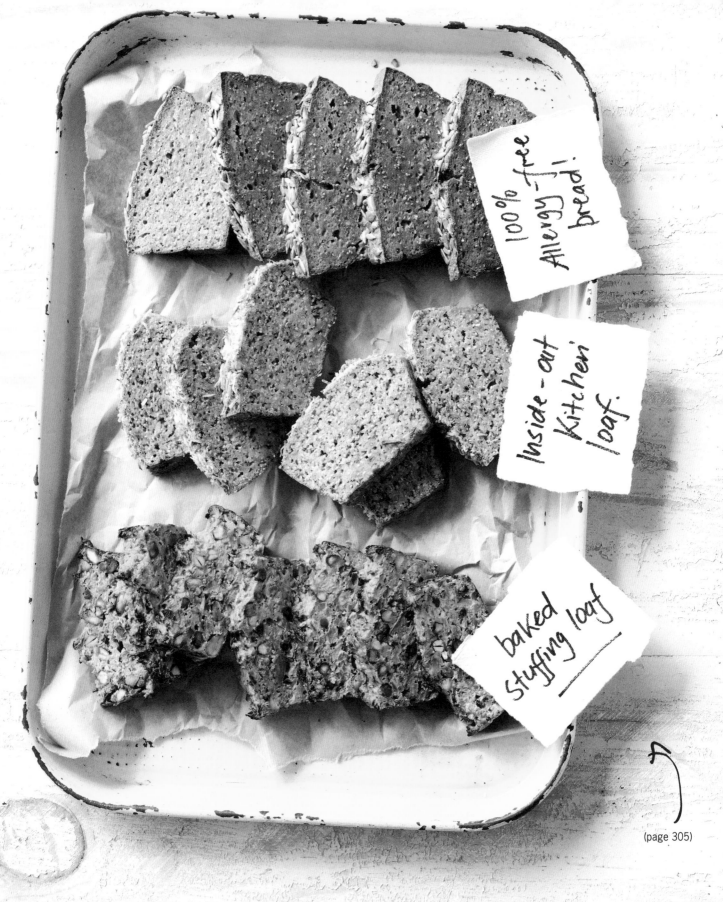

100% Allergy-free bread!

Inside-out Kitchen loaf.

baked stuffing loaf

(page 305)

MY ALLERGY-FREE BREAD

MAKES 1 LOAF ————————————————————————————————

This stuff suits most FODMAPs, paleo peeps, vegans, lactose intolerants, nut sensitives, gluten-frees and anyone in between or beyond.

2 cups (350 g) buckwheat groats

4 tablespoons chia seeds

1½ teaspoons gluten-free baking powder

1 cup (150 g) grated sweet potato

¼ cup (50 g) coconut oil

1 onion, chopped (if you're on FODMAP, use 2 tablespoons chopped chives or the green tops of spring onions and add ½ cup (75 g) extra sweet potato)

1 teaspoon sea salt

4 tablespoons sunflower seeds

Rinse the buckwheat well. Place in a large bowl or jar and cover amply with water. Allow to soak for at least 4 hours (preferably overnight).

Preheat the oven to 160°C (gas 3) and line a 23 cm × 13 cm loaf tin with baking paper.

Place the chia seeds in a glass jar with 1 cup (250 ml) water. Seal with the lid and shake every few minutes until a chia gel forms (about 10 minutes).

Drain the buckwheat using a sieve – it might be slimy, so ensure you rinse it well. Allow all the water to drain out.

Place the drained buckwheat, chia gel, baking powder, sweet potato, coconut oil, onion and salt in a food processor or high-powered blender and process until a thick paste forms. Spoon into the prepared loaf tin and sprinkle the sunflower seeds on top.

Place the bread on the middle shelf of the oven and cook for 1 hour. When cooled, remove from the loaf tin and allow to cool completely before cutting into 1 cm slices. Serve as is, or toasted and spread with coconut oil (or butter or olive oil, depending on your dietary needs).

This bread will last 4–5 days in the fridge. To freeze, cut into slightly thicker (1.5 cm) slices and layer between baking paper. It can be thawed and toasted very successfully.

INSIDE-OUT SPROUTED KITCHERI LOAF

MAKES 1 LOAF

This bread is great on your guts and wonderfully balanced to keep your doshas calibrated (see page 362). I've also sprouted the beans to reduce the phytic acid and make it even gentler on the guts – not a big deal if you don't have time, but it creates a more textured bread, so consider doing so. Why is it 'inside-out'? Well, I've taken my standard kitcheri recipe (from my second book) and put the toppers (the egg and coriander) and the sweet potato variation all on the inside of the bread to bring you a meal in one loaf.

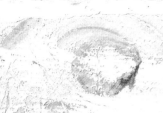

See my note on page 23 about the benefits of eating resistant starch in this way. →

1 tablespoon ghee or coconut oil, plus extra to serve (optional)

1 small red onion, finely chopped

1 teaspoon each of black mustard seeds, cumin seeds and fennel seeds

1 teaspoon each ground coriander seeds and ground turmeric

1 tablespoon grated ginger

1½ cups (150 g) sprouted mung beans or brown lentils (page 352)

1 cup (135 g) cooked basmati rice

1 cup (150 g) grated sweet potato

1 cup (125 g) arrowroot

1 teaspoon baking powder

1 teaspoon sea salt

3 eggs

4 tablespoons ground chia seeds

shredded coconut, to garnish

Homemade Cream Cheese (page 46), to serve

Preheat the oven to 180°C (gas 4). Grease and line a 23 cm × 13 cm loaf tin with baking paper.

Melt the ghee or coconut oil in a small frying pan over a medium–high heat. Add the onion and sauté for 1–2 minutes. Add the mustard, cumin and fennel seeds, spices and ginger, and sauté for 1–2 minutes until the mustard seeds start to pop and the onion is translucent. Set aside to cool.

Transfer the onion to a food processor with the sprouts, rice, sweet potato, arrowroot, baking powder, salt, eggs and chia seeds and process until combined. Pour into the prepared tin and smooth the top of the batter. Sprinkle with shredded coconut. Bake for 1 hour or until a skewer inserted in the middle comes out clean. Leave to sit for 5 minutes before transferring to a wire rack. Once the loaf is completely cool, cut into thick slices and store in a container (or wrapped in foil) in the fridge. It will keep for up to 5 days. Alternatively, slice and freeze for up to 1 month.

Serve the kitcheri loaf warm, spread with cream cheese, coconut oil or butter.

½ SERVE VEG + FRUIT PER SERVE

CARROT 'BACON'

Use as a vegan substitute on Abundance Bowls (pages 126–37) and beyond.

carrots – as many as you have to spare
coconut oil
sweet paprika, to serve
sea salt, to serve

Preheat the oven to 180°C (gas 4) and line a baking tray with baking paper. Using a veggie peeler, or a mandoline set at 2 mm, thinly slice each carrot lengthways to form long, even strips. Coat the carrot strips lightly in coconut oil (don't drench; you might like to use a spray). Place the carrot strips flat on the tray, making sure they don't overlap. Bake for 20 minutes, flipping them halfway or until you get your version of perfect crispiness. Use these as you would bacon (on burgers, in salads or as a snack). They keep for 1–3 days in an airtight container in the fridge (if they last that long!).

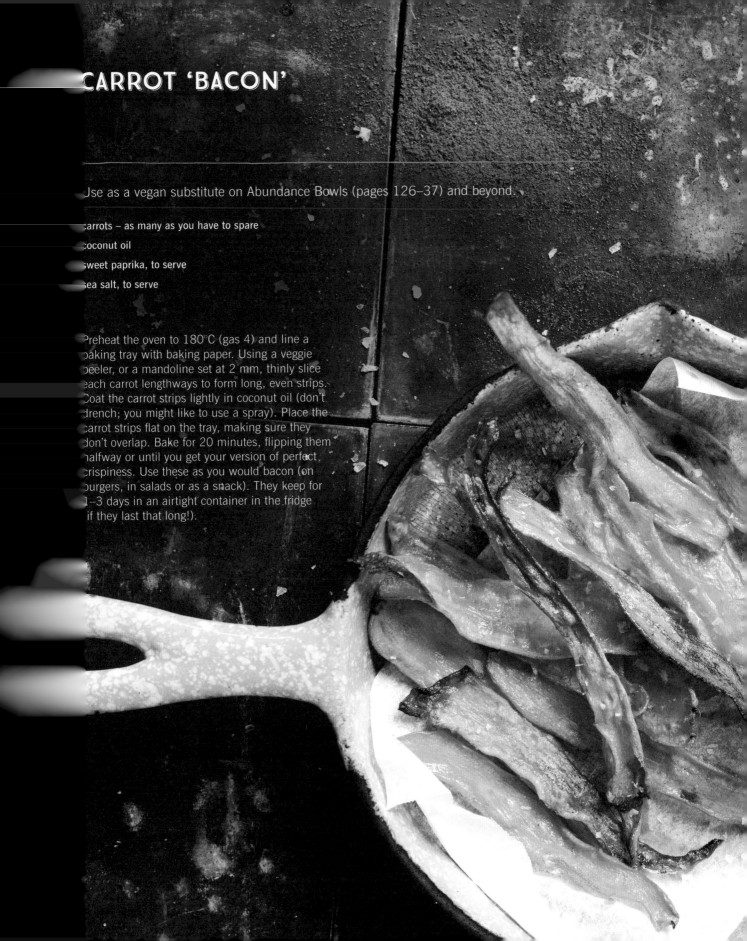

TWO-MINUTE DESK LUNCH NOODLES

SERVES 1

Pack this up in a big jar in layers, take it to work, add hot water and stir with a chopstick (or your pen). Done.

The frozen veggies keep things cool 'til lunch.

What prawns should you buy?

Look for Marine Stewardship Council–certified prawns (they certify prawns in 15 countries around the world).

Not too many.

All prawns have sustainability issues in part because the bycatch is shocking. Depending on where they are trawled, for every prawn caught, up to 27 other species are trapped in the bycatch and tossed away. *Please, pause on this.*

Go farmed rather than trawled, due to bycatch issues. Organic farmed prawns are very high quality. Or go local estuary or river prawns, which aren't trawled.

1–2 teaspoons red curry paste

1 teaspoon red miso paste

dash of fish sauce

small handful of rice noodles

¼ cup (60 ml) coconut milk or cream (or use 3 cubes frozen coconut milk or cream; page 25)

small handful of frozen peas (or thinly sliced mangetout)

½ cup (75 g) Par-Cooked 'n' Frozen broccoli (page 22)

5 cooked prawns, peeled and deveined, or a small handful of Shredded Chicken (page 214)

3–4 spring onions, thinly sliced on the diagonal

coriander leaves and lime wedges, to serve

Pop them in a separate zip-lock bag.

Place all the ingredients, except the coriander and lime, in a large jar in the order given above. Whack in the fridge when you get to work. At lunchtime, pour over enough boiling water to just cover everything, pressing the ingredients down. Cover and leave for 2 minutes, stirring once or twice. Top with the coriander and a squeeze of lime juice. Eat.

MAKE IT KIMCHI INSTANT NOODLES:
Use ½ cup (125 ml) of 'But the Kitchen Sink' Kimchi (page 337) instead of the pastes and sauce, and replace the prawns with Pulled Beef (page 223), Some Beefin' Good Jerky (page 209) or cubed tofu. Add some chilli sauce if you like.

MAKE IT ITALIAN 'PASTA' NOODLES:
Add, in this order: 1/3 cup (45 g) Cooked Quinoa (page 26); 1 courgette, sliced into thin strips; 1/3 cup (75 ml) Nomato Sauce (page 51); a small handful of Shredded Chicken (page 214) and the broccoli and peas (as per the recipe above). Serve with basil leaves or Leftovers Pesto (page 55).

2 SERVES VEG + FRUIT PER SERVE

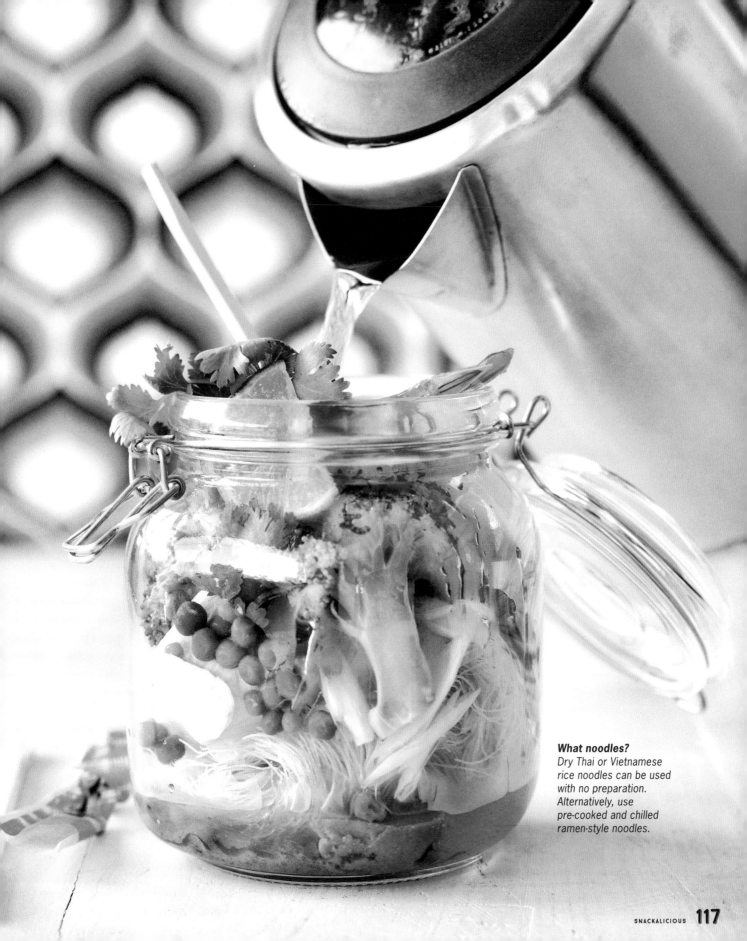

What noodles?
*Dry Thai or Vietnamese
rice noodles can be used
with no preparation.
Alternatively, use
pre-cooked and chilled
ramen-style noodles.*

A SUPER-GREENS
COUCH FONDUE

SERVES 6 ——

You can use any leftover leafy greens for this cheesy dipper dinner –
beetroot leaves work well! Eat on the couch with a DVD.

*Referencing outdated
technologies = sure
sign one is getting old.*

coconut oil, olive oil, butter or ghee,
for greasing

1 bunch Swiss chard, stalks removed,
leaves very finely chopped

1 onion, roughly chopped

2 cloves garlic, finely chopped

1½ cups (350 ml) sour cream

2 cups (225 g) grated vintage cheddar
(or your favourite hard cheese)

sea salt and freshly ground black pepper

Preheat the oven to 180°C (gas 4) and grease an ovenproof dish with oil, butter
or ghee.

Combine the chard, onion and garlic in a food processor and blitz until finely
chopped (not puréed). Add the sour cream and half the cheese, and season to
taste with salt and pepper. Blitz briefly to combine, then transfer to the prepared
dish. Sprinkle with the remaining cheese and bake for 15–20 minutes, or until
the cheese is melted and golden.

Serve with fun dipping things: scrubbed new carrots, sliced baby cucumbers,
sliced radish, chicory 'cups', fennel sticks, purple carrot sticks, sliced raw swede,
Socca wedges (page 106), seed crackers . . .

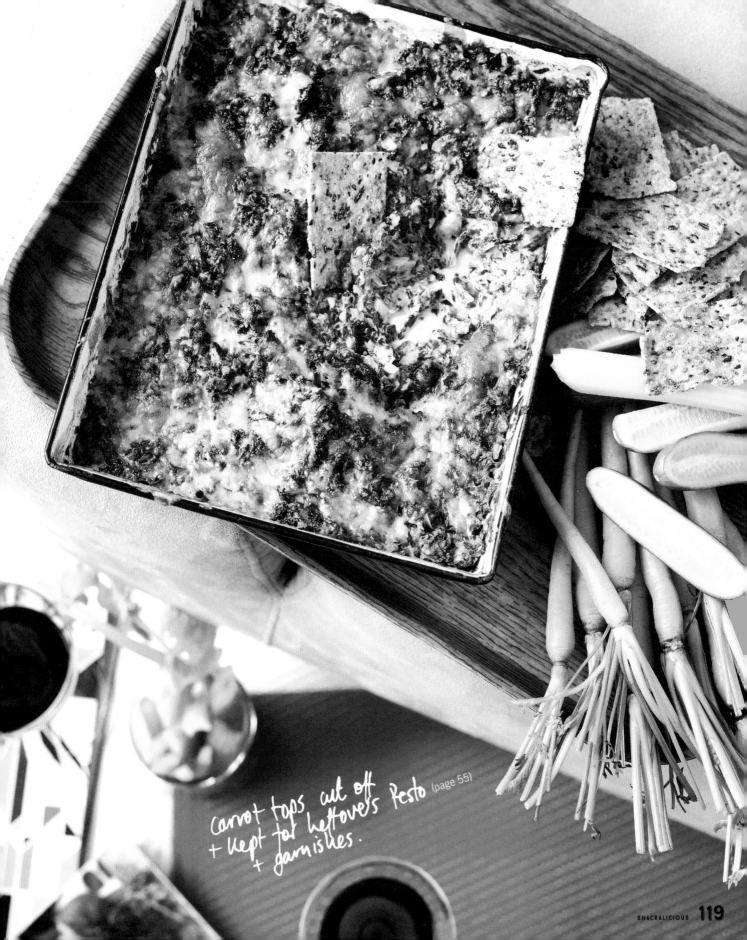

carrot tops cut off
+ kept for leftovers Pesto (page 55)
+ garnishes.

JUST a PAGE OF THREE-INGREDIENT SNACKS

Things I tend to eat for breakfast or for weekend "lunch-lites".

These are the three-ingredients-or-less things I 'snack' on,
often as part of my breakfast or a light weekend lunch.

Why I don't *really* snack

The concept of snacking
was developed by
nutritionists in the 1990s
to help treat the huge
numbers of people who
had developed diabetes
(and everyone else on the
planet riding a blood-sugar
rollercoaster and needing
to fuel themselves every
couple of hours). But we
are not designed to eat in
this way – it is inefficient
and taxing on our bodies.

Once you're off sugar for
a few months, you'll find
you don't need to snack
anyway – you'll be used
to eating full meals that
are nutritionally dense.

So, if I snack, it's directly
at the end of a meal if I
find myself still hungry.
Or in lieu of a meal if I'm
not that hungry.

1. **CHOC-NUT SPOON POPS**
Mix 1 tablespoon coconut oil with 1 heaped teaspoon raw cacao
powder and a big sprinkle of rock salt in a small cup (you can add
a tablespoon of nut butter as well and a drizzle of rice malt syrup
if you like). Pile onto a dessertspoon and freeze for 15 minutes.

2. **APPLE AND PEANUT BUTTER WITH PUMPKIN SPICE BUTTER**
Spread a slice of apple with natural peanut butter and a
dob of Pumpkin Spice Butter (page 80).

3. **UNTINNED SARDINES (PAGE 156) WRAPPED IN A LEAF**

4. **SWEDE CHEESEBURGERS**
Place slices of mature cheddar between thinly sliced raw swede.

*Ever tasted raw swede?
Oh, it's so good and sweet
and creamy-crunchy.*

5. **SOME BEEFIN' GOOD JERKY (PAGE 209) WRAPPED
IN A CABBAGE LEAF**

*I also like using radicchio
leaves.*

6. **MISOMITE IN A CUP**
Place a dollop of Misomite (page 54) in a chicory cup
or lettuce leaf.

7. **BRUSSELS SPROUT, HALOUMI AND SAUERKRAUT SLIDERS**

MAKES 16

40 g coconut oil

1 tablespoon tamari

½ teaspoon ground cumin

¼ teaspoon cayenne pepper

16 large brussels sprouts,
trimmed and halved

250 g haloumi

Simplicious Sauerkraut (page 337),
to serve

Preheat the oven to 200°C (gas 6) and line a large baking tray with
baking paper.

In a large bowl, combine 1 tablespoon of the coconut oil with the
tamari and spices. Toss through the sprouts until well coated. Place
them cut-side down on the baking tray and bake for 5 minutes.

Meanwhile, cut the haloumi in half lengthways and then into 5 mm
thick slices, giving you about 16 squares of haloumi, roughly the
size of your sprout halves.

Place on the oven tray with the sprouts and cook for another
10–15 minutes, turning halfway, or until everything is golden.

Assemble the sliders by layering a slab of haloumi and some
sauerkraut between two brussels sprout halves and securing with
a cocktail stick.

MICHAEL POLLAN

These are great at
cocktail dos, too

1.

witlof

3.

6.

a collard leaf

7.

4.

2.

5.

A WEEK of LUNCHBOXES: Five days of interesting food co that look cute in a box.

I appreciate that kids want more interesting lunches. But I also don't think parents should be spending all evening assembling them. Here are some quick fixes. In my experience, the best way to get your kids to eat the stuff in their lunchboxes is to have them make/assemble it with you.

KERMIT SLUSHIE ....
(page 125)

SUNFLOWER STRAWBERRY THUMBLES ....
(page 298)

MONSTER-MASH ROLL-UPS ....
(page 124)

HAM-WRAPPED CARROT STICKS ....

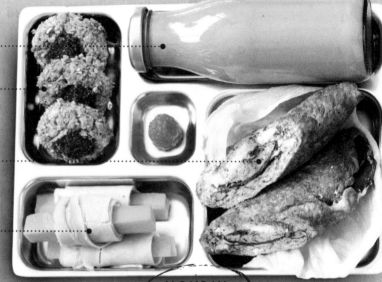

MONDAY

STRAWBERRY FROZEN YOGHURT ....
(page 125)

CHEESEBURGERS ....
Thread a leftover cooked meatball (page 144) and a chunk of cheese between two chunks of red pepper on a cocktail stick.

ORANGE AND THYME RAINBOW CHIPS ....
(page 95)

CARROT AND CUCUMBER STICKS ....

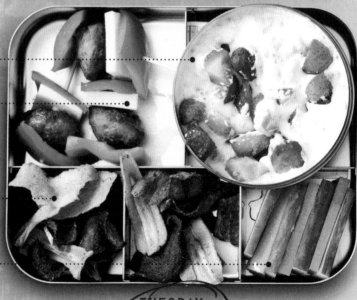

TUESDAY

CUCUMBER AND CARROT FLOWERS
You can make these with your kids; buy a bento cutter online or from an Asian supermarket. Use the leftover bits in your own smoothie or salad.

STRAWBERRY FROZEN YOGHURT
(recipe over page)

ROAST CHOOK 'MEFFINS'
(page 98)

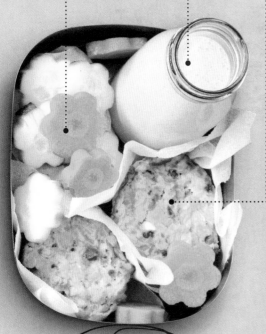

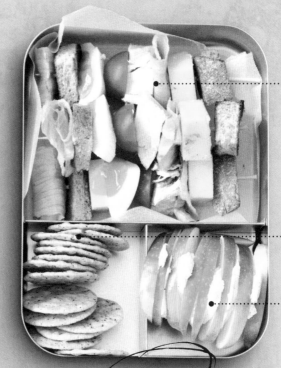

CHICKEN CAESAR ON A STICK
(recipe over page)

RICE CRACKERS OR SLICE 'N' BAKE MISO BUTTER BISCUITS
(page 96)

APPLE WEDGES AND CREAM CHEESE

WEDNESDAY

THURSDAY

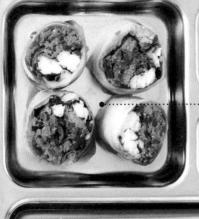

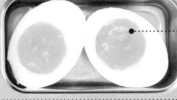

HARD-BOILED EGGS

check out my favourite egg-peeling trick (page 44)

RAINBOW ROLLS
(recipe over page)

KIWI AND RASPBERRY KEBABS

CREAM CHEESE-FILLED CELERY STICKS
(recipe over page)

FRIDAY

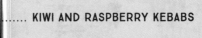
raisin-free + nut-free ants on a log

What should a healthy lunchbox contain?

This list is based on international dietary guidelines and works to the idea that a lunchbox contains about one-third to half of your kids' nutrition for the day.

2–3 serves VEGGIES
(1 serve = 1 cup (100 g) leafy greens or ½ cup/75 g other veggies)

1 serve FRUIT (1 serve = 1 peach or 2 kiwi fruit or ½ cup/75 g berries)

1 serve PROTEIN (1 serve = 2 eggs or 1 kid-sized handful of meat or 1 cup /75 g cooked legumes or 2 tablespoons nuts/seeds)

1 serve DAIRY (1 serve = 1 cup/250 ml milk or 2 slices cheese or ¾ cup/175 ml yoghurt)

Most guidelines also advise 2½ serves of grains. Which I don't feel needs to be factored in consciously. We get enough grains without trying.

MONSTER-MASH ROLL-UPS

SERVES 1–2

2 eggs

1 tablespoon chia seeds

1 tablespoon full-fat milk

1 tablespoon chopped herbs (try dill or basil) or ½ teaspoon dried herbs

1 teaspoon coconut oil

handful of baby spinach leaves

1 tablespoon crumbled feta

Whisk the eggs, chia seeds, milk and herbs together and leave to sit for 5 minutes. Heat the oil in a small frying pan over a medium–high heat. Pour in the egg mixture. Sprinkle with the spinach and feta. Reduce the heat to low–medium and cover with a lid (or a large plate or another pan). Cook for 2–3 minutes until the egg is set.

Lay a piece of baking paper on a flat surface. Slide the omelette onto the paper. Use the baking paper to tightly roll the omelette. Cut in half to serve.

MAKE IT EXTRA-NUTRITIOUS:
Add 1 teaspoon Fermented Turmeric Paste (page 340) to the eggs before whisking and lay a sheet of nori on top of the omelette before rolling.

1 SERVE VEG + FRUIT PER SERVE

RAINBOW ROLLS

MAKES 4

If you're organised, you can make this mixture the night before with the kids, and the next morning get them to help make the rolls.

1 beetroot, trimmed, scrubbed and grated

1 large carrot, grated

3 tablespoons chia seeds

⅓ cup (75 ml) Green Minx Dressing (page 54) or Whey-Good Mayo (page 50)

4 rice paper sheets (22 cm diameter)

½ cup (25 g) pea sprouts or green leaves (mint, spinach, watercress)

½ cup (65 g) Shredded Chicken (page 214)

Toss the beet, carrot, chia seeds and dressing or mayo in a bowl and let the chia work its soaking-up-the-sogginess magic for 5 minutes.

Set up a worktop with a chopping board, a plate and a large pan filled with warm water. Submerge a sheet of rice paper in the water for 30 seconds or until soft. Place on the chopping board and spread over 4 tablespoons of the beet mixture. Top with some sprouts or green leaves and some chicken. Fold one side in and then roll to form a log. Plonk one or two in each lunchbox.

1 SERVE VEG + FRUIT PER SERVE

What should a healthy lunchbox contain?

2-3 serves Veggies + 1 serve fruit + 1 serve protein + 1 serve dairy

CHICKEN CAESAR ON A STICK

MAKES 4 SKEWERS

2 hard-boiled eggs, halved

2 cherry tomatoes, halved

big wedge of iceberg lettuce, cut into cubes

1 slice bread, toasted and cut into cubes

1 cucumber, sliced

4 pieces Shredded Chicken (page 214) and/or cheddar

Thread the ingredients onto 4 skewers.

 ½ SERVE VEG + FRUIT PER SERVE

STRAWBERRY FROZEN YOGHURT

SERVES 4

1 cup (200 g) full-fat organic plain yoghurt

1 cup (150 g) frozen strawberries (or any other berries)

1 cup (60 g) coconut flakes

Place the ingredients in a blender and blend until smooth (or just mash with a fork). Transfer to containers with wide necks and firmly fitting lids, and freeze.

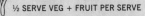 ½ SERVE VEG + FRUIT PER SERVE

KERMIT SLUSHIE

This little thing will keep lunch cool and thaw to become a slushie.

SERVES 4

1 frozen banana

2 cups (200 g) greens (baby spinach, cos lettuce, courgettes, mint)

1½ cups (350 ml) coconut water (or water)

3 cubes frozen coconut cream (page 25)

Place all the ingredients in a blender and blend until smooth. Place in a lunchbox brick or re-usable purée bag and freeze.

 ½ SERVE VEG + FRUIT PER SERVE

Peanuts V seeds

'Peanuts, tree nuts and nut products' are the focus for anaphylaxis policies in schools and are often banned. Seeds, however, are often suggested as good alternatives and are allowed in most schools.

Which is why I use tahini and seeds instead of nut butter and peanuts when creating my healthy lunchboxes.

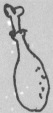

ABUNDANCE
BOWLS

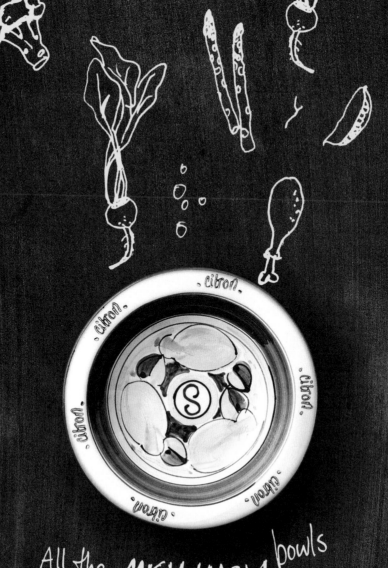

All the **MISH MASH** bowls
of <u>nutrient-dense</u> goodness I bore you
with on social media @_sarahwilson_ #sarahwilsoneats
#swmishmashmeals

HERE'S HOW I SHAPE MY BOWLS

These one-pan, two-minute mélanges are my standard lunch (or breakfast, or dinner) fare. I feel weird putting them into recipe format because I mostly make them on a whim, using what I've got (and a few too many lax cooking techniques). But I've been asked by my publisher to do so. So . . . here's how I shape my bowls:

Raw bowls V cooked bowls
Both have benefits.

The raw bowl argument:
Cooking reduces a food's enzymes and the fewer enzymes in a food, the more our own body's enzymes must be drawn upon to break down a meal. The more of our own enzymes we use, the quicker we age.

The cooked bowl argument:
Many of the vitamins and minerals in vegetables are embedded in the plant's cellulose cell walls, which require cooking to break them down. So many of the valuable nutrients in raw vegetables end up not being absorbed by the body.

In conclusion: I advocate a mix across a meal/your day of 70% cooked, 30% raw (varying a little from winter to summer). The best way to get your raw fix is via ferments (where the fermentation breaks down the tough cellulose walls) and eating vegetables that are meant to be eaten raw e.g. lettuce and cucumber.

Step 1: Start with 3 serves of veggies
Sauté in oil or sweat in 2 frozen stock cubes (page 25) or ferment brine (page 334).

1 serve → 1 cup (100 g) leafy greens
1 serve → ½ cup (75 g) all other veg

Step 2: Add 1 serve of protein
Deglaze, if required, with a big splash of ferment brine (page 334) or apple cider vinegar, or a squeeze of lemon juice.

2 eggs, a palm-sized portion of meat, or 1 cup (75 g) properly prepared legumes (page 28).

Step 3: Stir through 1–3 tablespoons of fat
As you all know, you need saturated fat to absorb essential vitamins A, E, K and D, and to digest meat protein. You're wasting your time without it.

Dressing, oil, cheese or avocado.

Step 4: Add an enzyme kick
1–2 tablespoons fermented veggies (page 334) or enzyme-rich food like sprouts (page 352) or bitter vegetables.

Step 5: Flavour-bomb
Soup Toppers (page 245), Seaweed Dukkah (page 45), Kale Flakes (page 179), Celery Leaf Salt (page 265), capers, dulse flakes, fresh herbs etc.

CLEAN BITTERS BOWL

2 handfuls of chopped radicchio, red chicory and/or red cabbage

½ cup (75 g) thinly sliced fennel or radish

1 celery stalk and leaves, thinly sliced

small handful of mint or coriander leaves, torn

¼ avocado, chopped

2 tablespoons Powerhouse Dressing (page 53)

½ cup (40 g) cooked puy or brown lentils (page 28)

smashed activated almonds (page 28), to serve

Toss together the radicchio, red chicory and/or red cabbage with the fennel or radish, celery and mint or coriander. Add the avocado, dressing and lentils, and top with the almonds.

ADD KICK: 2–3 tablespoons Pink Sauerkraut (page 337).

Big fennel V baby fennel
Large fennel bulbs are best for baking and soups, small ones are best for salads. But don't worry too much if you have the wrong one for the job. Both work.

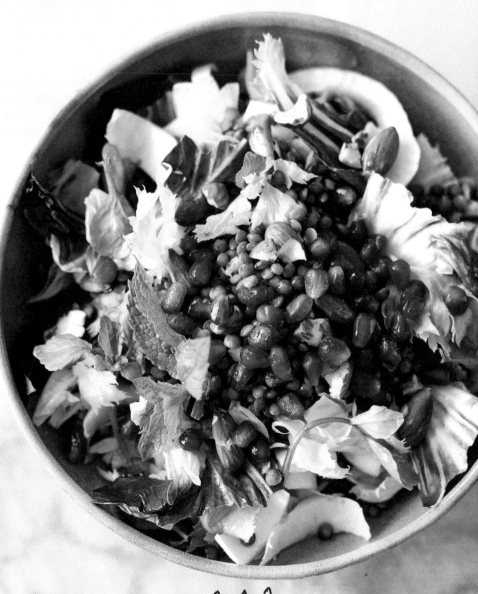

Add prettiness: a tablespoon of pomegranate seeds, half an APPLE or 4 strawberries

4½ SERVES VEG + FRUIT PER SERVE

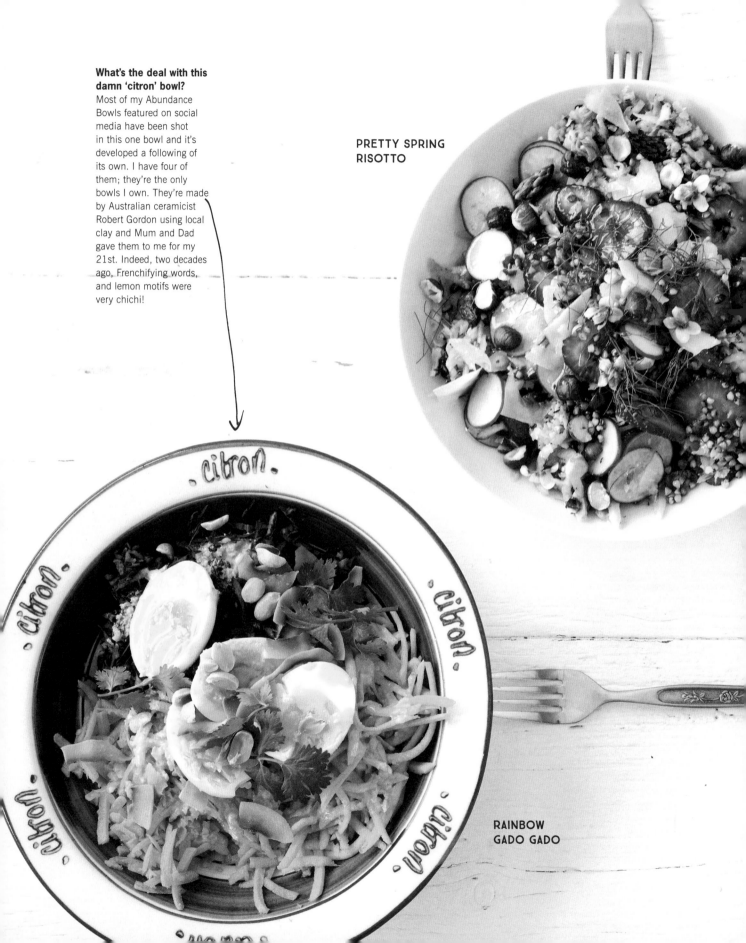

What's the deal with this damn 'citron' bowl?
Most of my Abundance Bowls featured on social media have been shot in this one bowl and it's developed a following of its own. I have four of them; they're the only bowls I own. They're made by Australian ceramicist Robert Gordon using local clay and Mum and Dad gave them to me for my 21st. Indeed, two decades ago, Frenchifying words, and lemon motifs were very chichi!

PRETTY SPRING
RISOTTO

RAINBOW
GADO GADO

TMT Dressing

NORI ROLL
IN A BOWL

fancy borage
flowers

seaweed dukkah

All recipes on the next page →

PRETTY SPRING RISOTTO

1 teaspoon olive oil, butter or ghee

3 cups (450 g) grated spring veggies (asparagus, courgettes, broccoli, fennel bulb and stalks)

1 frozen stock cube (page 25) or 1 tablespoon water

3 strawberries and/or radishes, sliced

shaved parmesan and chopped hazelnuts (preferably activated; page 28), to serve

Powerhouse Dressing (page 53), to serve

Heat the oil, butter or ghee in a skillet or small saucepan over a medium heat. Sauté the grated vegetable 'rice' for 1 minute, then deglaze with the stock or water. Serve with the sliced strawberries and/or radishes, a smattering of parmesan flakes and chopped hazelnuts and a good dollop of dressing.

ADD BULK: Sprinkle over ½ cup (85 g) Activated Groaties (page 27).

RAINBOW GADO GADO

1 cup (150 g) grated beetroot (or red cabbage)

1 cup (150 g) grated pumpkin

1 cup (150 g) grated carrot

2 boiled eggs, halved

4 tablespoons TMT Dressing (page 53) or 1 tablespoon each natural peanut butter, miso paste and coconut milk, whisked together

toasted peanuts and coriander leaves, to serve

Arrange the grated veggies in a bowl, top with the eggs and dressing and scatter over the toasted peanuts and coriander.

ADD KICK: 1–2 tablespoons of 'But the Kitchen Sink' Kimchi (page 337) or Simplicious Sprouts in a Jar (page 352), and a sprinkle of Seaweed Dukkah (page 45).

NORI ROLL IN A BOWL

4 asparagus spears

½ cup (75 g) Cooked Buckwheat (page 27), Cooked Quinoa (page 26) or Cauliflower Rice (page 23)

100 g Simplicious Smoked Salmon (page 160) or 90 g can pole-and-line-caught tuna

2 radishes, sliced

½ avocado, sliced

small handful of Simplicious Sprouts in a Jar (page 352)

1 nori sheet, crumbled, or 2 teaspoons Seaweed Dukkah (page 45)

TMT Dressing (page 53), to serve

1 teaspoon black sesame seeds

Blanch the asparagus in boiling water for a few minutes (or zap in the microwave if you're at work). Place the buckwheat, quinoa or cauli rice in a bowl. Top with the fish, radish, avocado, sprouts, nori or dukkah and asparagus. Spoon over the dressing and sprinkle with sesame seeds.

MAKE IT VEGETARIAN: Replace the fish with 100 g fried tempeh strips.

Why tempeh, not tofu?
I'm not a fan of soy, for a range of reasons, one of which is the phytic acid content. Tempeh, however, is fermented, which breaks down many of these problematic toxins.

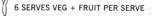 6 SERVES VEG + FRUIT PER SERVE

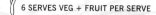 6 SERVES VEG + FRUIT PER SERVE

4 SERVES VEG + FRUIT PER SERVE

FOUR-INGREDIENT GREEN CHOOK SHRED-UP

1 bunch tenderstem broccoli, roughly chopped

1 frozen stock cube (page 25) or 1 tablespoon water

½ cup (65 g) Shredded Chicken (page 214)

1 tablespoon Leftovers Pesto (page 55)

½ avocado, chopped, or 3 tablespoons crumbled feta

In a skillet or small saucepan, sweat the broccoli in the stock or water for 1–2 minutes, adding a little more water if needed. Add the chicken. Mix the pesto with the avocado or feta and add to the pan, stirring to heat through.

ADD KICK: My Indian Kimchi (page 338) and Seaweed Dukkah (page 45).

ADD BULK: 1 portion Cooked Quinoa (page 26).

4 SERVES VEG + FRUIT PER SERVE

THE SIX-STAR WALDORF

1 cup Massaged Kale (page 23)

1 celery stalk and leaves, chopped

8 mangetout or sugar snap peas, sliced

½ peach, chopped

a dash of apple cider vinegar

2 tablespoons smashed pecans (preferably activated; page 28)

1–2 tablespoons crumbled feta

Toss the kale, celery, peas and peach with the apple cider vinegar. Top with the pecans and feta.

2 SERVES VEG + FRUIT PER SERVE

VATA BALANCING BOWL

Sweet Potato Chips (below), to serve

1 cup (100 g) Par-Cooked 'n' Frozen Swiss chard (page 22), thawed, or 2 cups (200 g) sliced chard

½ cup (65 g) Pulled Beef (page 223), Shredded Lamb (page 220) or Pulled Pork (page 222)

½ cup (75 g) frozen peas, thawed

steamed courgette rounds or yellow squash wedges, to serve

Make the sweet *Dead simple and fast* potato chips. ← *(due to secret tricks).* Remove from the pan and keep warm.

Deglaze the pan with a little water or ferment brine (page 334). Add the chard, meat and peas and cook for 2–3 minutes or until heated through. Serve with steamed courgette rounds or yellow squash wedges and sweet potato chips.

ADD KICK: A dollop of Pink Sauerkraut (page 337) and TMT Dressing (page 53).

3 SERVES VEG + FRUIT PER SERVE

SWEET POTATO CHIPS

Slice ½ sweet potato into 5 mm rounds. Heat a generous dollop of coconut oil in a small frying pan over medium–high heat. Add the sweet potato slices and sprinkle liberally with sea salt (this speeds up the cooking!). Cook both sides until dark golden (about 5 minutes all up).

1 SERVE VEG + FRUIT PER SERVE

PUTTANESCA FESTIVAL

small handful of watercress or radicchio leaves

1 courgette, carrot or parsnip, cut lengthways into thin ribbons with a veggie peeler or spiraliser

1 celery stalk and leaves, thinly sliced

4 cherry tomatoes, quartered

¼ red onion, thinly sliced

handful of pitted black olives

8 tablespoons Untinned Sardines (page 156) or 90 g can pole-and-line-caught tuna in brine or extra-virgin olive oil

1 tablespoon Leftovers Pesto (page 55)

4 tablespoons Activated Groaties (page 27) or toasted sourdough cubes

Place all the veggies and the olives in your bowl and toss. Top with the fish and pesto and scatter over the groaties or sourdough.

MAKE IT WARM:

If you have digestion or thyroid issues, you might like to sauté the vegetable ribbons (you can use the oil or brine from your fish), then add the other ingredients to heat through.

Courgettes in a salad
The great thing about using courgettes instead of cucumber or salad greens is that you can add the dressing in the morning and the whole thing marinates nicely – rather than going soggy – ready for lunch.

3 SERVES VEG + FRUIT PER SERVE

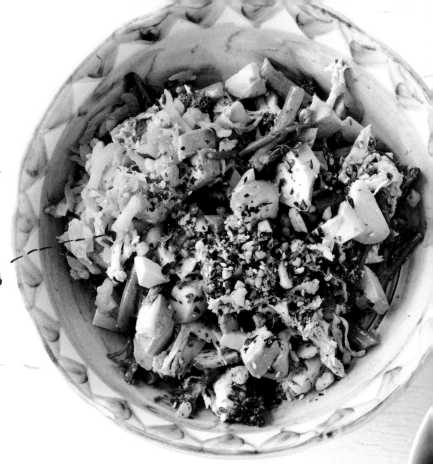

Recipes backover this way!

**FOUR-INGREDIENT
GREEN CHOOK
SHRED-UP**

Indian KIMCHI

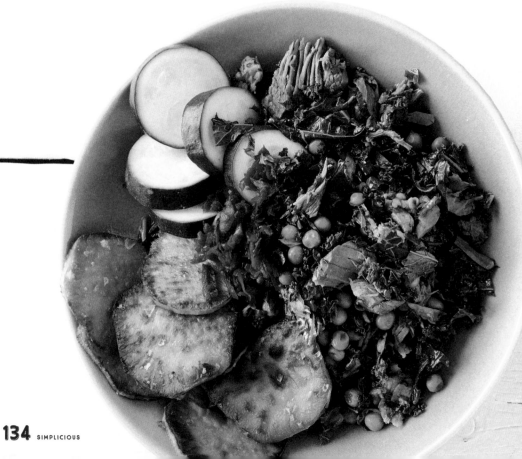

My "Anxi (great for

**VATA BALANCING
BOWL**
WITH PINK
SAUERKRAUT AND
SWEET POTATO CHIPS

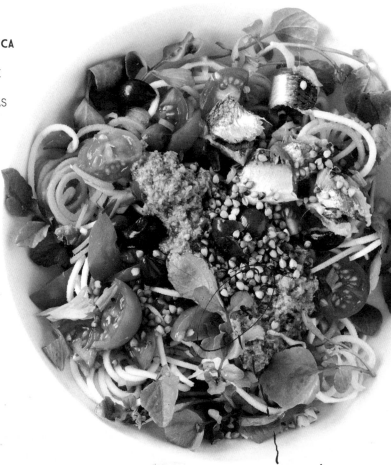

PUTTANESCA FESTIVAL
WITH SOME ACTIVATED GROATIES AS THE 'PASTA' ELEMENT

Activated GROATIES

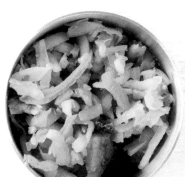

THE SIX-STAR WALDORF

BOWL"
E-Y DAYS)

INDIAN KIMCHI (PAGE 338)

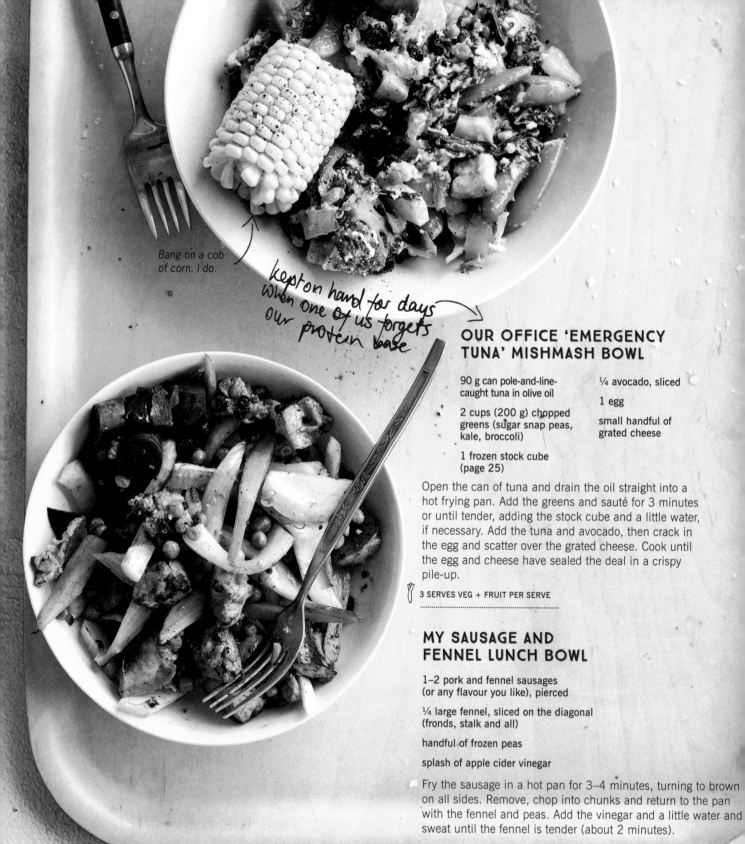

Bang on a cob of corn. I do.

Kept on hand for days when one of us forgets our protein base

OUR OFFICE 'EMERGENCY TUNA' MISHMASH BOWL

90 g can pole-and-line-caught tuna in olive oil

2 cups (200 g) chopped greens (sugar snap peas, kale, broccoli)

1 frozen stock cube (page 25)

¼ avocado, sliced

1 egg

small handful of grated cheese

Open the can of tuna and drain the oil straight into a hot frying pan. Add the greens and sauté for 3 minutes or until tender, adding the stock cube and a little water, if necessary. Add the tuna and avocado, then crack in the egg and scatter over the grated cheese. Cook until the egg and cheese have sealed the deal in a crispy pile-up.

3 SERVES VEG + FRUIT PER SERVE

MY SAUSAGE AND FENNEL LUNCH BOWL

1–2 pork and fennel sausages (or any flavour you like), pierced

¼ large fennel, sliced on the diagonal (fronds, stalk and all)

handful of frozen peas

splash of apple cider vinegar

Fry the sausage in a hot pan for 3–4 minutes, turning to brown on all sides. Remove, chop into chunks and return to the pan with the fennel and peas. Add the vinegar and a little water and sweat until the fennel is tender (about 2 minutes).

ADD KICK: 1–2 tablespoons Chopped Salad Pickle (page 335).

2 SERVES VEG + FRUIT PER SERVE

PRETTY IN PASTEL PINK PARSNIP PASTA

1 Cooked 'n' Frozen Beetroot (page 23), chopped into 1.5 cm cubes

½ cup (100 g) full-fat organic plain yoghurt

1 small clove garlic, crushed

big pinch of ground cumin

sea salt and freshly ground black pepper

½ teaspoon coconut oil or olive oil

2 parsnips, peeled and cut lengthways into long strips with a veggie peeler or spiraliser

small handful of walnuts (preferably activated; page 28), roughly chopped

small handful of flat-leaf parsley, roughly chopped

⅓ cup (75 ml) Green Minx Dressing (page 54), Watercress Sauce (page 176) or Leftovers Pesto (page 55) mushed with ½ avocado

Place a quarter of the beetroot in a food processor with the yoghurt, garlic and cumin. Season to taste with salt and pepper, then blend until smooth.

Heat the oil in a frying pan over a medium heat. Add the parsnip strips and fry for 1–2 minutes, or until just soft. Add the pink sauce and remaining beetroot cubes to the pan and heat through. Serve with the walnuts, parsley and dressing.

This one serves two for a light lunch

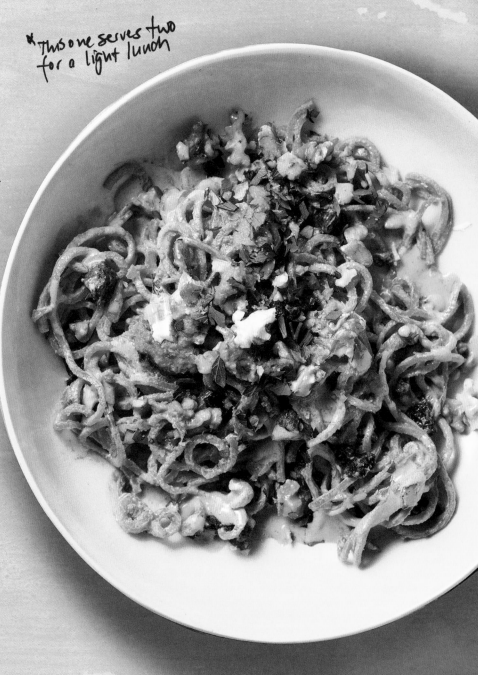

3 SERVES VEG + FRUIT PER SERVE

A CHAPTER DEDICATED TO
MINCE

It's cheap, easy to extend and
BOMBPROOF (culinarily speaking)

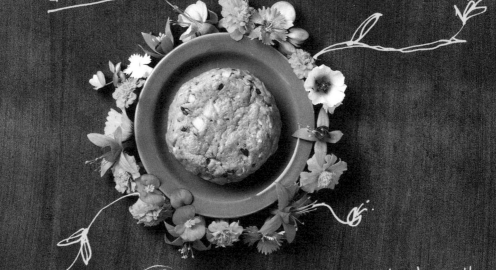

(P.S.) Most recipes in this chapter allow you
to use different minced meats interchangeably

SUPERFOODIE LASAGNE CAKE

SERVES 6

I don't subscribe to the notion of superfoods. Any meal laden with veggies and really low in toxins is super.

9 rice paper sheets
(22 cm diameter)

2 cups (200 g) spinach leaves
(or 1 cup/100 g) Par-Cooked 'n' Frozen
spinach or Swiss chard (page 22), thawed
and drained)

2 nori sheets, torn into large pieces
(or 1 tablespoon dulse flakes)

MEAT SAUCE

1 tablespoon coconut oil, olive oil,
butter or ghee

1 red onion, finely chopped

500 g mince (any meat)

2 cloves garlic, crushed

¼ teaspoon cayenne pepper,
or to taste

1 teaspoon Fermented Turmeric Paste
(page 340) or freshly grated turmeric
(or ¼ teaspoon ground turmeric)

1 cup (250 ml) Nomato Sauce (page 51)
or 1½ cups (300 g) diced tomatoes and
1 teaspoon dried oregano

2 cups (300 g) grated pumpkin
or 1 cup (250 ml) Pumpkin or Sweet
Potato Purée (page 23)

sea salt and freshly ground
black pepper

CHEESY CAULIFLOWER SAUCE

1 head cauliflower, chopped

2 tablespoons butter

½ cup (125 ml) milk (any kind)

½ cup (50 g) grated parmesan,
plus extra for the topping

sea salt and freshly ground
black pepper

Preheat the oven to 180°C (gas 4) and grease a 22 cm spring-form cake tin.

To make the meat sauce, heat the oil, butter or ghee in a large frying pan over a medium–high heat. Add the onion and mince and cook for 3–4 minutes. Stir in the garlic, cayenne and turmeric, and cook for 1–2 minutes. Add the Nomato Sauce or tomatoes, then reduce the heat and cook for 15–20 minutes, or until the sauce has thickened.

Meanwhile, to make the cheesy cauliflower sauce, steam or boil the cauli in a saucepan of water until tender (about 8 minutes). Drain. Add the butter, milk, parmesan, salt and pepper and purée with a stick blender until smooth and creamy (or use a food processor).

To assemble the lasagne, spread one-third of the meat sauce over the base of the cake tin, cover with three rice paper sheets, then top with one-third of the cheesy cauliflower sauce. Repeat for the remaining two layers, placing a layer of spinach, nori and pumpkin after the second and third layers of cheese sauce. Top the lasagne with the extra parmesan and a good grind of pepper. Cook for 40 minutes, or until the top is browned and the cheese is melted. Allow to sit for 10 minutes before serving.

3 SERVES VEG + FRUIT PER SERVE

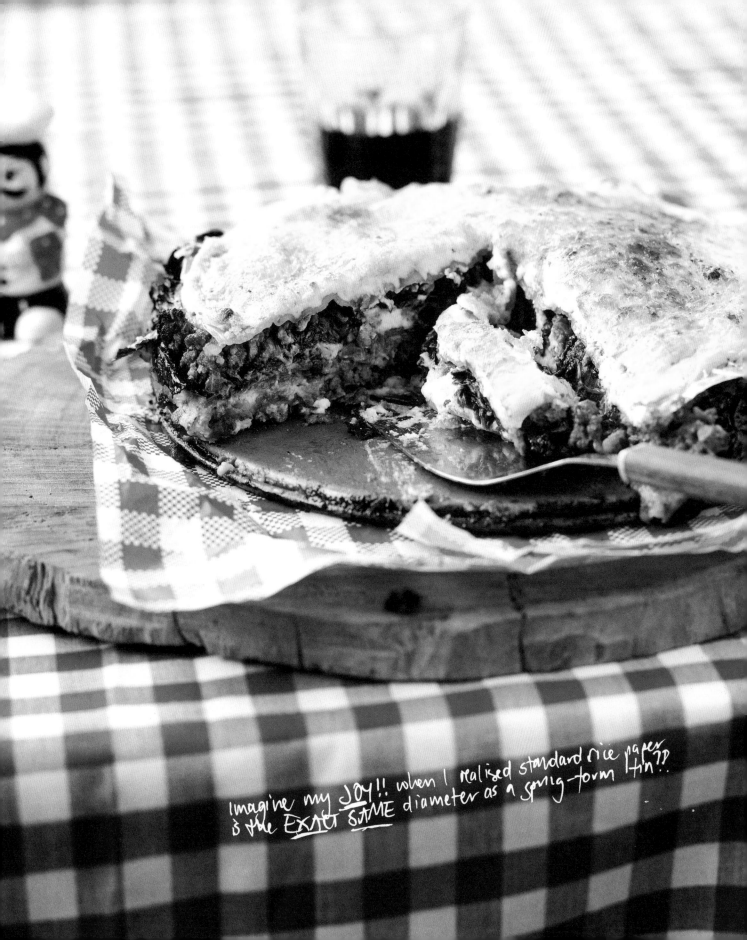

imagine my JOY!! when I realised standard rice paper
is the EXACT SAME diameter as a spring-form tin??

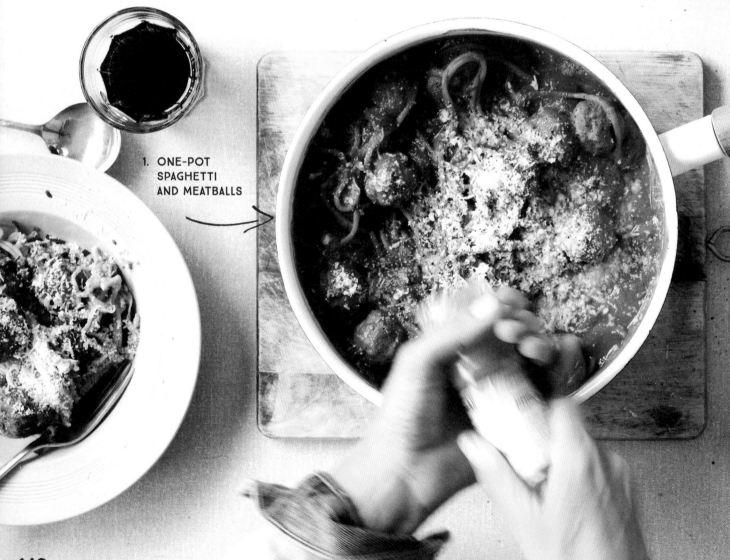

THREE WAYS with MEATBALLS:

Make in bulk, freeze raw +
use in these recipes...

1. ONE-POT
SPAGHETTI
AND MEATBALLS

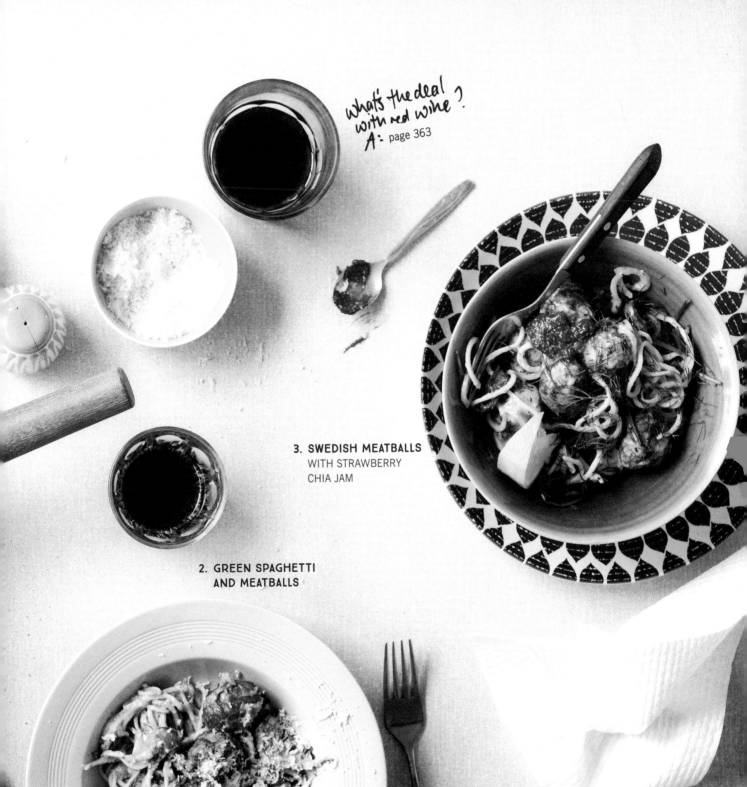

what's the deal with red wine?
A: page 363

3. **SWEDISH MEATBALLS**
WITH STRAWBERRY
CHIA JAM

2. **GREEN SPAGHETTI
AND MEATBALLS**

recipes over →

BASIC MEATBALLS

first make your ;

MAKES ABOUT 80 SMALL BALLS (16 SERVES)

2 kg fresh mince — *Use beef, chicken, lamb, turkey or pork.*

1 onion, finely chopped

½ bunch flat-leaf parsley or basil, leaves finely chopped

1 teaspoon each sea salt and freshly ground black pepper

olive oil, for frying

Place all the ingredients in a large bowl and, using your hands, mix until well combined. With wet hands, roll the mixture into walnut-sized balls.

To freeze: Line a baking tray with baking paper. Place the uncooked balls in a single layer on the tray and freeze for 2 hours or until frozen. Transfer to freezer-proof containers in meal-sized batches (5 per person) and return to the freezer.

To cook the meatballs now: Heat a little olive oil in a frying pan over a medium heat. Cook the meatballs on all sides (5–8 minutes in total). Remove from the heat, cover and allow to rest for a couple of minutes before serving.

MAKE IT YOUR OWN HOUSE MIX:

Add 1 teaspoon of cumin or fennel seeds (great with pork mince) or 1 teaspoon of oregano (great with lamb) to the recipe above.

A few mincey tips

* Buy in bulk when you see it on sale, divide into meal-sized portions and freeze.

* Your mince is brown? Forget it – it's fine. It's just that it's not been exposed to oxygen. Leave it on the worktop and it will go pink again.

* Freeze flattened out; thaw in the fridge and don't refreeze (unless you cook it first).

* Thinking of using a spatula to press down on that burger patty as it's cooking? Don't. You'll squeeze out all the juice and flavour. Ditto poking holes with a fork.

* RESPECT YOUR MINCE!

and then turn them into

1. ONE-POT SPAGHETTI AND MEATBALLS

SERVES 2

This recipe breaks *all* the cooking rules. Everything is cooked in the same pot: no boiling the pasta separately, no defrosting the meat first. The spag starch is not drained out so it makes for a slightly 'canned spaghetti' kind of vibe, which kids especially love.

2½ cups (600 ml) Nomato Sauce (page 51) or passata

1 teaspoon dried parsley (or 1 tablespoon chopped flat-leaf parsley)

If you use store-bought passata water it down (3:1) to reduce the sugar content.

1 teaspoon dried basil or oregano

¼ teaspoon fennel seeds

sea salt and freshly ground black pepper

10 frozen Basic Meatballs

100 g spaghetti (gluten-free, if desired)

finely grated parmesan, to serve (optional)

Place the Nomato Sauce or passata in a large saucepan with 1 cup (250 ml) water and bring to the boil over a high heat. Stir in the parsley, basil or oregano, and fennel seeds and season to taste with salt and pepper. Add the frozen meatballs and reduce the heat to medium–high. (The meatballs should just be covered by the sauce.) Allow to simmer, uncovered, for 20 minutes.

Break the spaghetti in half and add it to the pan, stirring to coat. Cook for 12 minutes, uncovered, or until the pasta is tender. (Be sure to stir the spaghetti to prevent it from sticking to the base of the pan.) If the sauce becomes too dry, add up to 1 cup (250 ml) boiling water. Serve topped with parmesan, if you like, and a good grind of pepper.

MAKE IT MORE NUTRIENT-DENSE:

Toss in 1–2 cups (150–300 g) of grated courgettes and a few cubes of frozen Pumpkin Purée (page 23) in the final 5 minutes of cooking.

 2½ SERVES VEG + FRUIT PER SERVE

2. GREEN SPAGHETTI AND MEATBALLS

SERVES 2

1 tablespoon coconut oil, olive oil, butter or ghee

10 Basic Meatballs, thawed

1/3 cup (75 ml) Leftovers Pesto (page 55) or Green Minx Dressing (page 54)

1 avocado

2–3 courgettes

sea salt and freshly ground black pepper

chilli flakes, to serve (optional)

parmesan shavings, to serve (optional)

Heat the oil, butter or ghee in a large frying pan over a medium–high heat. Cook the meatballs for 5–8 minutes, until browned and cooked through. Meanwhile, blend the pesto or dressing and avocado in a food processor (or use a stick blender and beaker) until smooth.

Use a spiraliser, julienne peeler, mandoline or grater to make courgette 'spaghetti'. Transfer to a saucepan and cover with boiling water for 1 minute (or leave raw if you like). Drain, then stir through the avocado sauce. Season with salt and pepper and a sprinkle of chilli flakes and parmesan, if desired.

MAKE IT MORE NUTRIENT-DENSE:
Toss in 1 cup (100 g) of chopped baby spinach leaves or a few cubes of Par-Cooked 'n' Frozen spinach or kale (page 22).

3. SWEDISH MEATBALLS

SERVES 2

1 celeriac, peeled

1 tablespoon butter

10 Basic Meatballs, thawed

1½ teaspoons caraway seeds

½ teaspoon ground allspice

1½ cups (350 ml) milk (any kind)

2 tablespoons cornflour

4 tablespoons chopped dill, plus extra to serve

sea salt and freshly ground black pepper

1 cup (100 g) baby spinach leaves

juice of ½ lemon, plus wedges to serve

Strawberry Chia Jam (page 57), to serve

steamed greens, to serve

Can't find celeriac? Use 2 or 3 parsnips instead.

When a recipe calls for a small amount of fresh dill, I generally use fennel fronds rather than buying a whole bunch of dill. Parsley will also do the job if you're stuck (or 1 tablespoon dried dill).

Cut the celeriac into several long chunks, then use a spiraliser, potato peeler or mandoline to make the noodles. (Exposed celeriac turns brown quickly, so if you're not cooking it immediately, immerse the slices in water and lemon juice.)

Heat 1 tablespoon of the butter in a large frying pan over a medium–high heat. Add the meatballs and cook for 5–8 minutes until browned. Sprinkle with the caraway seeds and allspice, and cook for a further minute until fragrant. Remove the meatballs from the pan.

Add the milk and cornflour to the pan and stir well. Cook, scraping up any brown bits from the bottom, for 1–2 minutes, or until thickened. Add the dill, celeriac noodles and meatballs to the pan and cook, covered, for 2–3 minutes or until heated through. Season with salt and pepper, then stir through the spinach. Remove from the heat and stir in the lemon juice. Serve with the jam, lemon wedges, steamed greens and a sprinkle of extra dill.

Celeriac V celery root
They're the same thing, but bear in mind some folks like to call the bottom of a bunch of celery 'celery root'. Ignore them. Possibly the ugliest-looking veggie around, celeriac tastes a bit like celery (with a dash of parsley, to my mind), is bursting with fibre, and can be found in the root-veggie section in winter (they keep quite well, so can be found into spring, too). Always choose heavy ones (the light ones are fluffy and sad to eat).

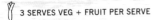
3 SERVES VEG + FRUIT PER SERVE

£1.69 PER SERVE

2 SERVES VEG + FRUIT PER SERVE

GREEK SAN CHOI BAU

1 tablespoon coconut oil, olive oil, butter or ghee, melted

10 frozen Basic Meatballs (page 144)

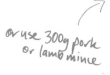

or use 300g pork or lamb mince

1 small aubergine, chopped into 1 cm cubes

1 teaspoon dried oregano

½ teaspoon ground cumin

½ teaspoon sweet paprika

juice of ½ lemon, plus wedges to serve

sea salt and freshly ground black pepper

½ savoy cabbage (or regular white or red cabbage)

½ cup (100 g) full-fat organic plain yoghurt

1 courgette or Lebanese cucumber, grated

TO SERVE

cherry tomatoes, quartered

mint leaves and/or flat-leaf parsley leaves, chopped

pine nuts, toasted (optional)

Heat the oil, butter or ghee in a large frying pan over a medium–high heat. Add the frozen meatballs and cook for 5 minutes, or until browned and the insides of the meatballs are slightly defrosted. (You can break them apart a little to aid cooking.) Add the aubergine, oregano and spices and cook for 2–3 minutes, until the aubergine is tender. Add the lemon juice and season to taste with salt and pepper.

Meanwhile, carefully separate the cabbage leaves, keeping them whole if you can, then steam for 5 minutes in your double steamer or in a bamboo steamer.

To make a tzatziki, combine the yoghurt and grated courgette or cucumber in a small bowl. Season with salt and pepper.

Serve the meatballs in the cabbage leaves topped with the cherry tomatoes, tzatziki, herbs, toasted pine nuts (if using) and a squeeze of lemon juice.

USE THE LEFTOVER CABBAGE:
Cook 1 cup (100 g) finely chopped cabbage with the aubergine and meatballs if you like.

4 SERVES VEG + FRUIT PER SERVE

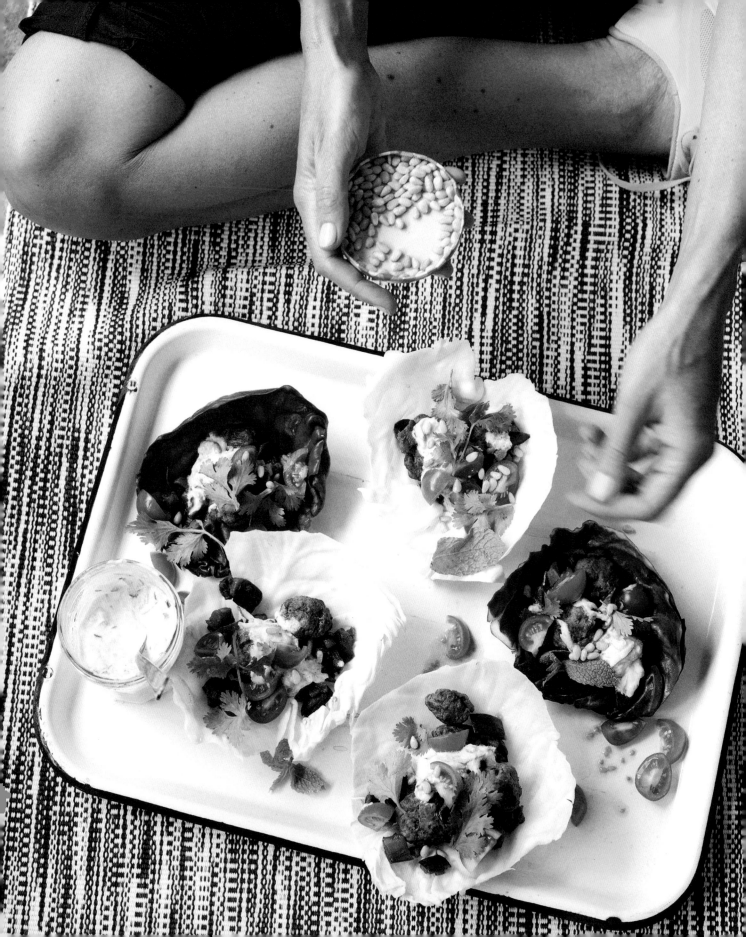

MIDDLE EASTERN AUBERGINE

1 large aubergine

2 tablespoons coconut oil, melted

1 small onion, chopped

250 g mince

Or 8 frozen Basic Meatballs

1 teaspoon ground allspice

2 teaspoons ground cinnamon

2 teaspoons ground cumin

sea salt and freshly ground black pepper

Or use 1½ tablespoons Ras el Hanout Mix (page 45).

3 tablespoons finely chopped mint and/or flat-leaf parsley, plus extra leaves to serve

¼ cup (50 g) full-fat organic plain yoghurt (preferably Greek-style), plus extra to serve

4 tablespoons pine nuts, toasted

TO SERVE

1 cup (100 g) baby spinach leaves

1 cup (150 g) green beans, steamed

Preheat the oven to 200°C (gas 6) and line a baking tray with baking paper.

Pierce the aubergine several times with a fork then halve it lengthways and lightly coat both sides with 1 tablespoon of the oil. Place the halves, cut-side down, on the prepared tray and bake for 20–30 minutes or until tender. Leave to cool slightly. Using a spoon, scoop the flesh from the aubergine halves, leaving a 1 cm border. Finely chop the flesh.

Meanwhile, heat the remaining oil in a frying pan over a medium heat and brown the onion and mince (about 3–4 minutes). Add the allspice, cinnamon and cumin to the pan and cook for 1–2 minutes. Add the aubergine flesh and season with salt and pepper. Stir in the herbs, yoghurt and pine nuts and remove from the heat.

Spoon the mixture into the aubergine shells and cover with foil. Bake for 10 minutes, then remove the foil and bake for a further 5 minutes to allow the mince to brown.

Serve with the spinach, beans, and the extra herbs and yoghurt.

4 SERVES VEG + FRUIT PER SERVE

£2.48 PER SERVE

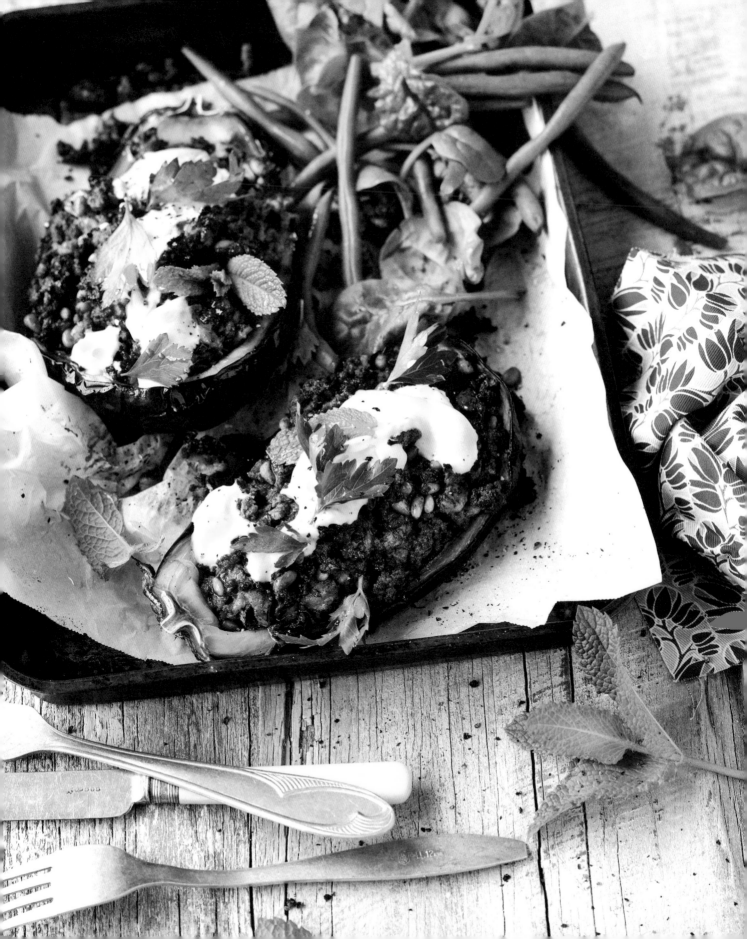

VIETNAMESE TURKEY PANCAKES

Pork or chicken mince is okay, too.

2 teaspoons coconut oil, plus extra for frying

300 g turkey mince

2 spring onions, thinly sliced

1 clove garlic, crushed

1 teaspoon finely grated ginger

1 long red chilli, thinly sliced

1 tablespoon fish sauce

juice of 2 limes

1 cup (40 g) coriander and/or mint leaves

½ red pepper, thinly sliced

lime wedges, to serve

steamed Oriental greens, to serve

RICE PANCAKES

½ cup (100 g) rice flour

2 tablespoons chia seeds

½ teaspoon ground turmeric

²/₃ cup (150 ml) milk (any kind; coconut milk works well)

½ cup (125 ml) iced water

If you've got some dosa batter in the fridge (page 89), use that instead.

To make the rice pancakes, mix all the ingredients together in a bowl and refrigerate while you prepare the mince mixture.

To make the mince mixture, heat the oil in a frying pan over a medium–high heat. Add the mince, spring onions, garlic, ginger and chilli. Cook for 5 minutes, breaking up any chunky bits with a wooden spoon, or until browned. Add the fish sauce and lime juice. Cook for a further 2 minutes. Remove from the heat.

To cook the pancakes, heat some oil in a skillet or frying pan over a medium–high heat. Stir the batter well. Add half the batter to the pan and swirl to cover the base. Cook for 3–4 minutes until golden, then flip and cook the other side for 2–3 minutes. Slide the pancake onto a plate. Repeat with the remaining batter.

Place half the mince mixture on each pancake. Top with half the herbs and pepper and fold to enclose. Serve with lime wedges and a side of steamed Oriental greens.

MAKE IT FASTER:
Use lettuce cups instead of rice pancakes.

2½ SERVES VEG + FRUIT PER SERVE

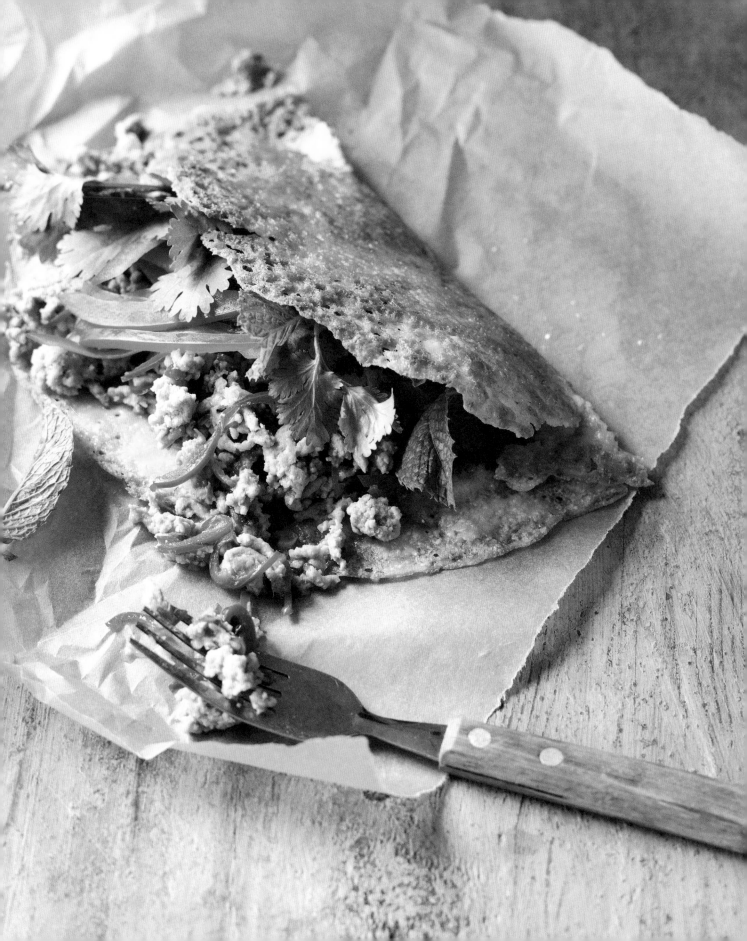

SUSTAINABLE FISH
IN A DISH

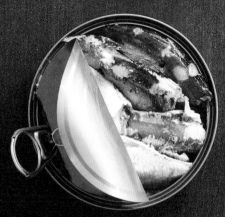

First choice   here's how as a few
                            dot pointers: ♡ SARDINES
1. small oily fish   vs. 1
2. fish offcuts (ask your monger to keep them
                          aside for you)
3. buy whole fish. And cook the carcass
4. white flesh fish
5. local
6. check out The Kit for helpful apps + consumer
                                              guides.

(see page 5)

let's get started with:

THREE WAYS with an OILY FISH:

want to cut to the omega 3 + sustainable chase?
Just eat small, oil-ful fish - Sardines, anchovies + mackerel
(herring, too!)

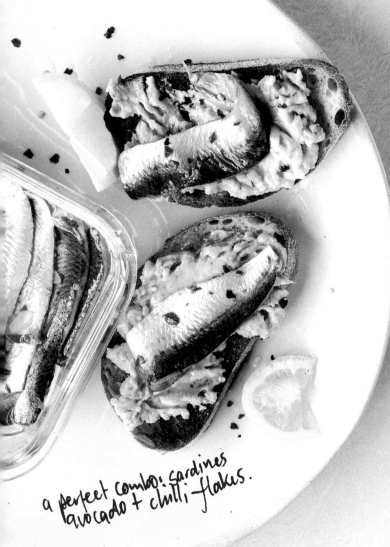

1. UNTINNED SARDINES
ON AVOCADO TOAST
WITH CHILLI FLAKES

**2. BAKED
MEDITERRANEAN
SUMMER SARDINES**

a perfect combo: sardines, avocado + chilli flakes.

I especially love eating the heads + tails of sardines. You don't? You should!

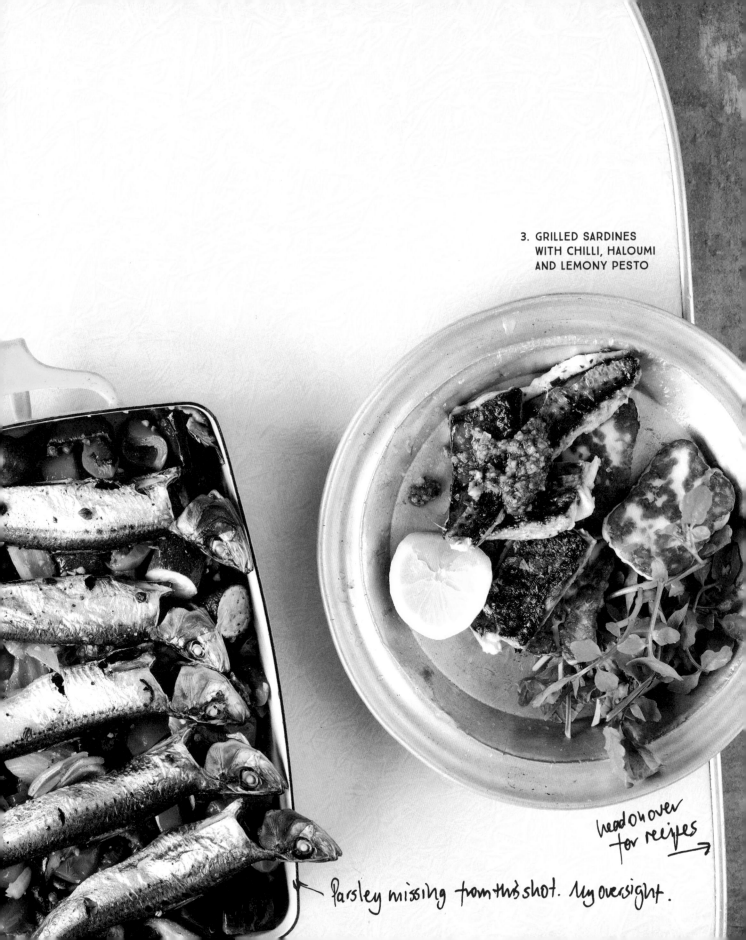

3. GRILLED SARDINES
WITH CHILLI, HALOUMI
AND LEMONY PESTO

head on over
for recipes →

Parsley missing from this shot. My oversight.

1. UNTINNED SARDINES

SERVES 6

I've played with various ways to preserve my oilies. Many fish fans work with vinegary cures or oil and/or salt, but these use a lot of ingredients that get tossed, which I'm not happy with. The recipe below is the most efficient, economical one and leaves you with condiments, too.

500 g filleted sardines, anchovies, herring or mackerel (cut the bigger fish into smaller pieces)

½ red onion, thinly sliced

½ baby fennel, including stalks and fronds if you like, sliced

2 bay leaves

½ teaspoon chilli flakes

3 tablespoons Homemade Whey (page 46) or apple cider vinegar

2 teaspoons sea salt

Don't worry if you're all out of big jars – a glass bowl or dish covered with cling film will do just as well.

In a large jar (broad enough for each fillet to lie flat), arrange the fish in layers with the onion, fennel, bay leaves and chilli. Add the whey or vinegar and salt along with 1 cup (250 ml) water.

Fill a smaller, clean jar with water, then seal and place inside the big jar (or bowl) as a weight to press the fish under the liquid (or use a plate). Drape a clean tea towel or cloth over the top and put the jar or bowl in a dark place for 24 hours to ferment.

Remove the water-filled jar or plate, pop a lid on your main jar (or if using a bowl, cover with cling film) and throw the jar or bowl in the fridge. It'll keep for 3–4 weeks.

MAKE IT 'YOU'RE A BIT GREEK':
Use garlic instead of onion and fresh oregano instead of bay leaves.

Why preserve your oily fish?

Oily fish can be hard to come by, due to the fact that they're seasonal and not wholly popular . . . yet (I'm working on it). So when you find them, it's worth buying a lot. But they oxidise quickly (see opposite). Kill two birds by preserving in bulk so you have them ready to fly whenever you get the briny incline.

FIVE WAYS TO EAT SARDINES:

1. As a soup topper.
2. Spread on toast with avocado and chilli flakes.
3. Stirred through an Abundance Bowl (hot or cold); see pages 126–37.
4. On a platter with radishes, Homemade Cream Cheese (page 46) and crackers.
5. Rolled up in a radicchio leaf or chicory cup. (I do this. For breakfast.)

Omega 3s: beware!

Bear in mind that while omega 3s are great, they easily oxidise to become inflaming omega 6s. There are a few tricks to combat this (all incorporated in these recipes):

✱ Eat fish the day you buy it. Or preserve it.

✱ Wash the fish well. It removes the bacteria that speed up degradation.

✱ Immerse it in acid (curing).

✱ Minimise heat contact: eating it 'cured' rather than cooked is best. And quick grills or pan-fries are appropriate too.

2. BAKED MEDITERRANEAN SUMMER SARDINES

SERVES 6

1 large aubergine, cut into 3 cm cubes

1 large red pepper, roughly chopped

2 courgettes, halved lengthways and roughly sliced

250 g cherry tomatoes, halved

1 red onion, cut into wedges

2 cloves garlic, finely chopped

40 g coconut oil, plus extra (melted) for drizzling

3 tablespoons apple cider vinegar or red wine vinegar

sea salt and freshly ground black pepper

12 fresh whole sardines (heads on), cleaned, scaled and gutted (or 700 g other filleted oily fish)

3 tablespoons capers

lemon wedges, flat-leaf parsley and sourdough, to serve

Preheat the oven to 200°C (gas 6) and line a large baking tray with baking paper.

Place the aubergine, pepper, courgettes, tomatoes, onion and garlic on the prepared tray and toss with the oil and vinegar. Season with salt and pepper. Bake for 15–20 minutes, until the vegetables are tender.

Meanwhile, prepare the fish by drizzling with oil and seasoning with salt and pepper. Remove the tray from the oven, top with the fish fillets and capers, and continue cooking for a further 20 minutes or until lovely and crisp-looking. Serve with lemon wedges, a sprinkling of parsley and some crusty sourdough.

3. GRILLED SARDINES WITH CHILLI, HALOUMI AND LEMONY PESTO

SERVES 6 AS A STARTER

½ cup (125 ml) Leftovers Pesto (page 55) or Watercress Sauce (page 176)

juice and zest of 1 lemon

6 fresh whole sardines or 12 fresh whole anchovies (heads on), cleaned and gutted, or 350 g mackerel fillets, skin left on, cut into 6 pieces

2 teaspoons coconut oil, olive oil, butter or ghee, melted

½ teaspoon chilli flakes

½ teaspoon sea salt

500 g haloumi, cut into 5 mm thick slices

watercress, to serve

lemon wedges, to serve (optional)

Make a lemony pesto by combining the Leftovers Pesto or Watercress Sauce with the lemon juice and zest. Set aside.

Preheat a grill, griddle pan or barbecue hotplate to medium–high. Rub the fish with the oil, butter or ghee and season with the chilli flakes and salt. Place the haloumi and fish under the grill, in the griddle pan or on the barbecue hotplate and cook, turning once, for about 2–3 minutes each side, until lightly charred. Serve with watercress, lemony pesto and lemon wedges.

MAKE IT A MAIN COURSE:

Triple the fish and serve atop The Green Counterbalance Salad (page 309) or some Massaged Kale (page 23).

2 SERVES VEG + FRUIT PER SERVE

£1.39 PER SERVE

MY BROTHER PETE'S ENTRÉE-AND-MAIN-IN-ONE KOKONDA

SERVES 6 PEEPS

Pete brought this cured fish recipe back from the Solomons, where he used to live, and made it for 15 of us at a family Christmas. I've kept the instructions in his original wording, sent to me via email, as much as I can.

When you go to the fish shop . . .

Bear in mind you use the whole fish for this two-part meal (entrée = fish stock, main = kokonda). Ask your monger to fillet and clean the fish, but ensure you get to take the carcass with you! Ask for an extra carcass or two while you're there to make a stronger stock.

Also, you're 'cooking' (or denaturing) the fish in lemon so it's important to use fish that's super-fresh.

Pete catches his an hour before dinner and fillets it himself; for the rest of us he advises telling the fishmonger it's for marinating not cooking so they can ensure you're getting fresh stuff.

600 g whole fresh white non-oily fish, filleted (reserve the carcass for the stock) and cut into 2 cm pieces

juice of 4–6 lemons (to cover the fish)

1 long red chilli, sliced

6 spring onions, thinly sliced

2 small yellow peppers, cubed

1 Lebanese cucumber, cubed

2 tomatoes, cubed

400 ml can coconut cream

sea salt and freshly ground black pepper

coriander leaves, to serve

Pete makes his own. See instructions in The Kit (see page 5).

The night or morning before: Place the fish in a glass or ceramic dish. Pour over the lemon juice, ensuring that the fish is completely covered by the juice. Cover and place in the fridge to marinate for at least 3 hours (preferably overnight). This method will 'cook' the fish, leaving it firm and opaque.

Meanwhile, use the carcass to make fish stock (page 42).

The next day or when ready to serve: Drain the fish (reserving the marinade; see below) and whack into a serving dish. Add the chilli, spring onions, pepper, cucumber and tomatoes and stir to combine. Pour over the coconut cream and season to taste with salt and pepper.

Gently heat the stock and serve it first in mugs. ← *'No need to get fancy.' – Pete*

Then, serve the kokonda with coriander leaves.

'Or with Usain Bolt's favourite, taro (unless you are paleo) to make it authentically South Pacific. And think yourself lucky.' – Pete x

USE THE LEFTOVER LEMON MARINADE:
Add it to the fish stock before you reheat it. Or use it to deglaze your next chicken or fish dish.

1½ SERVES VEG + FRUIT PER SERVE

£0.74 PER SERVE

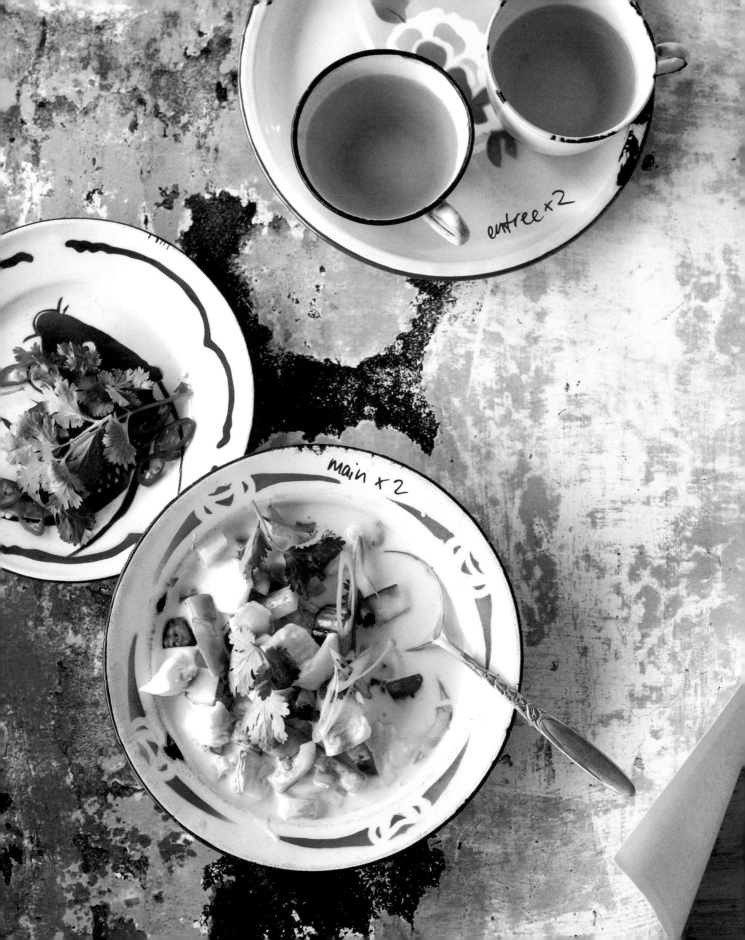

entree x2

main x2

SIMPLICIOUS
SMOKED SALMON

(WELL, KIND OF)

SERVES 12

About $40 if you were to buy the amount we make here (which cost me $16-50!)

I have a few issues with smoked salmon. It's expensive, it comes in a packet and the smoking part means it can contain carcinogenic guff. Not conclusive, but enough to suspend question marks over it. And so all roads lead to making your own gravlox (also called gravlax). Most are cured in sugar. Mine isn't. Most take several palaver-y steps. I skip these.

If the salt is too fine the moisture will dissolve the crystals and the fish will absorb too much salt too quickly.

Leaving the skin on makes it easier when you slice it later. And it wastes less.

400 g salmon fillets, bones removed, skin left on

4 tablespoons coarse sea salt

zest of 2 lemons

2 teaspoons white peppercorns, ground using a mortar and pestle (or 2 teaspoons allspice)

1 small bunch dill, chopped

Which salmon is best?
In Australia, wild-caught Australian salmon is best. The more commonly seen Atlantic salmon is farmed, and can be used as an occasional choice. Lots of small wild-caught fish are used to feed farmed salmon. So using wild-caught local fish is a better option.

Either way my take is that if you're going to eat the stuff, then you should eat it in small amounts and savour it respectfully.

Dry the fish well using kitchen paper. Combine the salt, lemon zest, pepper and dill and smother it over both sides of the fish (just use your hands, and make sure you cover it completely). Press the skinless sides of the fillets together and place in a large zip-lock bag, but don't completely seal it. You can also place it in a glass dish loosely covered with cling film. Leave it on the worktop for 2–6 hours.

Seal the bag properly (or tightly seal the cling film) and whack it in the fridge for 24–48 hours. Place a weight on top (such as a chopping board) to compress the fish.

Once done, the fish will be firm and sitting in a pool of liquid in the bag or bowl. Drain the fish and scrape off the excess salt mixture. If it's too salty, you can rinse it, but only JUST before you serve it (otherwise bacteria will grow). Slice it super-thinly and eat respectfully with eggs, on little rye squares with butter and radish discs.

It will keep in the fridge, covered, for 2–3 weeks.

MAKE IT WITH WHITE FISH:
Use 450 g (you might need to use 3–4 fillets), skin left on.

My preferred option!

MAKE IT PINK:
Blitz 1 large peeled beetroot to a purée and spread this mixture between the salted fish fillets before placing them in the bag.

This is a really pretty option, especially served with Pink Devilish Googie Eggs (page 253).

ONE-PAN MOROCCAN FISH PILAF

SERVES 2

This is the cleverest meal, truly. You cook your pilaf, vegetables and fish all in one hit.

1 cup (135 g) Cooked Quinoa (page 26)

1 cup (250 ml) Homemade Fish Stock (page 42)

2 carrots, quartered lengthways and sliced on the diagonal

½ cup (75 g) frozen peas

3 tablespoons almonds or pistachios

3 tablespoons chopped mint or coriander, plus extra to serve

1 tablespoon olive oil

sea salt and freshly ground black pepper

2 sustainable white fish fillets

½ teaspoon Ras el Hanout Mix (page 45) or ¼ teaspoon each ground cumin and coriander

lemon wedges, to serve

Preheat the oven to 220°C (gas 7). In a small baking dish or skillet, combine the quinoa, stock, carrots, peas, nuts, herbs and oil. Season with salt and pepper. Plonk the fish on top and sprinkle over the spice mix.

Cover (with lid or foil) and bake for 20 minutes. Serve with lemon wedges.

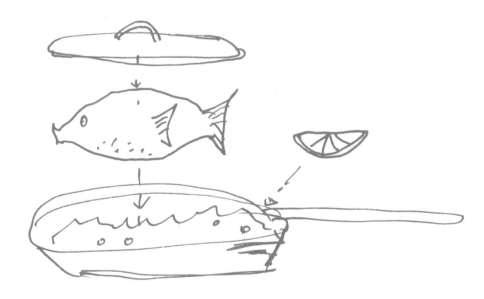

 2 SERVES VEG + FRUIT PER SERVE

£2.25 PER SERVE

SKILLET FISH 'N' SUPERSLAW

SERVES 2

This is my holier-than-thou version of fish 'n' chips
and coleslaw.

1 bunch tenderstem broccoli, chopped
into bite-sized pieces

250 g packet coleslaw mix
(or 1 large carrot and ¼ cabbage, grated)

2 baby new potatoes, very thinly sliced
(about 2 mm thick)

1 tablespoon chopped macadamias,
almonds or cashews (preferably activated;
page 28)

1 teaspoon apple cider vinegar

2 teaspoons coconut oil

sea salt and freshly ground
black pepper

300 g salmon fillet (see page 160),
skin left on

1 teaspoon smoked paprika

juice of ½ lemon, to serve

Preheat the oven to 200°C (gas 6) and line a skillet or baking tray with baking
paper.

In a large bowl, toss together the broccoli, coleslaw mix, potato, nuts, vinegar and
oil, and season with salt and pepper.

Cut the salmon fillet in half lengthways to create two even portions. Spread the
coleslaw mix over half of the prepared tray and place the fillets skin-side down
on the other. Sprinkle the salmon with the paprika. Bake for 12–15 minutes,
uncovered. Serve the salmon on top of the superslaw with a squeeze of lemon.

MAKE IT SUMMERY:
Replace the potatoes with peach slices.

3 SERVES VEG + FRUIT PER SERVE

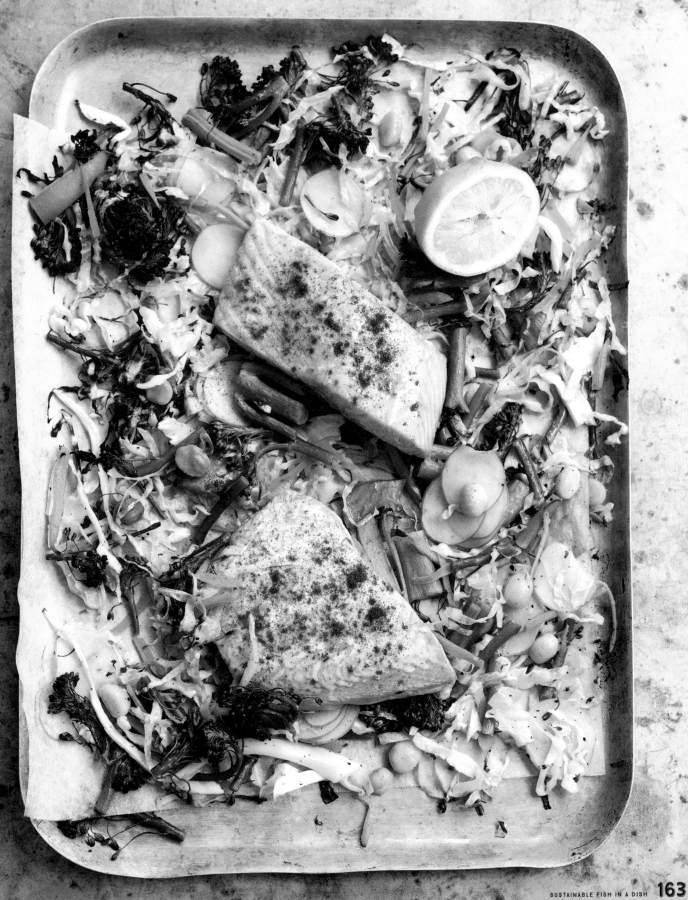

SUSTAINABLE SWEET FISH CURRY

SERVES 6

Too many people get scared if their fish has been sitting around in the fridge for more than a day or two. I don't. I make fish curry.

400 ml can full-fat coconut milk, unshaken

4 tablespoons Thai red curry paste (look for a brand that doesn't contain sugar – many do)

1 tablespoon finely chopped lemongrass (optional)

1 tablespoon grated fresh turmeric, Fermented Turmeric Paste (page 340) or ½ teaspoon ground turmeric

1 large onion, chopped

2 cups (300 g) chopped sweet potato or pumpkin (3 cm chunks)

½ cup (125 ml) Homemade Chicken Stock (page 42) or water

800 g sustainable firm white fish, cut into 4 cm chunks (offcuts are perfect)

3 cups (450 g) chopped veggies (beans, courgettes and cauliflower are a good combo)

1 cup (150 g) frozen peas

3 cloves garlic, finely chopped (optional)

1 tablespoon fish sauce or lime juice

6 kaffir lime leaves, cut into fine strips

I buy these in bulk and keep them in the freezer.

handful of mint, coriander or basil leaves

1 long red chilli, sliced (optional)

Heat a large frying pan or wok over a medium heat. Spoon the thick, top layer of the coconut milk into the pan. Add the curry paste, lemongrass (if using) and turmeric and stir-fry for 2–3 minutes. Add the onion and sweet potato or pumpkin and cook for 5 minutes. Pour in the remaining coconut milk and the stock. Add the fish, veggies, peas and garlic (if using).

Bring to a gentle boil. Simmer for 5 minutes or until the fish is just cooked through. Stir in the fish sauce or lime juice, kaffir lime leaves, herbs and sliced chilli (if using). Serve in bowls (it's quite soupy).

2 SERVES VEG + FRUIT PER SERVE

£2.29 PER SERVE

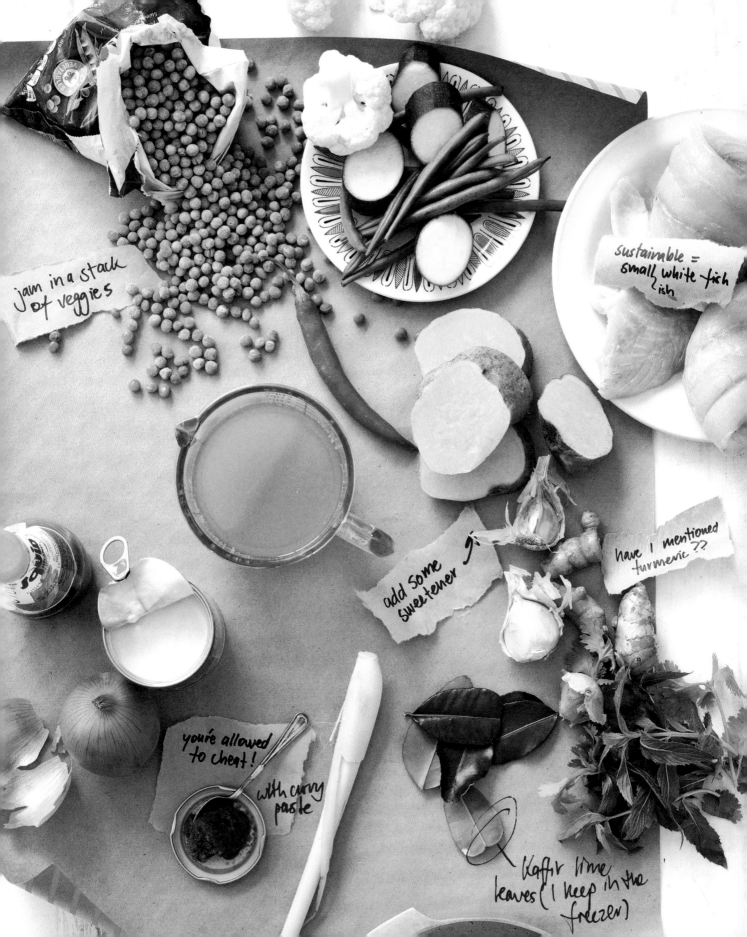

GIFT-WRAPPED
MISO 'COD'

The original miso cod, invented by Nobu restaurant, ain't a simplicious food. It's made with black cod, also known as butterfish or sablefish overseas, which is very sustainable in the US and parts of Europe, but not in Australia. It's also glazed in a cacophony of Oriental sugars, including mirin, rice wine and sweet miso. I cut out the sugar and use blue eye trevalla; if black cod is sustainable in your region, enjoy it as an occasional treat, or use line-caught or organically farmed sea bass fillets instead.

4 tablespoons red miso paste
(or 8 tablespoons white miso paste)

1 teaspoon rice malt syrup

2 teaspoons grated ginger

2 teaspoons toasted sesame oil

2 × 200 g black cod or sea bass fillets

150 g green beans, thinly sliced on
the diagonal

coconut oil, for drizzling

TO SERVE

2 spring onions, thinly sliced
on the diagonal

lemon wedges

1–2 teaspoons sesame seeds

In a glass (or other non-corrosive) bowl, combine the miso, rice malt syrup, ginger and sesame oil and stir until smooth. Add the fish fillets, douse and let sit for 5 minutes.

Preheat the oven to 200°C (gas 6). Lay two sheets of baking paper (each about 30 cm × 25 cm) side by side on your worktop. Place half of the beans in the centre of each sheet. Top each pile of beans with a fish fillet, spoon over the marinade and drizzle over some coconut oil. Wrap each into a parcel – gift-box style – making sure no juices can escape and no air can get in. This is super-important. Tie the parcels with kitchen string for extra measure.

Place the parcels on a baking tray and bake for 9–11 minutes. Serve with the spring onions, lemon wedges and a scattering of sesame seeds.

 ½ TSP ADDED SUGAR PER SERVE

1½ SERVES VEG + FRUIT PER SERVE

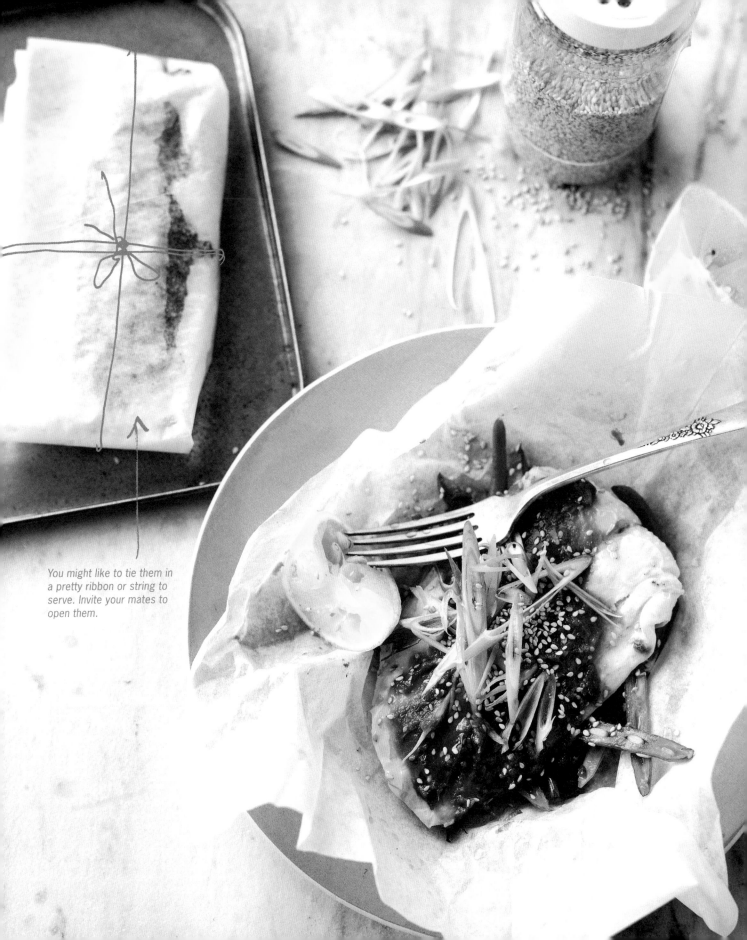

You might like to tie them in a pretty ribbon or string to serve. Invite your mates to open them.

SO I HAVE THIS STACK OF
VEGETABLES . . .

a chapter dedicated to using up that HEAD of [CAULI]
STACK of BROCCOLI and that heaving
and making the most out of the fact that
COURGETTES are ON SALE
right now + making
use of THAT
FROTHING of KALE
that's taking over my fridge.

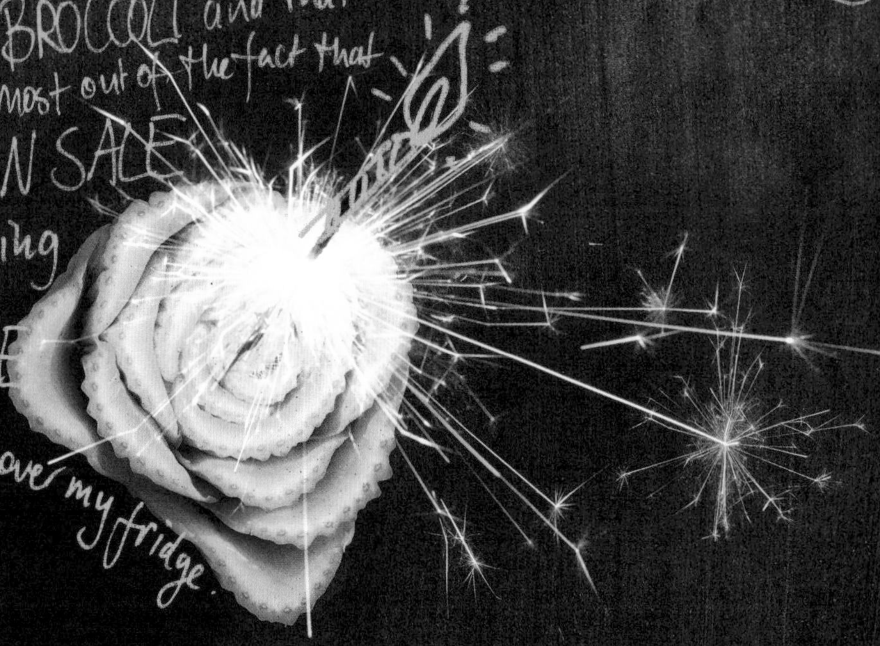

celebrating the
WHOLE VEGETABLE
since 2018

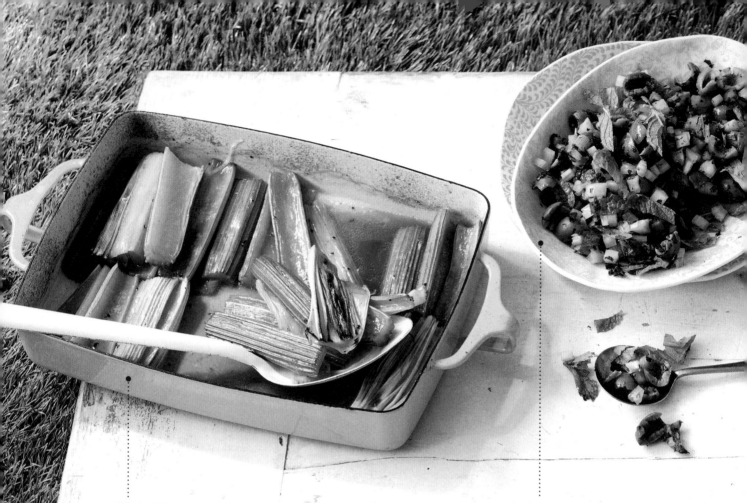

BRAISED CELERY AND
LEEKS WITH VANILLA

SERVES 6 AS A SIDE

1 bunch celery, stalks cut into
10 cm lengths (slice the wider
stalks in half lengthways)

1 leek, halved lengthways, then
cut into 10 cm lengths

40 g butter

1 cup (250 ml) Homemade
Stock (chicken or a veggie
variation; page 42)

¼ teaspoon pure vanilla extract
(or make your own; page 45)
or a pinch of pure vanilla
powder

sea salt and freshly ground
black pepper

Preheat the oven to 180°C (gas 4). Arrange the celery and
leek in a large baking dish. Dot with the butter. Combine the
stock and vanilla and pour over the veggies. Season with
salt and pepper. Cover with foil and braise for 30 minutes,
then remove the foil and roast for another 30 minutes or
until the liquid has reduced to a thick sauce. Serve.

1½ SERVES VEG + FRUIT PER SERVE

A SALAD OF
CRUSHED OLIVES

SERVES 6 AS A SIDE

1½ cups (250 g) green olives, pitted

½ bunch celery (including leaves),
finely chopped

½ bunch mint, leaves finely chopped

½ cup (125 ml) Powerhouse Dressing
(page 53)

*To be honest,
I rarely pit
olives; I just
warn guests to
pit their own –
the Italians do
this too. In this
recipe, though,
you need to.*

Toss the olives with the rest of
the ingredients in a serving bowl.
Feel free to prepare in advance to
slightly 'pickle' things a bit.

Pitting olives hack
*Place the olives on something flat and
use a sturdy coffee mug to press and
roll them firmly.*

1 SERVE VEG + FRUIT PER SERVE

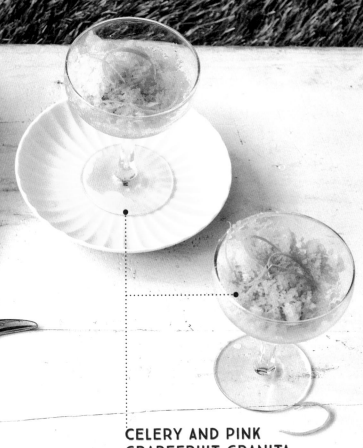

CELERY AND PINK GRAPEFRUIT GRANITA

SERVES 4–6

½ bunch celery, stalks only, roughly chopped

1 pink grapefruit, peeled, pith and pips removed, and segmented (zest finely sliced for garnish, if you like)

3 tablespoons rice malt syrup

Place the celery and grapefruit on a tray in the freezer for 1 hour. Heat the rice malt syrup in a small saucepan with 4 tablespoons water and boil for 3 minutes. Plonk the frozen celery and grapefruit in a blender with the syrup and whizz until smooth. Pour into a freezer-proof container and freeze for 2 hours, removing every 30 minutes to rake with a fork. Serve as an entrée or dessert in summer, garnished with zest, if you like. A drizzle of extra-virgin olive oil is nice, too.

USE THE LEFTOVER CELERY HEARTS:
Grow more celery (page 33).

🥄 1 TSP ADDED SUGAR PER SERVE

🍴 ½ SERVE VEG + FRUIT PER SERVE

CELERY SODA

SERVES 6

I personally don't use a juicer for a number of reasons (see page 34 for some of them). But if I did, I'd make this. So fresh.

½ bunch celery, juiced (reserve a few of the paler, inner leaves)

2 cups (500 ml) coconut water

2 cups (500 ml) soda water

mint sprigs, to serve (optional)

Mix all the ingredients in a large jug. Serve cold with a sprig of inner celery leaf (or a sprig of mint if you prefer).

USE THE LEFTOVER CELERY LEAVES:
Make Leftovers Pesto (page 55) or Celery Leaf Salt (page 265).

🍴 ½ SERVE VEG + FRUIT PER SERVE

BACK TO THE 70s
LETTUCE SOUP

SERVES 6

Cos (romaine) lettuce is best in this soup. Or use two little gem lettuces or an iceberg instead. A handful of rocket, if it's lying around, can be thrown in, too. I think what gives this the real 'crockery and copper-goblet spin' is the frozen peas. Yes?

¼ cup (50 g) butter

1 tablespoon flour (any kind)

1 leek or onion, chopped

2 cloves garlic, crushed

2 cups (500 ml) Homemade Stock (chicken or a veggie variation; page 42)

1 nice and big cos lettuce, chopped

2 cups (300 g) frozen peas

½ cup (20 g) mint leaves

juice of ½ lemon

½ teaspoon granulated stevia or 1–2 drops liquid stevia (optional)

sea salt and freshly ground black or white pepper

full-fat organic plain yoghurt and your favourite Soup Topper (page 245), to serve

Lettuce is lovelier with white pepper.

Heat the butter in a large saucepan over a low–medium heat. Stir in the flour. Add the leek or onion and the garlic and cook until soft (but not browned). Add the stock, 1 cup (250 ml) water, lettuce and peas and bring to the boil. Whack on a lid, reduce the heat and simmer for about 5 minutes. Remove from the heat. Add the mint, lemon juice and stevia (if using). Purée in the pan using a stick blender (or transfer to a blender) and season to taste with salt and pepper. Heat again to serve. Or cool, refrigerate and serve cold in summer! Serve with a blob of yoghurt or some soup toppers.

USE THE LEFTOVERS FOR A WORK LUNCH:
Pour into jars, freeze and either microwave in the office or, in summer, drink cold like a smoothie.

2 SERVES VEG + FRUIT PER SERVE

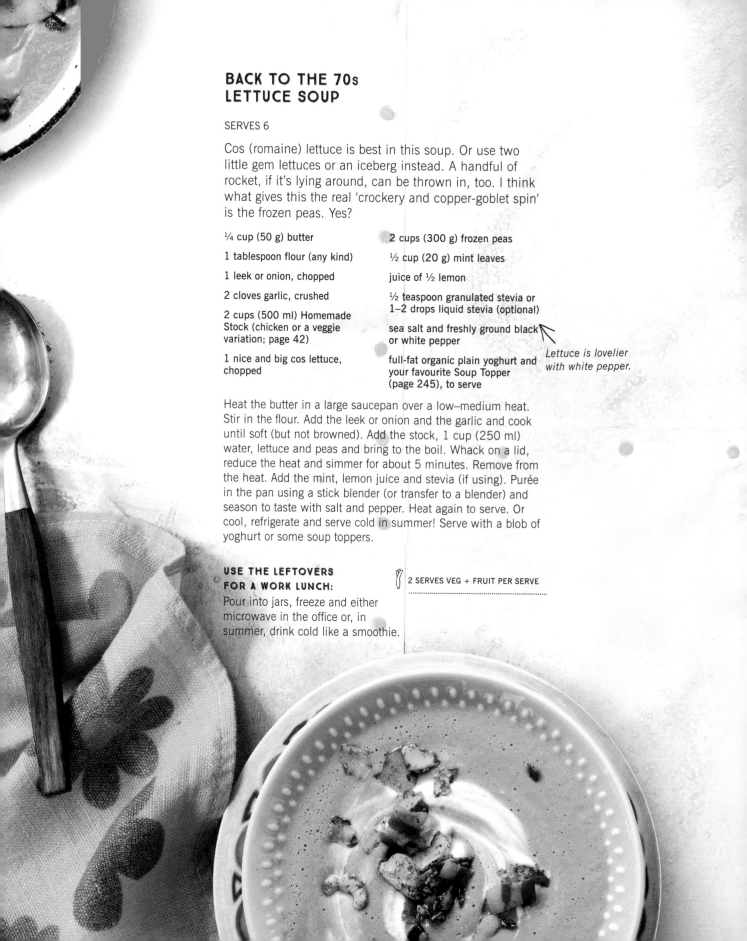

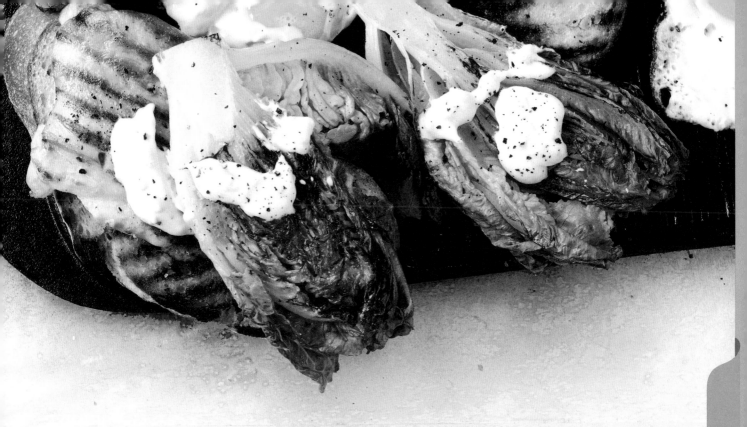

GRILLED CAESAR ON THE BARBIE

SERVES 4

Only trim the base of the lettuces so they don't fall apart when you cut them.

400 g chicken thigh fillets, cut into 8 pieces

sea salt and freshly ground black pepper

2 teaspoons olive oil

4 eggs

4 baby cos lettuces, trimmed and halved lengthways

4 slices leftover (stale) sourdough bread (optional)

CAESAR DRESSING

½ cup (125 ml) Whey-Good Mayo (page 50)

5 anchovies, finely chopped

1 clove Good for Your Guts Garlic (page 340), crushed

To make the dressing, combine the mayo, anchovies and garlic in a small bowl. Season with salt and pepper and mix well. Thin, if desired, with 1–2 teaspoons of water.

No barbie? Use a large frying pan.

Season the chook with salt and pepper. Preheat a barbecue hot-plate over a high heat. Reduce the heat to medium–high and grill the chicken for 3–4 minutes on each side or until lightly charred and cooked through. While the chook is cooking, add some oil to the hotplate and fry the eggs for 2–3 minutes or until set. Add the lettuce, cut-side down, and the bread (if using) and grill for 1–2 minutes. Serve drizzled with the dressing.

2 SERVES VEG + FRUIT PER SERVE

HAVE SOME LETTUCE WITH YOUR DRESSING

SERVES 6 AS A SIDE

Bring your salad to the dressing party with this dead-simple concept.

1 iceberg lettuce, chopped into 12 thick wedges

1 cup Green Minx Dressing (page 54)

Arrange the wedges on a platter and pour over the dressing.

½ SERVE VEG + FRUIT PER SERVE

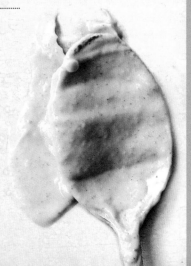

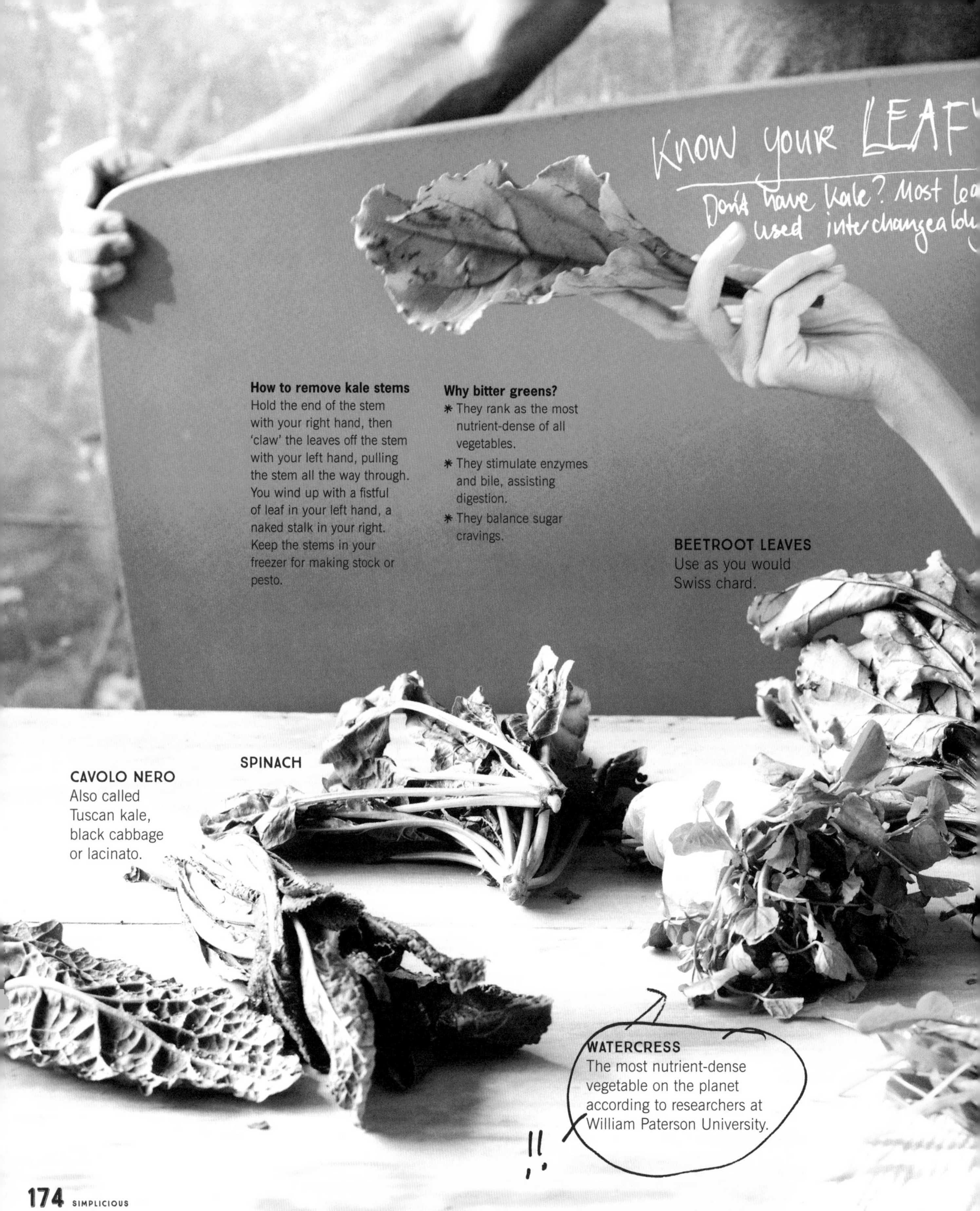

Don't have kale? Most lea[f]
used interchangeab[ly]

How to remove kale stems
Hold the end of the stem
with your right hand, then
'claw' the leaves off the stem
with your left hand, pulling
the stem all the way through.
You wind up with a fistful
of leaf in your left hand, a
naked stalk in your right.
Keep the stems in your
freezer for making stock or
pesto.

Why bitter greens?
* They rank as the most
  nutrient-dense of all
  vegetables.
* They stimulate enzymes
  and bile, assisting
  digestion.
* They balance sugar
  cravings.

BEETROOT LEAVES
Use as you would
Swiss chard.

CAVOLO NERO
Also called
Tuscan kale,
black cabbage
or lacinato.

SPINACH

WATERCRESS
The most nutrient-dense
vegetable on the planet
according to researchers at
William Paterson University.

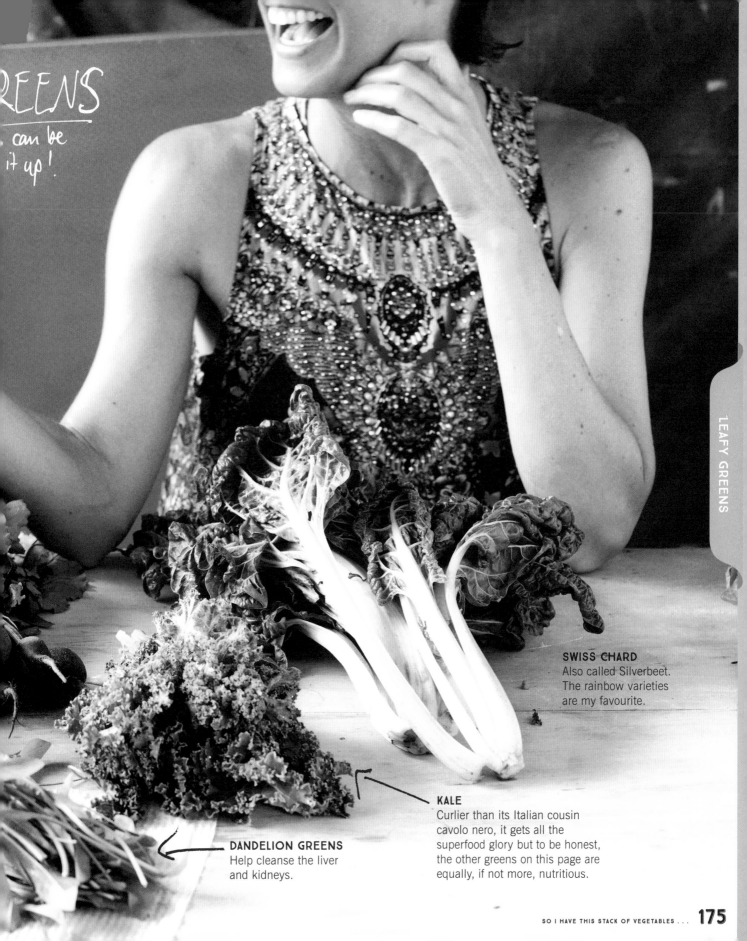

REENS

...can be
it up!

SWISS CHARD
Also called Silverbeet.
The rainbow varieties
are my favourite.

KALE
Curlier than its Italian cousin
cavolo nero, it gets all the
superfood glory but to be honest,
the other greens on this page are
equally, if not more, nutritious.

DANDELION GREENS
Help cleanse the liver
and kidneys.

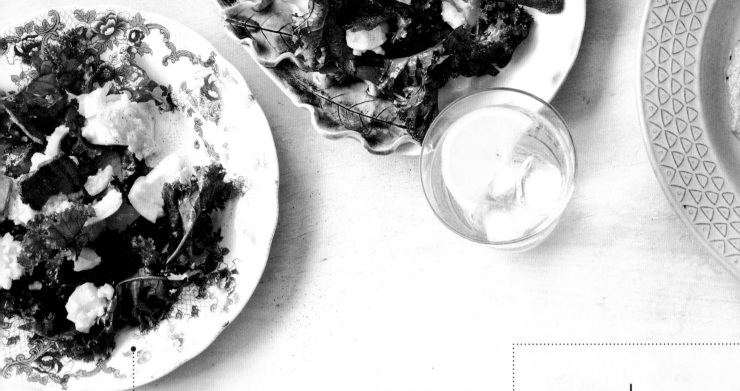

HIPSTER GRANDADDY SALAD

SERVES 6 AS A SIDE, 2 AS A MEAL

A salad with bacon, egg and white pepper always reminds me of my grandad who added white pepper and celery salt to everything. The massaged kale gives this old-school salad a modern edge.

1 batch of Massaged Kale (page 23)

4 hard-boiled eggs, roughly chopped

¾ cup (about 12 tablespoons) Bacon Bits (page 44; optional)

1 teaspoon ground white pepper

Celery Leaf Salt (page 265) or sea salt, to taste

Toss your kale with the eggs, bacon, pepper and salt.

WATERCRESS SAUCE AND SOME EGGS

SERVES 2

⅓ cup (75 ml) extra-virgin olive oil

1 onion, thinly sliced

2 cloves garlic, finely chopped

1 bunch watercress, washed, dried and chopped

sea salt

4 hard-boiled eggs, halved

Heat 1 tablespoon of the olive oil in a small frying pan over a low–medium heat. Add the onion and sauté until translucent. Add the garlic and cook for a further 2 minutes or until fragrant. Add the watercress and allow to wilt until the stems are softened (about 5 minutes).

Transfer to a blender with the remaining oil and ⅓ cup (75 ml) water. Blend until smooth. Season to taste with salt. To serve, place the eggs on a plate and drizzle with watercress sauce.

Reminder!

To dry watercress, place in a clean, sealable laundry bag in your washing machine and run on the last spin cycle for 30 seconds or so to remove water by centrifugal force.

2 SERVES VEG + FRUIT PER SERVE

2 SERVES VEG + FRUIT PER SERVE

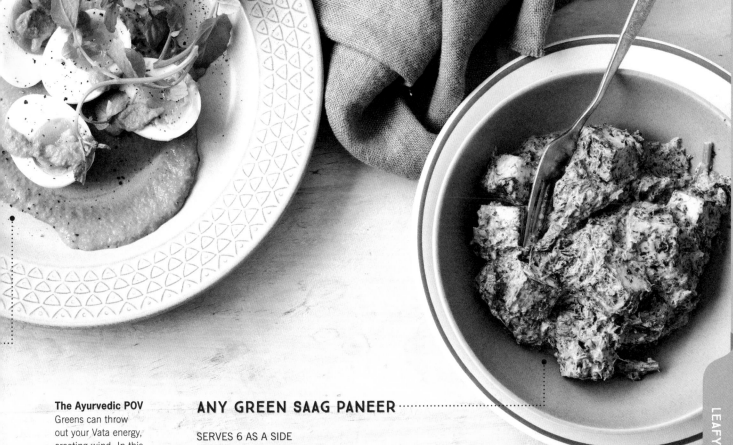

The Ayurvedic POV

Greens can throw out your Vata energy, creating wind. In this dish, paneer, a fresh cheese much like haloumi, comes to the rescue along with some good-quality fat and gently warming spices, reducing your Vata without aggravating your Pitta. Got it?

ANY GREEN SAAG PANEER

SERVES 6 AS A SIDE

40 g ghee (or coconut oil, though ghee is best)

250 g Homemade Paneer (page 48) or haloumi, cut into 2 cm cubes

1 large onion, chopped

2 cloves garlic, finely chopped

2 cm knob of ginger, finely chopped

2 teaspoons freshly chopped turmeric or Fermented Turmeric Paste (page 340) or ½ teaspoon ground turmeric

3 teaspoons Ras el Hanout Mix (page 45) or 1 teaspoon each ground coriander, ground cumin and cayenne pepper

½ teaspoon freshly ground black pepper

500 g greens, rinsed and chopped

big pinch of sea salt

2–3 tablespoons full-fat organic plain yoghurt (optional)

Green options: 2 small bunches of spinach (older, tougher spinach is best – baby leaves won't get the same result) or 1 small bunch of Swiss chard or 1 bunch of dandelion greens, beetroot leaves, kale or watercress with ½ bunch of spinach.

Heat half the ghee or oil in a large saucepan over a medium–high heat and cook the paneer or haloumi until golden. Set aside on a plate. Heat the remaining ghee or oil in the same pan and sauté the onion, garlic and ginger until soft. Add all the spices and sauté until very golden (about 5 minutes). If the spices start to catch, add a little water. Add the greens and salt, cover and cook for 5–10 minutes. (If your pan isn't big enough, add the greens gradually.) Once cooked, purée using a stick blender or food processor. Stir through the yoghurt only if you're after a creamier texture. Add the paneer or haloumi and heat for 5 minutes before serving.

MAKE IT VEGAN:

Use tofu instead of cheese.

 1 SERVE VEG + FRUIT PER SERVE

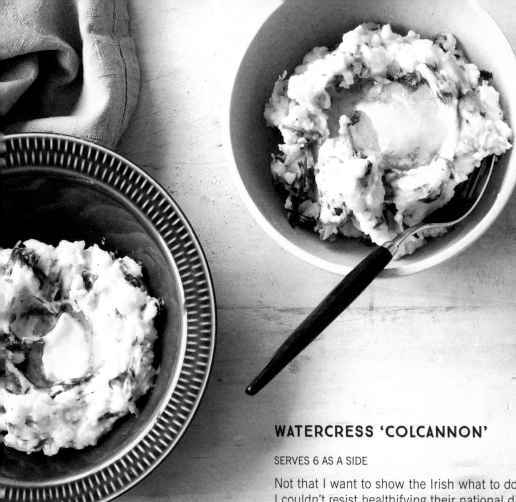

WATERCRESS 'COLCANNON'

SERVES 6 AS A SIDE

Not that I want to show the Irish what to do with a spud, but I couldn't resist healthifying their national dish (usually made with potatoes and cabbage) just a little.

Just scrub the spuds; no need to peel. →

1 kg 'white' veggies (potatoes, cauliflower, parsnips, celeriac, swede), chopped

⅓ cup (75 g) butter, plus extra to serve

1 leek, chopped

1 bunch watercress, dandelion greens or Swiss chard, roughly chopped

1 cup (250 ml) milk

sea salt and freshly ground black pepper

Place the white veggies in a stockpot or large saucepan with enough water to cover. Bring to the boil, covered, over a high heat. Reduce the heat and simmer for 15 minutes or until soft. Drain.

Meanwhile, melt the butter in a large stockpot over a medium heat. Add the leek and cook for 3–5 minutes or until soft. Add the greens and cook for 5 minutes, or until the leaves are wilted and the stems are soft. Add the milk and heat until it bubbles. Add the cooked white veggies and season with salt and pepper. Mash with a potato masher or fork, leaving a few clumpy bits.

To serve, mound the mash into bowls. Use the back of a spoon to make an impression in the centre and fill with a pad of softened butter. Once the butter melts, each forkful should be dipped into the well of butter before eating.

MAKE IT ORANGE:
Replace half the white veggies with sweet potato and carrot.

MAKE IT MEATY:
Add 3 rashers of bacon, chopped, when cooking the leek.

MAKE IT SUMMERY:
Mash in 1 cup (150 g) peas and ½ bunch of mint.

 3 SERVES VEG + FRUIT PER SERVE

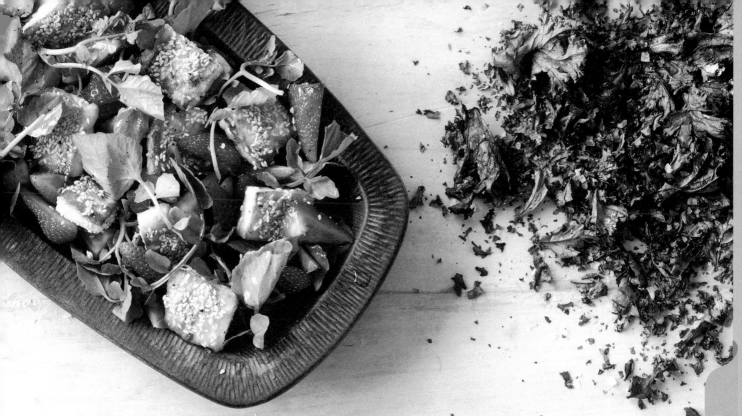

SESAME-CRUSTED HALOUMI AND STRAWBERRY SALAD

SERVES 6 AS A SIDE

4 tablespoons sesame seeds
(white is best, but use what you've got)

sea salt and freshly ground black pepper

250 g haloumi (or Homemade Paneer; page 48),
cut into 3 cm squares, 5 mm thick

40 g coconut oil, melted

250 g strawberries, hulled and quartered

1 bunch watercress, tough stems removed
and leaves torn into bite-sized bits

½ cup (125 ml) Powerhouse Dressing (page 53)

Sprinkle the sesame seeds on a plate and
season to taste with salt and pepper. Place
the haloumi or paneer in a bowl with the
coconut oil and toss gently to coat. Roll the
cheese squares in the sesame seeds until
evenly coated.

Cook the haloumi or paneer in a frying pan
over a medium–high heat until lightly browned
on both sides. Toss the remaining ingredients
in a bowl and top with the cooked haloumi
or paneer.

½ SERVE VEG + FRUIT PER SERVE

KALE FLAKES

Use these salty green flakes as a
salad-, soup- or stew-topper or mix
them with toasted sesame seeds and
Activated Groaties (page 27) for a
nutrient-dense snack.

1 bunch kale or cavolo nero,
stems removed and leaves torn

1 teaspoon sea salt flakes

Preheat the oven to 200°C (gas 6).
Place the leaves on a baking tray in a
single layer (you may need two trays)
and sprinkle with salt. Bake for 10–15
minutes until crispy and crunchy.

When cool, crumble in your hands into
small flakes or process briefly in a food
processor. Store in an airtight container
for up to 1 week.

2 SERVES VEG + FRUIT PER SERVE

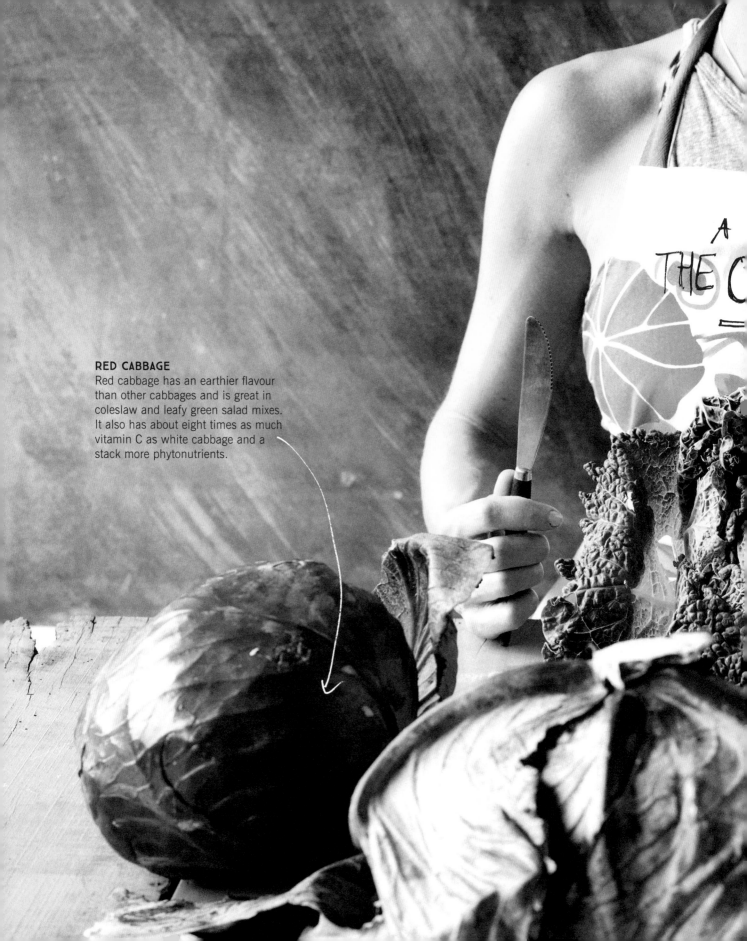

RED CABBAGE
Red cabbage has an earthier flavour
than other cabbages and is great in
coleslaw and leafy green salad mixes.
It also has about eight times as much
vitamin C as white cabbage and a
stack more phytonutrients.

SAVOY
Leaves are tender, even when eaten raw. This makes them perfect for salads and wraps, and as a bed for other dishes. Savoy also lacks the sulphur-like pong when cooked, if that matters to you.

WHITE CABBAGE
Also known as patta gobi, it's held in high esteem as it works well in a multitude of dishes. Use it raw in salads or boiled or braised.

CHINESE LEAVES
Also called napa, it's widely used in East Asian cuisine. Great raw in salads and cooked in dumplings and spring rolls.

Other cabbages (not pictured): brussels sprouts, pak choy, choy sum

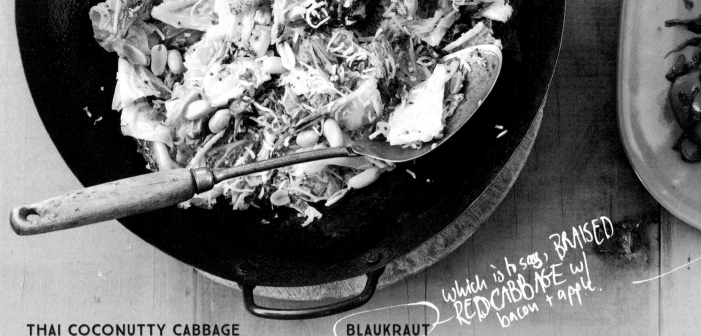

Handwritten note: which is to say, BRAISED RED CABBAGE w/ bacon + apple.

THAI COCONUTTY CABBAGE

SERVES 2

40 g coconut oil

2 teaspoons mustard seeds

4 cloves garlic, finely chopped

1–2 green chillies, sliced

1 teaspoon ground turmeric or 3 tablespoons Fermented Turmeric Paste (page 340)

1 teaspoon ground cumin

½ teaspoon freshly ground black pepper

½ head cabbage (savoy or Chinese leaves), coarsely chopped

big pinch of sea salt

½ cup (40 g) shredded coconut

chopped peanuts, to serve (optional)

handful of coriander leaves, chopped, to serve (optional)

Heat the oil in a large wok or saucepan over a medium–high heat and cook the mustard seeds until they start to pop. Add the garlic, chilli, turmeric, cumin and pepper and sauté for another minute. Add the cabbage and salt and turn down the heat to very low. Cook, covered, until the cabbage has softened (about 8 minutes). If the cabbage is still quite liquid-y, cook for a few more minutes, uncovered. Remove from the heat and add the coconut. Serve sprinkled with chopped peanuts and coriander, if desired.

MAKE IT A MEAL:
Add 1 cup (200 g) basmati rice and 2½ cups (600 ml) Homemade Stock (page 42) and cook for an additional 15 minutes. Or toss through some Shredded Chicken (page 214).

BLAUKRAUT

SERVES 6 AS A SIDE

6 rashers bacon, cubed

1 onion, halved and thinly sliced

2 apples, green or red, cored and cut into 2 cm wedges

1 red cabbage, cored, quartered and thinly sliced

sea salt and freshly ground black pepper

1 tablespoon caraway or fennel seeds, lightly crushed using a mortar and pestle

1 tablespoon apple cider vinegar

1–2 tablespoons rice malt syrup or ½–1 teaspoon granulated stevia

½ cup (125 ml) Homemade Chicken Stock (page 42) or water

4 tablespoons red wine (or additional stock or water)

chopped hazelnuts (preferably activated; page 28), to serve

Cook the bacon in a stockpot or large saucepan over a medium heat, stirring occasionally, until the fat renders and the bacon is crisp (about 8 minutes). Add the onion and apple and cook, stirring, until the onion softens (4–6 minutes). Stir in the cabbage and season with salt and pepper. Add the caraway or fennel seeds and deglaze with the apple cider vinegar. Add the rest of the ingredients and bring to the boil. Reduce the heat, cover, and simmer until the cabbage is tender (20–25 minutes). Serve sprinkled with the hazelnuts.

½ TSP ADDED SUGAR PER SERVE

1 SERVE VEG + FRUIT PER SERVE

1½ SERVES VEG + FRUIT PER SERVE

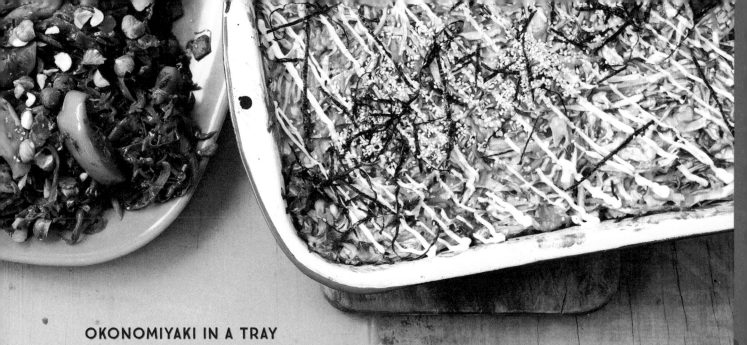

OKONOMIYAKI IN A TRAY

SERVES 6 AS A LIGHT MEAL

Okonomiyaki, usually served as a pancake for one, has always struck me as a fiddly dish crying out for a dumping of leftover veggies. So I bulked it up, packed in whatever I had in the fridge and whacked it in a tray. Bam.

3 cups (300 g) finely shredded cabbage and/or brussels sprouts

2 cups (300 g) grated sweet potato or carrot (or another colourful veggie like leftover peas, corn etc)

½ bunch spring onions, thinly sliced

6 eggs, whisked

3 tablespoons tamari

1 cup (120 g) buckwheat flour (or any flour)

1 cup (250 ml) Whey-Good Mayo (page 50)

3 tablespoons sesame seeds

4 tablespoons 'But the Kitchen Sink' Kimchi (page 337; optional)

1 nori sheet, cut into thin strips

Preheat the oven to 180°C (gas 4) and grease a large baking dish. Place the cabbage, grated veggies and spring onions in a large bowl and toss. Stir through the eggs, tamari and flour until a batter forms. Dump the mixture into the baking dish. Bake for 30 minutes, or until the top starts to brown and the eggs have cooked through. Remove from the oven. Place the mayo in a zip-lock bag or small plastic bag and trim one corner (or use a piping bag) and squeeze out in even lines over the pancake. Sprinkle over the sesame seeds, kimchi and nori strips (if using). Freeze the unused okonomiyaki in per-serve portions for up to 3 months.

2 SERVES VEG + FRUIT PER SERVE

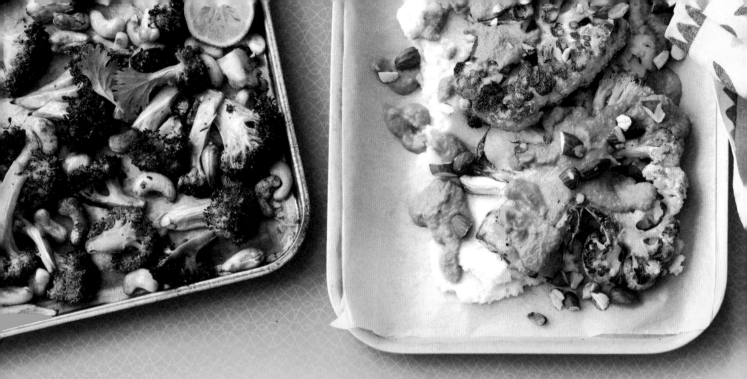

ASIAN CASHEW CRISP

SERVES 2

¼ cup (50 g) coconut oil or ghee, plus extra for greasing

1 large head broccoli or cauliflower (or a combo of both), cut into small florets, including the stalk

½ teaspoon chilli flakes

⅓ cup (40 g) cashews (preferably activated; page 28)

1 tablespoon fish sauce

lime wedges, to serve

coriander leaves, to serve

Preheat the oven to 220°C (gas 7). Line a baking tray with baking paper and brush (or spray) with oil. Toss all the ingredients together in a large bowl until well coated. Spread over the prepared tray. Bake, turning once or twice, until the florets have crunchy blackened bits (about 20–30 minutes). Serve with lime wedges and fresh coriander.

CAULIFLOWER TARTINES WITH GREEN GODDESS DRESSING AND HAZELNUTS

SERVES 2

1 head cauliflower

1 tablespoon coconut oil, plus extra for greasing

sea salt and freshly ground black pepper

a sprinkle of ground cumin

4 tablespoons chopped almonds or hazelnuts (preferably activated; page 28)

1 tablespoon butter

2 tablespoons grated parmesan

½ cup (125 ml) Leftovers Pesto (page 55) blended with ½ avocado or ½ cup (125 ml) Green Minx Dressing (page 54)

Preheat the oven to 220°C (gas 7). Line a baking tray with baking paper and brush (or spray) with oil.

Remove any outer leaves from the cauliflower, but keep the stem intact. Place the cauli on a chopping board, stem-side down. Cut two 3 cm thick slices from the centre of your cauli, ensuring they're nice and straight. Reserve the rest of the cauliflower for the purée, below.

Place the cauli steaks on the prepared tray and rub with oil. Season generously with salt, pepper and cumin. Roast for 25–35 minutes, gently turning after 15 minutes, until the cauli is browned and the stems feel tender when pierced with a knife. In the final 10 minutes add the nuts to the tray.

Meanwhile, steam (or microwave) the reserved cauliflower until soft. Place in a deep bowl with the butter and parmesan. Using a stick blender, whizz until smooth.

Spoon the purée onto a serving plate and top with the steaks. Drizzle over the dressing and scatter with the toasted nuts.

You can also barbecue or pan-fry your cauli steaks – 4–5 minutes each side should do the job.

3 SERVES VEG + FRUIT PER SERVE

4 SERVES VEG + FRUIT PER SERVE

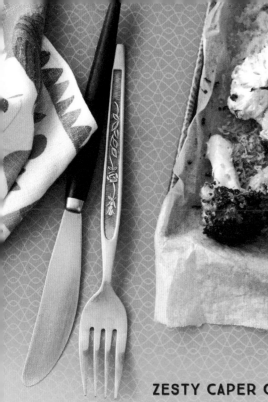

ZESTY CAPER CRUNCH

SERVES 2

¼ cup (50 g) coconut oil or ghee,
plus extra for greasing

1 large head broccoli or cauliflower
(or a combo of both), cut into small
florets, including the stalk

1 red onion, halved and sliced into
thin wedges

5 cloves garlic, thinly sliced

4 tablespoons baby capers
(preferably in salt)

½ teaspoon chilli flakes

½ teaspoon sea salt

½ cup (about 70 g) Cooked Quinoa (page 26)
or Cooked Buckwheat (page 27)
or 25 g breadcrumbs

¼ cup (25 g) grated parmesan

2 tablespoons lemon zest

*If you use a combo of
cauliflower and broccoli,
cut your cauli florets smaller
than your broccoli ones!*

Preheat the oven to 220°C (gas 7). Line a
large baking tray with baking paper and brush
(or spray) with oil. In a large bowl, toss the
broccoli and/or cauli with the onion, garlic,
capers, oil, chilli and salt, then spread over
the prepared tray. Bake, turning once or twice,
for 15 minutes. Sprinkle with the quinoa,
buckwheat or breadcrumbs and bake for a further
5–10 minutes, or until golden. Serve sprinkled
with parmesan and lemon zest.

4 SERVES VEG + FRUIT PER SERVE

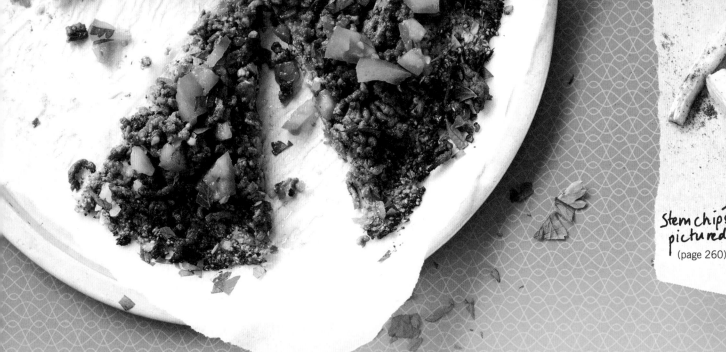

stem chips
pictured h
(page 260)

LEBANESE ROLL PIZZA

SERVES 2

1 head broccoli, roughly chopped (including the stalk)

180 g cheddar (or any hard cheese)

4 tablespoons chia seeds

sea salt and freshly ground black pepper

40 g coconut oil, melted

½ red onion, chopped

1 clove garlic, chopped

250 g lamb or beef mince

1 teaspoon chilli flakes

1 teaspoon ground coriander seeds

TO SERVE

½ cup (20 g) roughly chopped flat-leaf parsley

1 large tomato, chopped

½ teaspoon finely chopped Good for Your Guts Garlic (page 340)

lemon wedges

Preheat the oven to 210°C (gas 6) and line a baking tray with baking paper.

Blitz the broc in a food processor to form small chunks, then transfer to a bowl. Place the cheese in the processor and pulse to form rough crumbs. Add the cheese to the broccoli, stir in the chia seeds and season with salt and pepper. Press the mixture onto the prepared tray to make a thick 'pizza' base. Drizzle with 1 tablespoon of the coconut oil and bake for 15 minutes.

Meanwhile, heat the remaining coconut oil in a large frying pan over a medium heat. Add the onion and sauté for a couple of minutes. Turn up the heat to medium–high, add the garlic and mince and cook for 2 minutes. Add the chilli and coriander and cook for a further 2 minutes or until most of the liquid has evaporated.

Remove the pizza base from the oven and scatter over the meat and onion mixture. Return to the oven and bake for 5 minutes. To serve, scatter over the parsley, tomato and garlic, and squeeze over some lemon juice.

MAKE IT VEGAN:

Use Vegan 'Mince' (right) instead of the lamb or beef mince.

4 SERVES VEG + FRUIT PER SERVE

VEGAN 'MINCE'

MAKES 4 CUPS (1 LITRE)

Use in tacos, on pizza, or sprinkled over spaghetti. Just don't add it to a sauce as it will dissolve.

1 head cauliflower, roughly chopped (including the stalk)

2 cups (225 g) walnuts

40 g coconut oil

3 cloves garlic, finely chopped

½ teaspoon smoked paprika

2 teaspoons ground cumin

1 teaspoon each sea salt and freshly ground black pepper

3 tablespoons tamari, soy sauce or coconut aminos

Preheat the oven to 180°C (gas 4) and line a baking tray with baking paper. Blend the cauli and nuts in a blender to a rice consistency (not a powder). Plonk in a large bowl and add the remaining ingredients, kneading with your hands to combine. Dump the mixture onto the baking tray and spread out evenly. Bake for 45–75 minutes, tossing every 20 minutes or so to ensure the whole lot browns. Cool, then divide into ½ cup (125 g) portions and freeze for up to 3 months.

Yes, you read right – this ar no frankenfoo and the smok meaty taste i really rather remarkable!

1 SERVE VEG + FRUIT PER SERVE

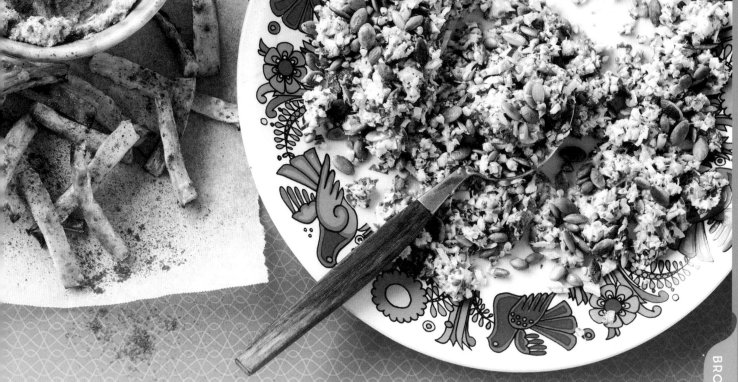

THE WHOLE BRASSICUS HUMMUS

MAKES 3 CUPS (725 ML)

This recipe ingeniously creates a hummin' hummus and some tasty stem chips to go with.

1 head broccoli or cauliflower (or a combo), chopped (reserve stems/stalks if you're making chips (page 260), or just bang them in too)

3 cloves garlic

4 tablespoons coconut oil, olive oil, butter or ghee, melted

½ cup (125 ml) TMT Dressing (page 53) or 4 tablespoons tahini mixed with the juice and zest of 1 lemon

½ teaspoon ground cumin

sea salt and freshly ground black pepper

Sweet Paprika Stem Chips (page 260), to serve (optional)

If you're not making the chips, feel free to steam the cauli and/or broc lightly instead of baking, and wring it out in a tea towel to remove all the moisture. Saves turning on the oven!

Preheat the oven to 180°C (gas 4). Place the broc and/or cauli and garlic on a baking tray. Drizzle over 2 tablespoons of oil, butter or ghee and roast for 20 minutes, turning halfway. Transfer to a food processor or blender with the remaining oil and the dressing and cumin. Process until well combined. Add more oil if it's too dry, or some chia seeds if it's too moist. Season with salt and pepper. Store in a jar in the fridge for up to 1 week.

MAKE IT BULKIER:

Add 1 cup (160 g) cooked chickpeas, and some extra dressing.

1 SERVE VEG + FRUIT PER SERVE

CRUNCHY BROCCOLI BUCKWHEAT TABBOULI

SERVES 6 AS A SIDE

1 large head broccoli, roughly chopped (including the stalk)

4 tablespoons pumpkin seeds (preferably activated; page 28)

½ cup (85 g) Activated Groaties (page 27)

1 cup (40 g) finely chopped flat-leaf parsley

1 cup (40 g) finely chopped mint

½ red onion, finely chopped

½ cup (125 ml) Whey-Good Mayo (page 50) whisked with the juice and zest of 1 lemon

small handful of something small, red and lovely: pomegranate seeds, edible flowers, redcurrants, goji berries (very optional)

Process the broccoli in a food processor to a rice consistency. Transfer to a large heatproof bowl and pour over enough boiling water to cover. Set aside for 3–4 minutes. Drain, allow to cool and return to the bowl. Dry-roast the pumpkin seeds in a small skillet or frying pan over a medium heat and add to the broccoli, along with the remaining ingredients.

MAKE IT A MEAL:

Add hard-boiled eggs, halved, or Shredded Chicken (page 214).

1½ SERVES VEG + FRUIT PER SERVE

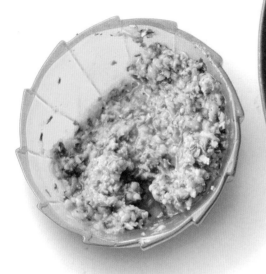

QUICK COURGETTE TZATZIKI

MAKES ABOUT 2 CUPS (500 ML)

1 cup (150 g) grated fresh or frozen courgettes

1 cup (200 g) full-fat organic plain yoghurt

2 cloves Good for Your Guts Garlic (page 340) or 2 teaspoons finely chopped garlic or other ferment

1 tablespoon brine (see page 334) or lemon juice

Combine all of the ingredients in a glass jar and store in the fridge for 2–3 days.

COURGETTE NO-CARBONARA

SERVES 2

500 g courgettes (3–4 medium ones)

sea salt

1 egg, plus 1 egg yolk

¼ cup (25 g) finely grated parmesan, plus extra to serve

freshly ground black pepper

20 g butter

8 tablespoons Bacon Bits (page 44) or 3–4 rashers bacon, rind removed, diced

Using a spiraliser or julienne peeler, slice the courgettes into noodles and place in a colander. Sprinkle with a little salt and leave for 10 minutes to drain. Blot gently with a tea towel to remove excess moisture if required.

In a small bowl whisk together the egg, egg yolk and parmesan until well combined. Season with freshly ground black pepper (the more the better!). Heat the butter in a large frying pan over a medium–high heat. Cook the Bacon Bits for 1–2 minutes or until hot; if using fresh bacon, cook for longer. Add the courgettes and cook for 1 minute. Add the egg mixture, tossing briefly to coat. Serve immediately, sprinkled with the extra parmesan.

USE THE LEFTOVER EGG WHITE:
Make an omelette. You can freeze it in the meantime by popping it in an ice-cube tray and then transferring the cube to a zip-lock bag. Or simply use 2 whole eggs and deal with a runnier sauce!

Pasta-making tip
The strips made from the centre part of the courgette tend to break more easily. If you want perfect-looking pasta, don't use the centre parts (freeze them to make Courgette Butter, right).

 ½ SERVE VEG + FRUIT PER SERVE

 1½ SERVES VEG + FRUIT PER SERVE

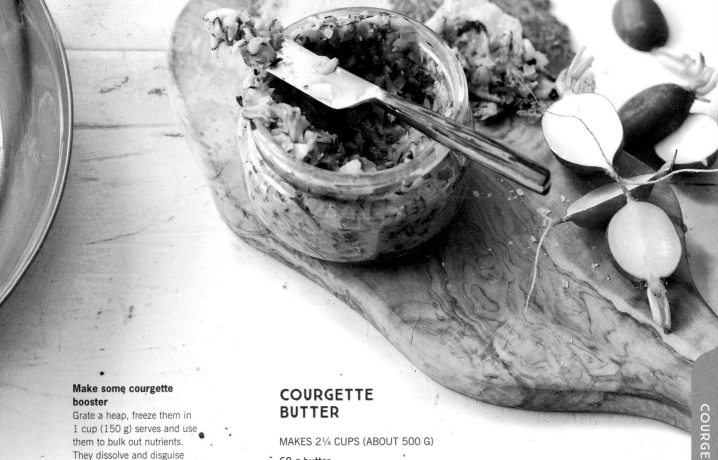

Make some courgette booster

Grate a heap, freeze them in 1 cup (150 g) serves and use them to bulk out nutrients. They dissolve and disguise themselves very easily, fooling most kids. Add to stews, pasta sauces, salads, smoothies (true story), muffins, cakes . . . You get the drift.

Note, however, that they will increase the liquid content of baked goods. So be sure to strain after grating (wring them robustly with your hands or in a clean tea towel).

COURGETTE BUTTER

MAKES 2¼ CUPS (ABOUT 500 G)

60 g butter

2–3 shallots (or 1 small onion), finely chopped

2 tablespoons thyme leaves

1 kg courgettes (4–5 big ones), coarsely grated and squeezed to remove the juices

sea salt and freshly ground black pepper

Heat the butter in a large frying pan over a medium–high heat. Sauté the shallots or onion for 15 minutes until caramelised. Add the thyme and courgettes and season with salt and pepper. Cook, stirring a little, for 20 minutes or until the courgettes have reduced by more than half. This will keep in the fridge for up to 1 month.

FIVE WAYS TO EAT COURGETTE BUTTER:

1. On a wedge of Socca (page 106).

2. Spread on toast.

3. As a soup topper.

4. Dolloped on pasta.

5. Added to a Salad of the Scoundrel (pages 252–3).

½ SERVE VEG + FRUIT PER SERVE

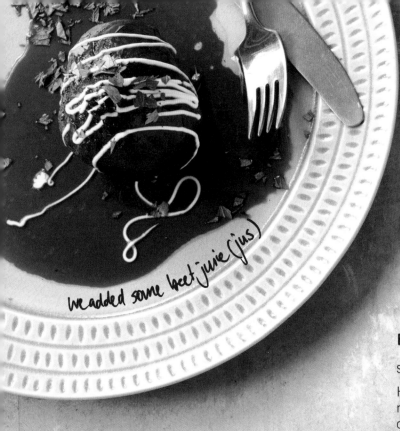

we added some beet juice (jus)

A REALLY FAT BEET
PLONKED PRETTILY ON A PLATE

SERVES 6

6 large beetroots

coconut oil, melted, for drizzling

sea salt and freshly ground black pepper

chopped basil, to garnish

Preheat the oven to 180°C (gas 4). Wash and dry the beets and place them in a baking dish. Drizzle with coconut oil and season with salt and pepper. Roast for 30–40 minutes. You can check if they're done after 30 minutes by sticking a knife in the centre of the largest beet; if it slides in easily, they're done. Let them cool. Trim the stalks and peel the beets if you like – the skins will slip right off. Pour the beet juice into a small saucepan and heat over a medium–high heat until reduced. Serve with the beets.

MAKE IT PRETTIER:
Drizzle with Whey-Good Mayo (page 50) or Homemade Cream Cheese (page 46) – use a piping bag or an old zip-lock bag with one corner snipped – and scatter with edible flowers.

. I eat the skins or put into a sandwich

2 SERVES VEG + FRUIT PER SERVE

BEET HALWA

SERVES 6

Halwa is an Indian dessert mostly made with sweetened condensed milk. I provide, forthwith, a far more nutritionally grounding version.

⅓ cup (75 g) ghee or butter

3 large beetroots, trimmed, scrubbed and grated

2½ cups (600 ml) milk (any milk, but full-fat dairy is best)

4 tablespoons rice malt syrup

1 teaspoon ground cardamom

1 cup (125 g) pistachios or cashews, activated (page 28) or toasted and chopped

Melt the ghee or butter in a heavy-based saucepan over a low heat. Add the beetroot and sauté gently for 5 minutes. Add the milk and bring to the boil. Reduce the heat and simmer for about 20 minutes (it might take longer, depending on how much liquid's in your beets), stirring occasionally, until the mixture thickens and begins to look glossy.

Add the rice malt syrup and stir for a few minutes. Keep stirring throughout to prevent catching. Add the ground cardamom and continue to simmer, stirring constantly, until all of the liquid has evaporated and the mixture is thick and glossy and starts to pull away from the side of the pan. Pour into serving bowls, sprinkle with nuts and serve warm or chilled.

1 ½ TSP ADDED SUGAR PER SERVE

1 SERVE VEG + FRUIT PER SERVE

feel free to reduce the amount of rice malt syrup, or use 1 tsp stevia instead.

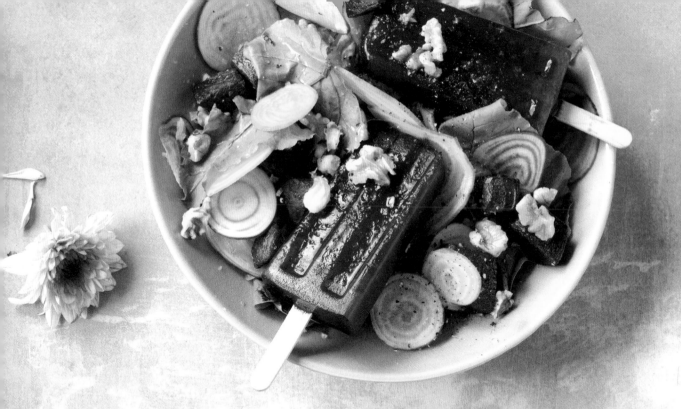

BEET THAT POPSTICK SALAD

SERVES 6

I made this at my 40th birthday, based on a dish I'd seen done by notoriously recalcitrant chef Colin Fassnidge at his sustainably minded restaurant 4Fourteen. As he told me via Twitter, he uses my first cookbook as a doorstop. I took it as a compliment.

USE THE LEFTOVER BIGGER, COARSER BEET LEAVES:
Make Massaged Beet Greens (page 23) – my favourite, or Leftovers Pesto (page 55).

3 red beetroots, trimmed, peeled and chopped into 2 cm chunks

¾ cup (100 g) frozen raspberries

2 tablespoons lemon juice

2 yellow or other coloured beetroots (if you can't find any, use 2 large carrots)

3 handfuls of baby beetroot leaves or rocket leaves

4 tablespoons walnuts (preferably activated; page 28), roughly chopped

1 tablespoon apple cider vinegar

1 tablespoon extra-virgin olive oil

pinch of sea salt

If you'd like your beets a little crispier, pan-fry quickly in a little coconut oil.

Place the red beetroot in a saucepan with enough water to cover. Bring to the boil (with the lid on) and cook for 20 minutes or until cooked through, but not mushy. Strain, reserving the precious bright-red beet water. Place 1½ cups (350 ml) of the beet water in a blender with the raspberries and lemon juice and blitz until smooth. Pour into six ice-block moulds and place in the freezer to set for 6 hours.

Slice the yellow beets into super-thin rounds (with a mandoline if you have one) or peel the carrot into long ribbons with a vegetable peeler (or mandoline). Place in a serving bowl with the cooled red beetroot chunks, leaves and walnuts. Toss gently with the vinegar, olive oil and salt.

To serve, remove the beet popsticks from the moulds by running them under hot water and place them on top of the salad.

2 SERVES VEG + FRUIT PER SERVE

JUST LIKE

GRANDMA

USED TO MAKE

B.T.W. If I was stuck on an Island, the one food I'd choose to have with me would be OFFAL — it's up to 100 times more nutritious than muscle

A chapter of OFFAL + cheap cuts:

liver   kidney
        sweetbreads

cheeks
brisket
skirt
chuck
thighs

because a lot of the time Nana really did know BEST.

MUM'S STEAK AND KIDNEY STEW WITH HERBY DUMPLINGS

SERVES 6

Mum's original recipe comes from a little cookbook that her local butcher gave her when she got married at 21. It espoused using cheap cuts, and eating a little meat at each meal, including breakfast (with carbs and sugar limited). These principles were very much pivotal in my early eating.

I've tweaked her recipe a little, tossing in some mushrooms, which can help to 'disguise' the kidneys if you're not used to them, and adding dumplings for an extra granny effect.

Why Mum made us eat kidneys
* They're high in iron: One kidney (about 85 g) = RDI of iron for women = 5 bags of baby spinach.
* They are one of the richest sources of selenium, an antioxidant that aids thyroid function and helps prevent tissue damage.
* And they're stupidly cheap.

Buy your kidneys already skinned from your butcher.

1 onion, sliced

1½ cups (115 g) cubed mushrooms (any variety is fine)

2 cloves garlic, sliced

1 kg stewing beef, cubed

2–4 lamb's kidneys (or 1 ox kidney), cored (remove the gristle on the inside with a small knife) and cubed

2 tablespoons plain flour (gluten-free if desired)

¼ teaspoon sea salt

½ teaspoon freshly ground black pepper

½ teaspoon dried mixed herbs or dried rosemary

¾ cup (175 ml) Homemade Beef Stock (page 42) or water

6 cups (about 750 g) steamed greens (beans, courgettes, broccoli or frozen peas), to serve

HERBY DUMPLINGS

25 g butter

2½ cups (300 g) self-raising flour (gluten-free if desired) mixed with ½ teaspoon sea salt

1 tablespoon chopped thyme

1 tablespoon chopped flat-leaf parsley

1 tablespoon full-fat milk

Place the onion, mushrooms, garlic, beef and kidneys in a slow-cooker insert. Add the flour, salt, pepper and herbs and stir to coat the meat and kidneys. Pour over the stock or water, cover and cook on low for 8–10 hours or on high for 4–5 hours.

To make the herby dumplings, rub the butter into the flour and salt with your fingertips until the mixture resembles fine breadcrumbs. Add the herbs and milk and mix to a soft dough. Roll into small balls.

Half an hour before serving, remove the slow-cooker lid and place the dumplings on top of the hot stew. Lay baking paper over the top and replace the lid. Cook on high for 30 minutes until the dumplings are cooked. Serve with steamed greens.

 1½ SERVES VEG + FRUIT PER SERVE

 £3 PER SERVE

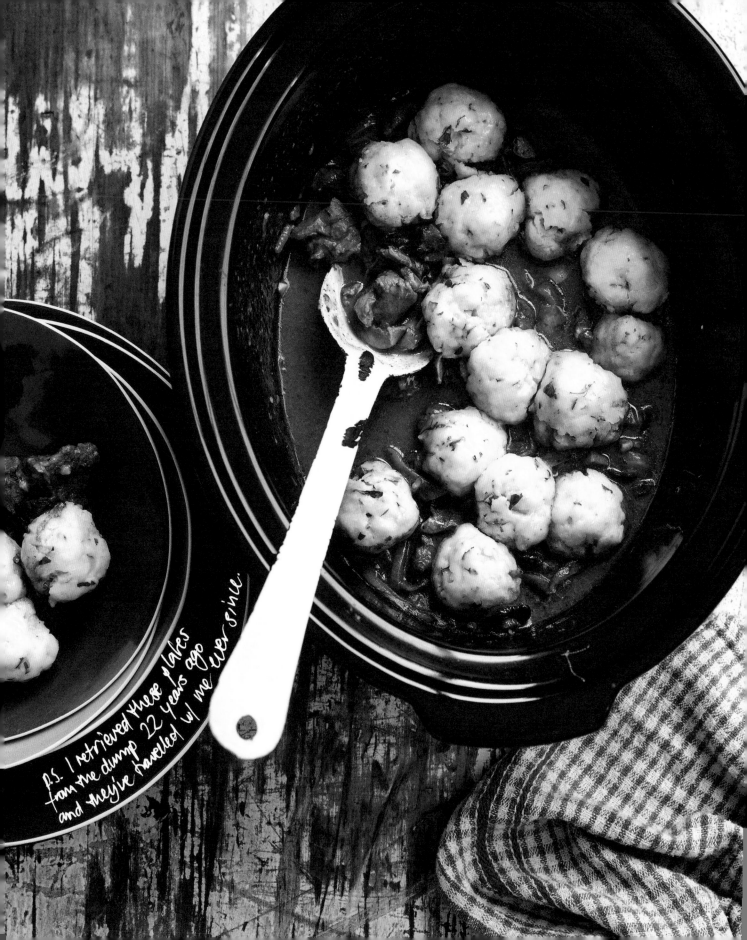

P.S. I retrieved these plates from the dump 22 years ago and they've travelled w/ me ever since.

BEGINNER'S COQ AU VIN PÂTÉ

MAKES 3 CUPS (ABOUT 700 G)

New to liver? This is the dish for you. Sexify your first time (or your fiftieth) with bacon and pad things out a tad with mushrooms. These particularly Frenchie flavours work mostly because, well, the French do flavour fabulously.

I wrap this pâté in a lettuce leaf and have it for breakfast many mornings. True story.

Ask your butcher to do the cleaning. They'll probably be thrilled to help out a new liver-lovin' customer.

500 g cleaned chicken livers or duck livers (or a combo)

100 g butter

1 rasher bacon, chopped

1 small onion (or 1 leek or ¼ bunch spring onions), chopped

250 g mushrooms (any kind; I like portobello), chopped

2 cloves garlic, chopped

1 tablespoon chopped thyme

2 teaspoons chopped sage

sea salt and freshly ground black pepper

½ cup (125 ml) dry white wine (or vermouth, scotch or brandy)

This is wonderfully gruesome work. Revel in it.

Liver: the ONLY superfood

This stuff is the most nutrient-dense food on the planet. It contains more nutrients, gram for gram, than any other food:

* 3 times as much choline as an egg;

* 17 times more B12 than red meat;

* 1400 times more vitamin A than red meat.

Trim the livers of any tough connective tissue and ensure the butcher hasn't left any green material (on chicken liver it's gallbladder and on duck liver it's bile).

Melt the butter in a frying pan over a medium heat. Add the bacon and onion, leek or spring onions and cook, stirring occasionally, until they start to turn lovely and golden. Add the mushrooms, liver, garlic and herbs and season to taste with salt and pepper. Cook, stirring occasionally, until the livers have browned and are only slightly pink on the inside (about 5 minutes). Transfer the lot to a blender (or a stick-blender beaker).

Add the wine to the pan and bring to the boil, scraping up the browned bits. Boil for about 1 minute to reduce slightly, then pour into the blender with the liver mixture. Process until very smooth.

Spoon the pâté into a bowl or jar. Allow to cool, then cover with cling film, pressing the wrap against the surface of the pâté so that it doesn't oxidise. Serve with raw veggie sticks, crackers or simply roll it up in a green leaf. The pâté will keep in the fridge for up to 3 weeks and in the freezer for up to 3 months.

You can cover the top of the pâté with a little melted butter to prevent it browning if you like, but I don't bother.

Total cost = £6.54
store-bought = £15.14

½ SERVE VEG + FRUIT PER SERVE

Frenchie
Coq au vin

thyme
+
sage.

onion
garlic

R vin

because bacon makes
liver better!
everything

mushrooms

CHINESE BEEF CHEEKS

SERVES 6

This dish is super-rich and loaded with flavour, turbo-charged by being marinated in the fridge overnight. Serve it with rice or quinoa and plenty of steamed green veggies to balance out the richness.

Beef cheeks are brimful of gelatine – super-good for gut health.

5 beef cheeks (1–1.3 kg)

1 bunch spring onions, finely chopped (reserve several green tops for garnish)

5 cloves garlic, thinly sliced

4 cm knob of ginger, grated

1 red bird's-eye chilli, thinly sliced

1 teaspoon five-spice mix

½ teaspoon granulated stevia (optional)

4 tablespoons Chinese rice wine or dry white wine

4 tablespoons soy sauce or tamari (preferably low-salt)

2 cups (150 g) sliced mushrooms (shiitake or portobello)

½ cup (125 ml) Homemade Beef Stock (page 42)

Cooked Quinoa (page 26) or steamed rice, to serve

6 cups (about 750 g) steamed greens

The night before: Trim the fat from the outside of the beef cheeks (it can be quite thick) and cut each cheek into two or three even-sized pieces. Place in the insert of the slow cooker along with all the ingredients except the mushrooms, stock, greens and reserved spring onion tops, and toss to combine. Cover and refrigerate overnight.

In the morning: Place the mushrooms on top and pour over the stock along with 1½ cups (350 ml) water. Cook on low for 7 hours or on high for 3½ hours.

Just before serving, slice the reserved green spring onion tops into long, thin strips and plunge into iced water for a minute to make them curly (if desired). Garnish the beef with the spring onion tops, and serve with quinoa or rice and steamed greens.

2½ SERVES VEG + FRUIT PER SERVE

£1.85 PER SERVE

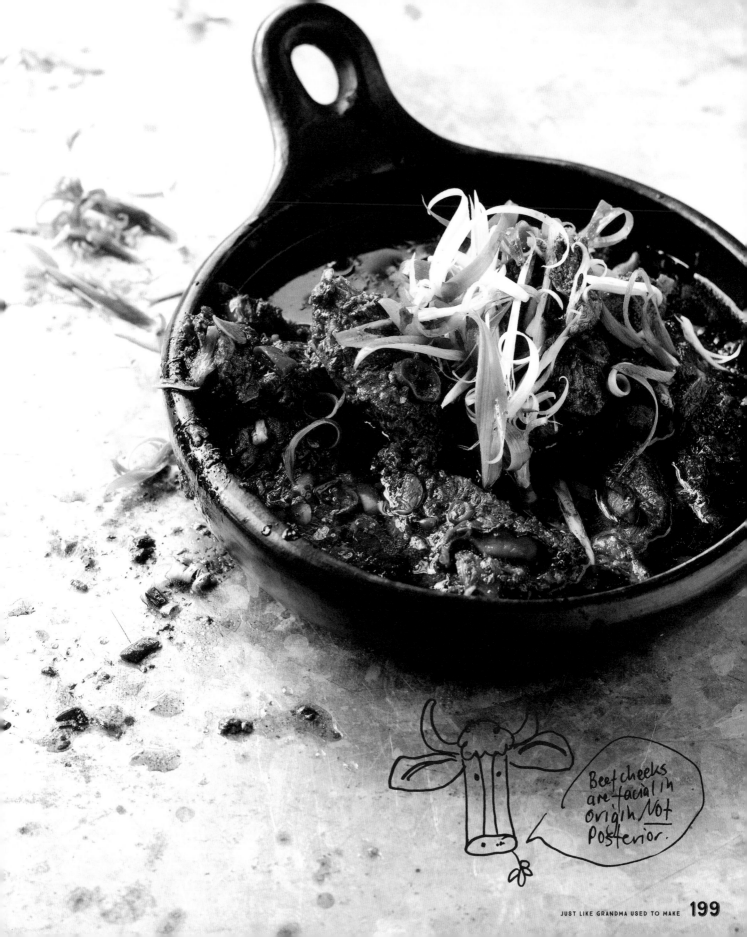

Beef cheeks are facial in origin Not Posterior.

'SWEET' TACOS
WITH EASY SLAW

SERVES 6

These use sweetbreads, the culinary name for the pancreas and thymus glands of various animals. (No need to tell the kids this.) Sweetbreads are definitely sweet and very moist and add great flavour and bulk to robust, salty dishes like tacos. Most good butchers sell them, or will get them in for you.

Sweetbreads

These morsels are rich in trace minerals such as zinc and selenium, said to reduce inflammation and to improve immunity, digestive processes and blood sugar signalling.

Sweetbreads cook quickly and actually are quite forgiving since they can't really be overcooked. To counteract the richness of the meat, many recipes serve sweetbreads with an acidic sauce featuring lemons or capers.

2 onions, finely chopped

4 cloves garlic, crushed

1 green pepper, chopped

1 bunch coriander stems, finely chopped (reserve the leaves for garnish)

1 kg beef brisket

400 g sweetbreads, cut into 1.5 cm cubes

1½ tablespoons tomato purée

1 teaspoon cayenne pepper

1 teaspoon dried oregano

1½ teaspoons ground cumin

¾ cup (175 ml) Homemade Beef Stock (page 42)

2 courgettes, grated *or use courgette ice cubes (page 24)*

12 taco shells or burrito wraps

TO SERVE

sliced avocado

Easy Slaw (see below)

sour cream, full-fat organic plain yoghurt or grated cheese

Place the vegetables and coriander stems in a slow-cooker insert. Place the brisket and sweetbreads on top. Add the tomato purée, cayenne pepper, oregano and cumin then pour the stock over the lot. Cover and cook on low for 8–9 hours or on high for 4–5 hours.

Remove the brisket and shred. Return the shredded meat to the slow-cooker insert with the courgettes and cook on high, lid off, for 20 minutes. Place the meat, avocado, slaw, sour cream and coriander leaves (or whatever sides you prefer) in serving dishes in the centre of your table. Heat the tacos (or warm the burritos) and have everyone 'load' their own.

EASY SLAW

500 g packet coleslaw mix or 2 large carrots and ½ red or white cabbage, grated

½ cup (125 ml) dressing (Whey-Good Mayo (page 50), Powerhouse Dressing (page 53) or whatever you have)

Mix together and off you go.

2 SERVES VEG + FRUIT PER SERVE

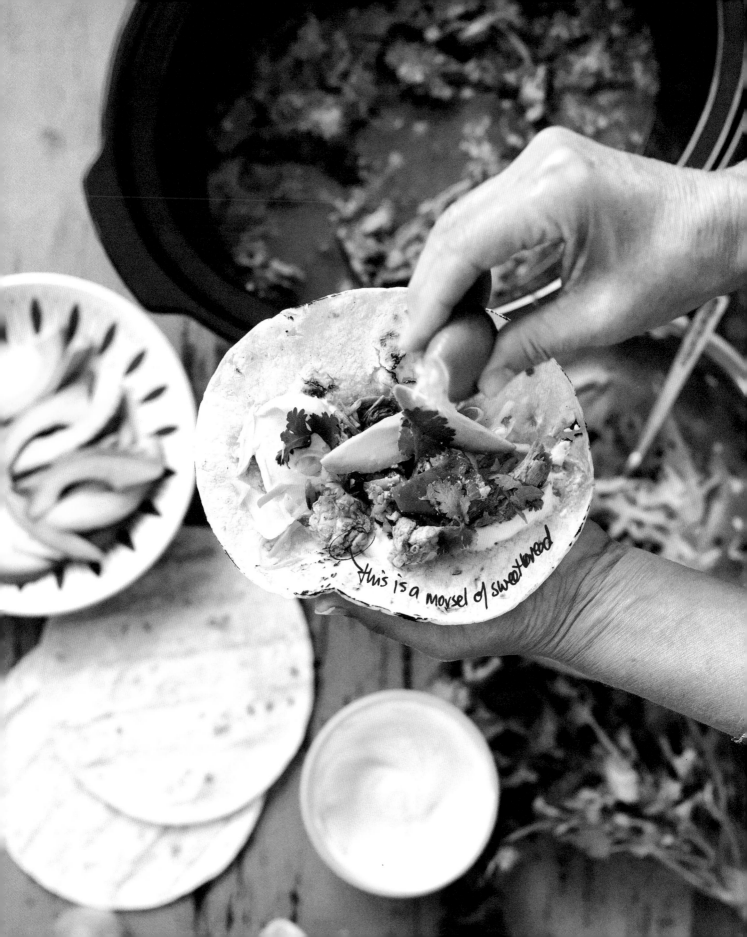

this is a morsel of sweetbread

LAMB'S FRY AND PEAR MEATLOAF

SERVES 6

Mum used to make us lamb's fry (livers cooked with bacon and mushrooms) on weekends. I really rather loved it. Liver needs to be cooked quickly or it goes feathery, which means it often has to be eaten by itself (that is, as a slab of offal). If that sounds off-putting, try a tip my butcher gave me: he minces some lamb and lamb's liver together, fresh. Yours will do the same, I'm sure. And then you can package it all up into this derivative loaf.

Be mindful we're talking about lamb's livers here. In the US, 'lamb fries' (note the absence of the possessive apostrophe) refers to lamb testicles; in the UK 'lamb's fry' refers to a mixture of all kinds of entrails. Got it?

Awfully good offal

* Organ meats are 10–100 times higher in nutrients than muscle meats.

* Those claims that meat is linked to cancer and early death? It's the methionine in muscle meat (bone- and organ-free cuts) that such grimness is linked to. Offal (as well as meat bones and skin), however, has high levels of glycine, which effortlessly balances the excessive methionine in muscle meats.

* Offal is also super-high in vitamins B6 and B12, folate, betaine and choline which work together synergistically to balance methionine.

* Eat the whole beast is the lesson here, people.

If your mixture is quite moist (my team's least favourite word) add 1–2 tablespoons of chia seeds (or extra almond meal) and allow to sit for 10 minutes to let the seeds do their soaking-up thing.

butter or ghee, for greasing

3 tablespoons almond meal

500 g lamb's livers minced with 500 g lamb or pork

1 courgette, grated and squeezed in a clean tea towel to remove moisture

1 pear or apple, peeled, cored and grated, plus extra slices for garnish

1½ cups (115 g) diced mushrooms (any kind)

1 onion, finely diced

1 tablespoon chopped sage or thyme, plus extra sage leaves for garnish

1 teaspoon ground mustard seeds or 1 tablespoon 'Bucha Mustard (page 336) or Dijon mustard

2 cloves garlic, finely chopped

2 large eggs

sea salt and freshly ground black pepper

4 rashers bacon

Shaved Sprouts and Pecorino Salad (page 305) or any leafy salad, to serve

Preheat the oven to 200°C (gas 6) and lightly grease a 23 cm × 13 cm loaf tin.

Place all of the ingredients except the bacon in a large bowl and mix well. Press the mixture into the greased loaf tin. Lay the bacon rashers across the top, tucking them in at the ends if they are too long. Arrange the extra sliced pear or apple on top, and sprinkle over the extra sage leaves. Bake for 45 minutes. Serve hot or cold with Shaved Sprouts and Pecorino Salad (or any green salad from this book). Freeze leftover slices of meatloaf between pieces of baking paper for up to 3 months.

MAKE IT FOR LATER:
Double the mixture and place it in two loaf tins. Freeze one of the tins (covered with a freezer-proof bag) for up to 3 months. When ready to use, simply plonk in your preheated oven and bake for 1–1½ hours.

2 SERVES VEG + FRUIT PER SERVE

After cooking + slicing this I ate the skin chips wrapped in radicchio with sprigs of CARROT TOPS and it was a Taste sensation.

carrot tops are a boon of a garnish.

sweet potato skin chips
(page 23)

CHICKEN CRACKLE SALT

In my quiet moments I sometimes wonder, 'What the hell happens to all that chicken skin that's criminally removed from chickens in poultry shops for all those folk insisting on skinless breasts?' Sadly, it's tossed. Happily, however, I have a fix for this travesty. My mate Aaron from ethical catering company Studio Neon in Sydney got me onto this when he made some for my 40th birthday. Gosh it made me happy . . . fat, salt and leftovers all in the one mix! The other thing I like about this recipe is that it entails going to your butcher or local chicken shop and asking them to do you a favour – to keep aside some skin. Forced mindful human engagement: this is what real food and real eating is about.

200g chicken skin

200g good-quality sea salt

Bring a small saucepan of water to the boil over a high heat. Add the chicken skin, reduce the heat and simmer for 10 minutes. Drain, and allow the skin to cool slightly. While it's still warm use a spoon or a butter knife to scrape off any excess fat that may be on the underside.

 Stretch and flatten the chicken skin on a wire rack placed over a baking tray. Place another wire rack on top of the chicken skin (this stops it from flying around as it crisps up if you have a fan-forced oven). Bake for 10–15 minutes or until brown and crispy. The skin will continue to crisp up as it cools.

Slightly break up the chicken skin and crush it with the salt using a large mortar and pestle (or use a stick blender, though be careful not to turn it into a fine powder – we want texture). Place in a sealable glass or plastic container and store in the pantry for up to 2 weeks.

MAKE IT A SOUP TOPPER:
Skip the salt and blitz stage and serve broken shards atop a soup or salad.

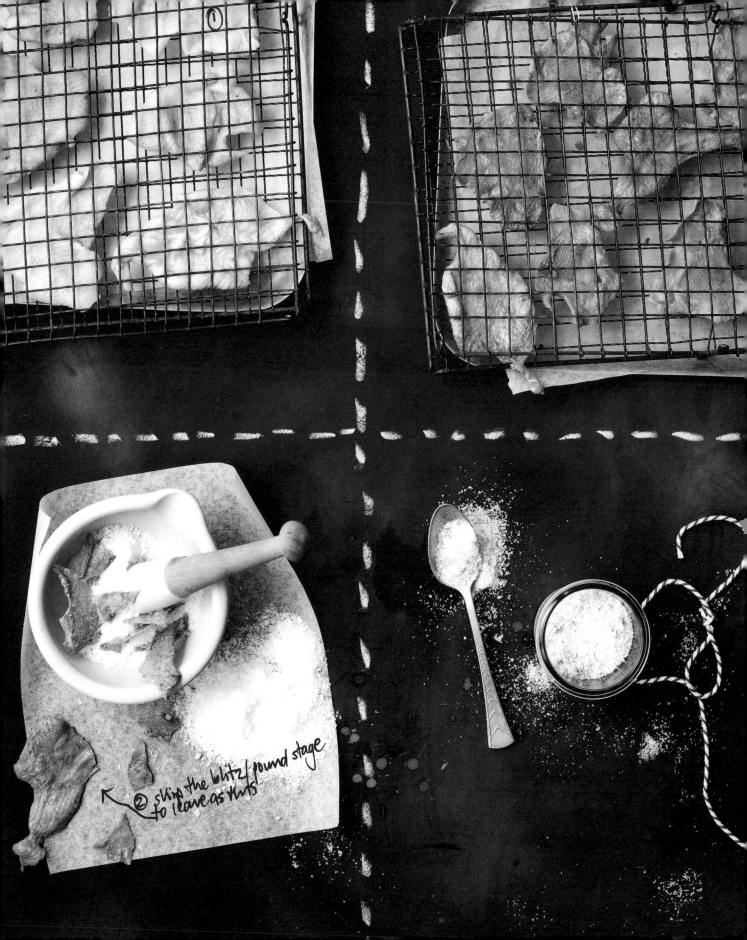

② skip the blitz/pound stage
to leave as this!

BLOKE BEEF 'N' BEER WITH MASH

SERVES 6

The local pub on a plate, brewed masterfully in the one pot
(2½ minutes of washing up entailed).

Beer + Meat = Good
A recent study has found
that when you marinate meat
with beer, it greatly reduces
the carcinogens that are
produced (yes, really) in the
cooking process.

600 g parsnips (or potatoes
or sweet potatoes), peeled and
chopped into 3 cm chunks

2 onions, finely diced

1–1.2 kg beef brisket,
excess fat trimmed

1½ tablespoons Dijon mustard

good pinch of sea salt

freshly ground black pepper

3 sprigs thyme

2 bay leaves

½ cup (125 ml) beer (preferably one with a
malty flavour)

3 big handfuls of green beans, trimmed

large knob of butter

Place the parsnips, potatoes or sweet potatoes and the onions in the base of your
slow-cooker insert. Coat the brisket in the mustard, season with salt and pepper
and place on top of the veggies. Add the thyme and bay leaves and pour over the
beer. Cover and cook on low for 8–10 hours or high for 4–5 hours.

In the last 15 minutes of cooking, place the beans on top of the meat. Cover
again and cook on high until the beans are tender.

*Feel free to thicken the
sauce by heating it in
a small saucepan and
stirring in 1 tablespoon
of arrowroot or other
flour.*

Remove the meat and the steamed beans from the slow cooker and set aside.
Using two forks, shred ('pull') the brisket. Drain most of the sauce from the insert
and set aside.

Add the butter to the insert and season with salt and pepper. Use a potato masher
to mash the veggies until smooth, adding extra sauce as needed. Serve the meat
with the mash and steamed beans. Drizzle the remaining sauce over the top.

2 SERVES VEG + FRUIT PER SERVE

£1.71 PER SERVE

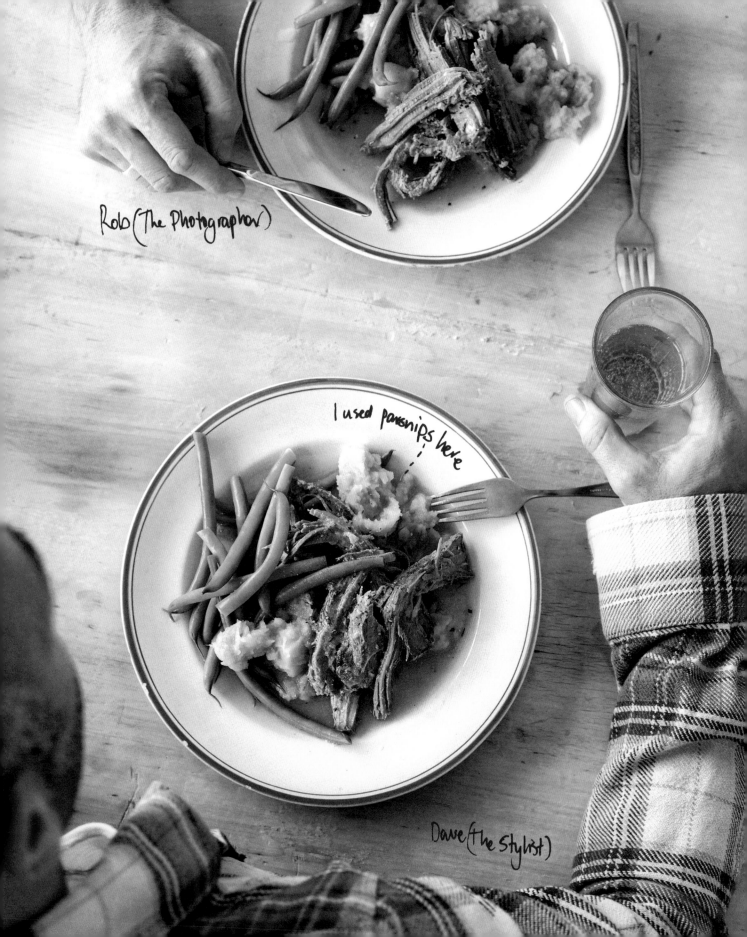

HOMEMADE BACON

MAKES 800 G

Some people get upset about nitrates in their bacon. The science says it's not really doing any harm. Similarly, some get upset about the sugar used to cure bacon. Don't. It's generally rinsed off. So why make your own? It saves money and gets your hands dirty! Plus it means you can experiment with flavours.

Nitrates in bacon

The nitrite in our saliva accounts for 70–90% of our total nitrite exposure; your spit contains far more of the stuff than anything you could ever eat. Also, the study that originally linked nitrates and cancer risk has since been discredited after being subjected to a peer review. And, indeed, more recent research suggests that nitrates and nitrites may not only be harmless, they may be beneficial, especially for immunity and heart health.

1.2–1.5 kg pork belly, rind left on

4 tablespoons sea salt

1 tablespoon freshly ground black pepper

1 tablespoon coriander seeds, fennel seeds or dried rosemary (or a combo)

½ teaspoon ground cinnamon or ground nutmeg

1 clove garlic, finely chopped

Rinse the pork belly and pat it dry. Combine the remaining ingredients in a small bowl and rub all over the pork. Place the pork and any remaining seasoning in a big re-usable plastic bag on a flat tray with a weight on top. Refrigerate for 1 week, flipping the bag every day or so. Liquid will build up – don't fret (it's the salt drawing moisture from the meat); throw it out.

Preheat the oven to 90°C (gas ¼). Rinse the pork, pat it dry and place in a baking dish. Roast uncovered for 2 hours. Remove from the oven and once cool to the touch, transfer the bacon to a chopping board and slice off the skin. Let the bacon cool to room temperature, then wrap it in greaseproof paper and refrigerate. Slice as you need it. It will keep for 2 weeks in the fridge. Or cut it into cubes and freeze for 3–6 months.

USE THE LEFTOVER RIND:
Add it to any of your freezer stock bags (page 32) to make a tastier stock.

SOME BEEFIN' GOOD JERKY

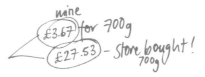

nine
£3.67 for 700g
£27.53 – store bought!
700g

MAKES 700 G

This jerky is seriously easy to make and will leave you feeling a little bit 'frontier'. It's great for lunchboxes. I fiddled around with this recipe to get a smoky–sweet 'processed meat' vibe. Here she goes . . .

Beef is best, and ensure it's lean in just this instance!

1 kg mince

1½ teaspoons sea salt

½ teaspoon black pepper

1 teaspoon garlic powder
(or 3 cloves garlic, finely chopped)

1 teaspoon ground cumin

1 teaspoon smoked paprika

If your oven only goes down as far as 90°C (gas ¼) that's dandy, but note the different cooking time.

Preheat the oven to 70°C (gas, on pilot light) and line two baking trays with baking paper. Use your hands to mix all the ingredients together in a big bowl. Take half the mixture and press it out on the first tray to 5 mm thick (use a rolling pin or bottle). You can work to a neat rectangle (though I like to keep it an organic shape and then break it into shards later). Repeat with the rest of the mixture on the second tray.

Dry for 6 hours in the oven (about 4 hours if using a 90°C (gas ¼) oven), pouring the juices into a jug every hour or so. (Keep the jug in the fridge – see below.)

Flip the jerky in the final hour. The stuff is done when you break off a piece, let it cool and it no longer leaks any moisture when squeezed.

Once done, allow the jerky to cool completely on a wire rack, then snap into shards (or cut with scissors) and store in an airtight container in the fridge for up to 2 months.

USE THE LEFTOVER MEAT JUICES:
Pour the juices into an ice-cube tray, freeze and use them to braise vegetables, add to soups or stews, or to make gravy.

While the oven is on at this low temperature it's a good time to make Good for Your Guts Garlic (page 340) or to dry some activated nuts (page 28), if you don't mind them infused with a meaty flavour. If your oven only goes to 90°C (gas ¼), why not make Homemade Bacon (opposite) at the same time?

A BUNCH OF

SUNDAY COOK-UPS

✡

BIG
COSY
MEALS
to
BULK-COOK often using a
slow cooker
on a
LAZY WEEKEND

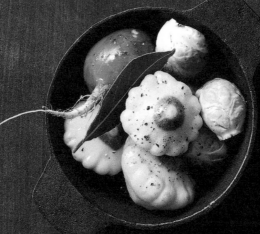

leaving you with leftover meat 'n' bits
that extend for yonks.

THE CHEAPEST STEW EVER

SERVES 6 + 8 PORTIONS OF LEFTOVER BEEF OR STOCK

Seriously, I costed this one out at 79p a serve. Drastically cheaper than chips. I've designed it so it can be served as a stew with leftover stock or a hearty soup with lots of leftover meat.

2 onions, chopped

2 large carrots, cut into 3 cm chunks

2 large parsnips, cut into 3 cm chunks

2 swedes or potatoes, cut into 3 cm chunks

2 celery stalks, chopped, leaves reserved

2 bay leaves

½ teaspoon dried oregano

2 cups (500ml) Homemade Beef Stock (page 42)

1 parmesan rind (if you have one in your freezer)

1.5 kg stewing beef (blade, chuck, brisket – whichever's cheapest), cut into 2 cm cubes

1 tablespoon English mustard

½ teaspoon sea salt

freshly ground black pepper

2 cups (200 g) Par-Cooked 'n' Frozen Swiss chard or kale (page 22)

Place all the ingredients, except the chard or kale, into the slow-cooker insert. Cover and cook on low for 8–10 hours or high for 4–5 hours. Remove and discard the bay leaves and parmesan rind (if using).

To serve as a stew: Remove half of the meat and 2 cups (500 ml) of stock from the slow-cooker insert and set aside (see below). Add the chard or kale and all but a few of the reserved celery leaves and heat through. Serve topped with the few remaining celery leaves and a big glug of olive oil.

To serve as a soup: Remove all of the meat from the slow-cooker insert, add the Swiss chard or kale and reserved celery leaves (keep a few for garnish) and heat to make soup. (Purée it with a stick blender if you prefer.) Serve sprinkled with the remaining celery leaves and some sliced sourdough or Socca wedges (page 106) on the side.

USE THE LEFTOVER STOCK:
If you have reserved 2 cups (500 ml) of stock, either drink it as a broth, or freeze it in 1 cup (250 ml) portions to make another soup.

USE THE LEFTOVER MEAT:
Divide any leftover beef cubes into ½ cup (65 g) portions and freeze for up to 3 months.

MAKE IT AN AUTOIMMUNE STEW:
When I'm inflamed and my immune system is cranky with me, I amend The Cheapest Stew Ever a touch to make this cytokine-pacifier. I swap the onions for 1 fennel bulb, chopped, ditch the potato and use swede or sweet potato, and serve with steamed courgettes or asparagus and a HUGE glug of olive oil.

If you're really serious about adjusting your diet to help manage an AI disease then you might like to try avoiding fructans (e.g. onion and garlic) and deadly nightshades (e.g. potato, tomato, aubergine, pepper and chilli).

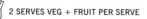

2 SERVES VEG + FRUIT PER SERVE

£0.79 PER SERVE

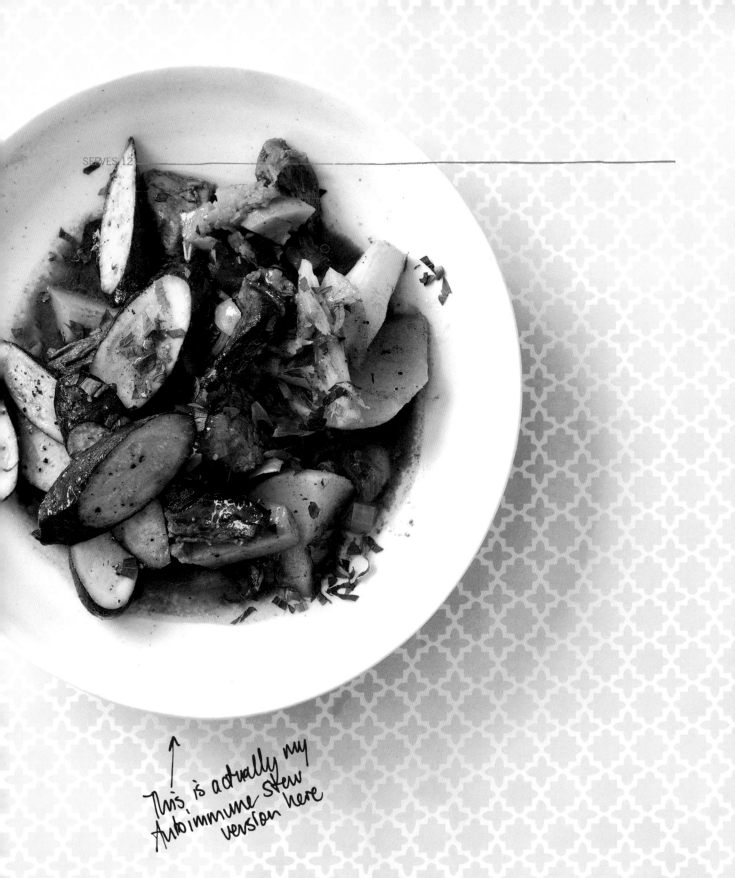

SERVES 12

This is actually my
Autoimmune Stew
version here

THREE WAYS with CHICKEN POT AU FEU.

This French classic ("pot on fire") sums up many things I love about French cooking + eating. It maximises the potential of the meat + veg while also!! requiring a mindful eating ritual.

1. BASIC POT AU FEU

SERVES 6 + LEFTOVER SHREDDED CHICKEN + STOCK

1 whole chicken

1 teaspoon peppercorns (black or white)

2 teaspoons sea salt

2 bay leaves

5 sprigs thyme

1 bunch new carrots, trimmed (or 3 large ones, halved lengthways, then cut into 5 cm long batons)

6 small parsnips, halved lengthways

2 turnips or swedes, scrubbed and cut into 6 wedges

1 fennel bulb, trimmed and cut in half lengthways, or 2 celery sticks, cut into 5 cm lengths

2 onions, peeled and quartered

1 head garlic, halved crossways, outer leaves peeled

TO SERVE

Homemade Aioli (page 50)

'Bucha Mustard (page 336; optional)

Leftovers Pesto (page 55; optional)

Investing in an organic one is non-negotiable for this dish as we'll be boiling the bones.

Remember to reserve all the veggie scraps for the second batch of stock.

Plonk the chook, leg-side down, in a big stockpot. Sprinkle over the peppercorns, salt and herbs. Cover the whole lot with water. Place the lid on the pot and bring to a gentle boil. Reduce to a simmer and cook for 45–60 minutes, skimming off the grey 'scum' a few times. Once the chicken is cooked (the legs pull away easily and the juices run clear when you cut into it), transfer to a chopping board to cool a little.

Add all the vegetables to the pot, cover and cook until soft (about 20–30 minutes).

Meanwhile, carve the chook into portions, reserving some for shredding (see below) and keeping the carcass and any excess skin.

To serve, divide the veggies between large serving bowls and top with the chicken pieces. Ladle over some stock, avoiding the herbs floating about. Serve with bowls of aioli, mustard and/or pesto in the centre of the table.

USE THE LEFTOVER CARCASS, BONES AND VEGGIE SCRAPS:
Make Homemade Chicken Stock (page 42).

USE THE LEFTOVER CHICKEN SKIN:
Make Chicken Crackle Salt (page 204).

USE THE LEFTOVER CHICKEN STOCK:
Drink it as a broth, or freeze it in 1 cup (250 ml) batches for up to 3 months.

SHREDDED CHICKEN

Shred any leftover chicken, divide it into ½ cup (65 g) portions and freeze for up to 3 months.

2½ SERVES VEG + FRUIT PER SERVE

£2.21 PER SERVE

…ito aioli

'boucha
mustard.

eftovers pesto

ot au Feu

Fini!

Use leftover chook skin to make chicken
Salt + drink the leftover stock for
lunch tomorrow

2. SOOTHING ASIAN POACHED POT

SERVES 6 + LEFTOVER SHREDDED CHICKEN + STOCK

1 whole chicken (yep, organic)

1 small (or ½ large) chinese leaves, cut into 6 wedges (don't remove the core as this will keep the wedges intact)

4 celery stalks, cut into 10 cm lengths

1 bunch spring onions, cut into 10 cm lengths

12 shiitake mushrooms, stems removed and sliced (or dried ones, soaked in boiling water for 20 minutes, the soaking liquid reserved)

½ bunch coriander, leaves picked, roots and stems left intact

4 cloves garlic, peeled and left whole

4 star anise

1 cinnamon stick

5 cm knob of ginger, sliced

dash of tamari or soy sauce (or a big shake of dulse flakes)

1 teaspoon peppercorns (preferably white)

2 teaspoons sea salt

Follow the instructions for Basic Pot au Feu (page 214), using the ingredients here, but add the coriander roots and stems only to the stockpot – the coriander leaves are for serving.

3. PRETTY SPRING POT

SERVES 6 + LEFTOVER SHREDDED CHICKEN + STOCK

1 whole chicken (organic once again)

2 bay leaves

5 sprigs thyme

1 teaspoon peppercorns (black or white)

2 teaspoons sea salt

rind of ¼ lemon, sliced

4 cloves garlic, peeled and left whole

1 leek, halved lengthways and cut into 5 cm lengths

3 baby yellow beetroots, quartered (or 1 bunch new carrots, trimmed)

1 fennel bulb, trimmed and cut into 6 wedges lengthways, fronds reserved

1 bunch asparagus, trimmed

2 cups (300 g) peas (mangetout or sugar snap peas, podded; or fresh broad beans, double-podded)

After podding, blanch them in boiling water to slip them out of their skins.

TO SERVE

6 poached eggs

You can cook your poachies in the stock after you've removed the veggies, rather than pulling out a new pot. Follow the instructions on page 44.

Follow the instructions for Basic Pot au Feu (page 214), adding the lemon rind with the herbs, salt and pepper. Add the garlic, leek, beetroot or carrots and fennel after removing the chicken. Add the asparagus just 5 minutes before serving, and the peas or broad beans only 1 minute before. Serve with a poachie on top and a sprig or two of fennel frondage.

1 SERVE VEG + FRUIT PER SERVE

2 SERVES VEG + FRUIT PER SERVE

SLOW-COOKED GREEN PEAS AND HAM

SERVES 6 + LEFTOVER HAM HOCK CHUNKS

This singular slow-cooked effort stretches to 10–12 portions. Eat it as a ham-flavoured soup and reserve the meat for later, or as a dense meaty stew, reserving the lush stock for later. It's best made in a slow cooker. Slow and low will better extract the collagen-y goodness from the ham.

Why ham on the bone?
It's cheaper, even bearing in mind the extra weight of the bone, more gelatinous, and it can be used for making a second batch of stock.

Unsmoked is better, but smoked is okay, too.

1.5–1.8 kg ham bone/hocks

500 g green split peas (or any legume, though peas are best), soaked overnight

3 carrots, finely chopped

3 celery stalks, finely chopped (keep a few leaves for garnish)

1 onion, finely chopped

I soak all beans, even split peas (page 28).

3 cloves garlic, finely chopped

2 bay leaves

2 tablespoons chopped thyme or 2 teaspoons dried thyme

2 big crunches each of sea salt and black pepper

Because of the gelatinous nature of the ham, your soup will solidify when cooled. This is a glorious thing. Simply heat to liquefy.

Place everything in a slow-cooker insert with 2 litres of water. Cook for 8–10 hours on low or 6–7 hours on high. Chuck out the bay leaves. Remove the ham hocks and reserve to make Ham Hock Chunks (see below).

Purée the soup using a stick blender or leave it as is if you like to keep things chunky. Serve with a few chunks of ham and some celery leaves on top.

HAM HOCK CHUNKS

Once the ham hocks are cool enough, pull the meat from the bones and chop it into chunks. Divide into ½ cup (65 g) portions and freeze for up to 3 months.

MAKE IT ON THE STOVETOP:
In a large saucepan, gently sauté the carrots, celery, onion and garlic in 1 tablespoon of olive oil for 10 minutes. Add the rest of the ingredients. Cover and bring to the boil, then reduce the heat and simmer for 1½–2 hours.

1½ SERVES VEG + FRUIT PER SERVE

£1.25 PER SERVE

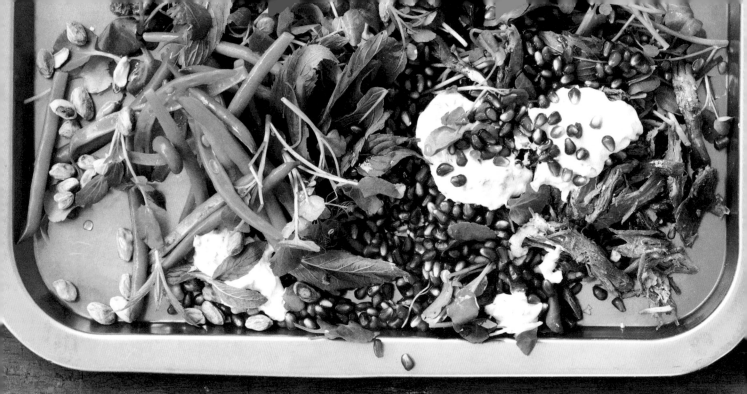

PERSIAN LAMB SALAD

CHEAT ROAST DINNERS
→ Pork, lamb, beef + shredded leftovers.

Roasts are great one-panners, but they can be temperamental, requiring thermometers to ensure a quality result, and I find them fiddly to serve (crook carving can create carnage). Plus, they tend to rely on primary cuts of meat. I get around all this by using secondary cuts that are foolproof to cook, and can be served as a 'pulled' roast (no carving!).

Plus, the recipes herewith are designed to leave you with leftover pulled meats for later. Yeah, thank me later.

GREEK LAMB SALAD

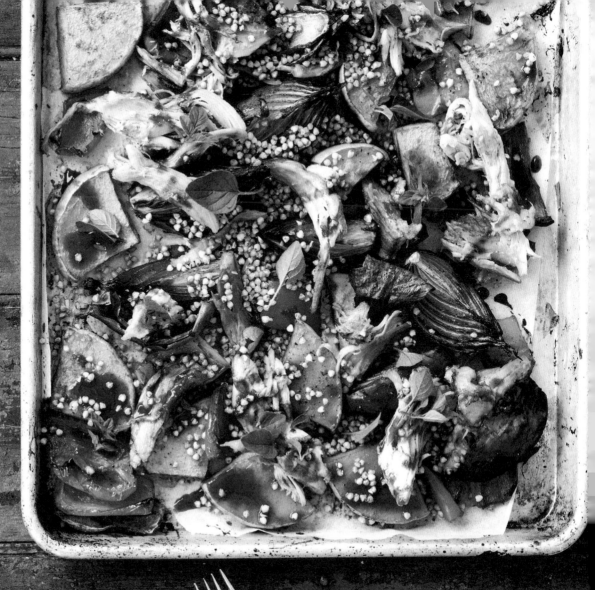

JERK PORK
SHOULDER ROAST

I garnished this with carrot tops.

a reader made these forks for me!

head on over for recipes

ROAST LAMB SHOULDER *with Shredded Lamb* ⟍

SERVES 6 + LEFTOVER SHREDDED LAMB

A versatile summer roast that can be
served as a variety of salads.

1.8 kg lamb shoulder, bone in,
fat trimmed

5 cloves garlic, sliced

5 sprigs oregano or 1 tablespoon
dried oregano

4 tablespoons olive oil

juice of 1 lemon

sea salt and freshly ground
black pepper

1 onion, cut into wedges

4 tablespoons Homemade Beef Stock
(page 42) or water

3–4 tablespoons arrowroot (for
gluten-free and paleo) or cornflour,
mixed to a paste with cold water

Make about twenty 1 cm deep cuts all over the lamb shoulder and place in the
slow-cooker insert. Poke the garlic and oregano into the slits and rub the lot with
the olive oil, lemon juice, and salt and pepper. ⟵

Put the onion in the slow-cooker insert and plonk the lamb on top. Pour over
the stock, then cover and cook on low for 8–9 hours, or high for 4–5 hours.

*Feel free to
marinate it for
a few hours or
overnight.*

Remove the meat, cover and leave to rest before shredding (see below).
Meanwhile, make a chunky gravy from the juices and onion by adding the flour
slurry to the insert. Stir it well, leave the lid off and cook on high for 20 minutes
or until the sauce thickens into a gravy. Serve as a salad (see right) with the gravy
on the side.

SHREDDED LAMB

When the meat has cooled, place in a bowl and shred with two forks.
Divide leftovers into ½ cup (65 g) portions and freeze for up to 3 months.

*You could marinate
your lamb in the
same dish to save
washing up.* ⟶

MAKE IT IN THE OVEN:
Preheat the oven to 200°C (gas 6). Heat
a dash of oil in a large, deep ovenproof
dish on the stovetop over a medium–
high heat. Add the marinated lamb and
sear for 5 minutes on each side. Add the
onion, half the stock and any marinade
juices and cover with foil. Place in the
oven, reduce the heat to 160°C (gas 3)
and cook, covered, for 3–4 hours until
the meat falls away from the bone.
Remove the meat and make the gravy
with the remaining stock.

**Eating meat on the bone
(and with the skin)**
This will provide your body with
the amino acid glycine, which
neutralises the methionine
in muscle meat – the bit that
gives meat-eating its bad
carcinogenic rap.

GREEK LAMB SALAD

SERVES 6

1 bunch Massaged Kale (page 23)
or 6 cups (300 g) baby spinach leaves

⅓ cup (50 g) kalamata olives

100 g feta, cubed

½ red onion, finely chopped

250 g cherry tomatoes, halved

⅓ cup (75 ml) olive oil

2 tablespoons lemon juice

sea salt and freshly ground black pepper

3 cups (500 g) Shredded Lamb (see left)

full-fat organic plain yoghurt
or Quick Courgette Tzatziki (page 188), to serve

Combine all of the ingredients in a large bowl.
Toss gently and top with the yoghurt or tzatziki.

PERSIAN LAMB SALAD

SERVES 6

1 bunch watercress

3 cups (350 g) green beans, steamed
(or blanched)

½ cup (20 g) mint leaves

seeds from ½–1 pomegranate

4 tablespoons pistachios

3 cups (500 g) Shredded Lamb (see left)

DRESSING

1 cup (200 g) full-fat plain organic yoghurt

3 tablespoons lemon juice

1 tablespoon tahini

½ teaspoon rice malt syrup
or a tiny pinch of granulated stevia

½ teaspoon ground cumin

To make the dressing, combine the ingredients in a
small bowl and mix well. Toss the watercress, beans,
mint leaves, pomegranate seeds, pistachios and lamb
in a large serving bowl. Dollop the dressing on top.

1½ SERVES VEG + FRUIT PER SERVE

1½ SERVES VEG + FRUIT PER SERVE

JERK PORK SHOULDER ROAST *plus Pulled Pork* ↓

SERVES 6 + LEFTOVER PULLED PORK

A full Caribbean meal with all the trimmings in one fell swoop. I like to make this one in the oven (see below).

1.7–2 kg pork shoulder, bone in, fat trimmed

400 g pumpkin or squash, cut into small wedges (roughly the size of the onion quarters), skin on

2 red onions, quartered

2 large peppers (red, yellow or green), seeds removed, cut into eighths

mint or oregano leaves, to garnish

steamed green beans or okra, to serve

Cooked Quinoa (page 26) or Cooked Buckwheat (page 27), to serve

JERK MARINADE

1 tablespoon ground allspice

2 teaspoons ground nutmeg

1 small red chilli, roughly chopped

6 spring onions, roughly chopped

4–5 sprigs thyme, leaves picked, or 1 tablespoon dried thyme

1/3 cup (75 ml) apple cider vinegar

4 cloves garlic, peeled

3 tablespoons rice malt syrup

3 tablespoons olive oil

good pinch of sea salt

freshly ground black pepper

juice of 3 limes

For the marinade, place all of the ingredients in a small blender or food processor and blitz until combined (or grind them to a paste using a large mortar and pestle).

Make about ten 1 cm deep cuts all over the pork shoulder and place in the slow-cooker insert. Pour over three-quarters of the marinade and massage into the pork, ensuring it gets into the cuts. Cover and place in the fridge for at least 2 hours (preferably overnight).

Toss the pumpkin, onions and peppers in a large bowl with the remaining marinade. Cover and place in the fridge – also for 2 hours (or overnight).

Cook the pork for 7 hours on low or 4 hours on high. Lift the pork out of the slow cooker, place the vegetables in, then turn the pork over and place it on top of the veggies. Cover and continue cooking on high for 2 hours, or until the meat falls away from the bone.

Remove the pork and shred (see below). Return half of the meat to the slow cooker and mix it in with the vegetables. Serve with mint or oregano leaves, green beans or okra and a side of cooked quinoa or cooked buckwheat.

← *I like to toss a few Activated Groaties (page 27) over the top.*

PULLED PORK

Place the pork in a bowl and, using two forks, shred ('pull') the meat, discarding the bone. Divide any leftover meat into 1/2 cup (65 g) portions and freeze for up to 3 months.

MAKE IT IN THE OVEN:
Preheat the oven to 200°C (gas 6). Place the marinated pork in a baking dish and cover with foil. Place in the oven, reduce the heat to 160°C (gas 3) and cook for 3–4 hours until the meat falls away from the bone. In the last 30–40 minutes, scatter the marinated vegetables in another baking dish and bake until done (feel free to pop the pumpkin in earlier to cook a little longer than the other veggies).

 ¾ TSP ADDED SUGAR PER SERVE

2 SERVES VEG + FRUIT PER SERVE

COFFEE AND CACAO-CURED PULLED BEEF

This 'roast' will leave you with some smokin' Texan brisket to play with.
Use it in salads, sandwiches, tacos and so on. To eat as a meal, serve
with a medley of sides (see below).

1.8–2 kg beef brisket

SPICE RUB

3 tablespoons finely ground dark roast instant coffee

3 tablespoons rice malt syrup

2 tablespoons raw cacao powder

1 tablespoon sweet smoked paprika

1 tablespoon garlic powder

2 teaspoons ground cumin

2 teaspoons chilli powder

2 teaspoons sea salt

Place the brisket in the base of the slow-cooker insert. Combine the spice-rub ingredients and pour over the top. Massage into the beef, ensuring every part is coated. Cover and refrigerate for at least 2 hours (preferably overnight).

Cook the brisket on low for 9 hours or high for 5 hours, or until the meat is tender. Shred the brisket (see below). Serve with your choice of Easy Slaw (page 200), Blaukraut (page 182), Crunchy Broccoli Buckwheat Tabbouli (page 187) and/or some sliced avocado.

PULLED BEEF

Place the brisket in a bowl and shred ('pull') with two forks. Divide leftover meat into ½ cup (65 g) portions and freeze for up to 3 months.

¾ TSP ADDED SUGAR PER SERVE

£1.57 PER SERVE

SWEET PERSIAN TAGINE
and Shredded Lamb or Pulled Pork !

SERVES 6 + LEFTOVER SHREDDED LAMB OR PULLED PORK

This is a great all-in-one meal for the cooler months, or if you're a Vata type. Again, we cook up extra meat to freeze and use later.

2 kg lamb or pork shoulder, bone in

2 tablespoons Ras el Hanout Mix (page 45) or 2 teaspoons each of sweet paprika, ground cumin and ground cinnamon

2 teaspoons ground turmeric

2 teaspoons ground ginger

pinch of granulated stevia (optional)

1 cup (170 g) dried chickpeas

1 onion, thinly sliced

½ can (200 g) diced tomatoes

1 kg sweet potato or carrots, chopped into 3 cm chunks

1 cup (250 ml) Homemade Stock (page 42) or water

1 tablespoon harissa paste

2 handfuls of green beans, halved

4 apricots, quartered and stones removed

2 tablespoons lemon zest or 4 tablespoons chopped leftover lemon from Lemon and Turmeric Tonic-ade (page 347)

½ cup (75 g) pitted green or black olives

TO SERVE

mint leaves, torn

⅓ cup (50 g) whole blanched almonds

Moroccan Cauliflower, Chickpea and Quinoa Bake (page 238)

Place the lamb or pork in a slow-cooker insert. Sprinkle over the spices and stevia and rub into the meat, making sure it is well coated. Cover and leave overnight in the fridge. Place the chickpeas in a bowl with plenty of water and leave overnight on the worktop.

Drain and rinse the chickpeas and add to the slow-cooker insert with the onion, tomatoes, sweet potato or carrot, stock or water and harissa paste. Cover and cook on low for 8 hours or high for 5 hours.

Forty-five minutes before serving, remove half of the lamb or pork, then shred (see below). Add the green beans, apricots, lemon and olives to the slow cooker and cook for 30 minutes or until the apricots have softened. Serve topped with mint leaves and almonds, with a side of Moroccan Cauliflower, Chickpea and Quinoa Bake.

SHREDDED LAMB OR PULLED PORK

Transfer the lamb or pork to a large bowl and shred the meat with two forks, discarding the bone. Return half to the cooker and divide the remaining lamb or pork into ½ cup (65 g) portions and freeze for up to 3 months.

3 SERVES VEG + FRUIT PER SERVE

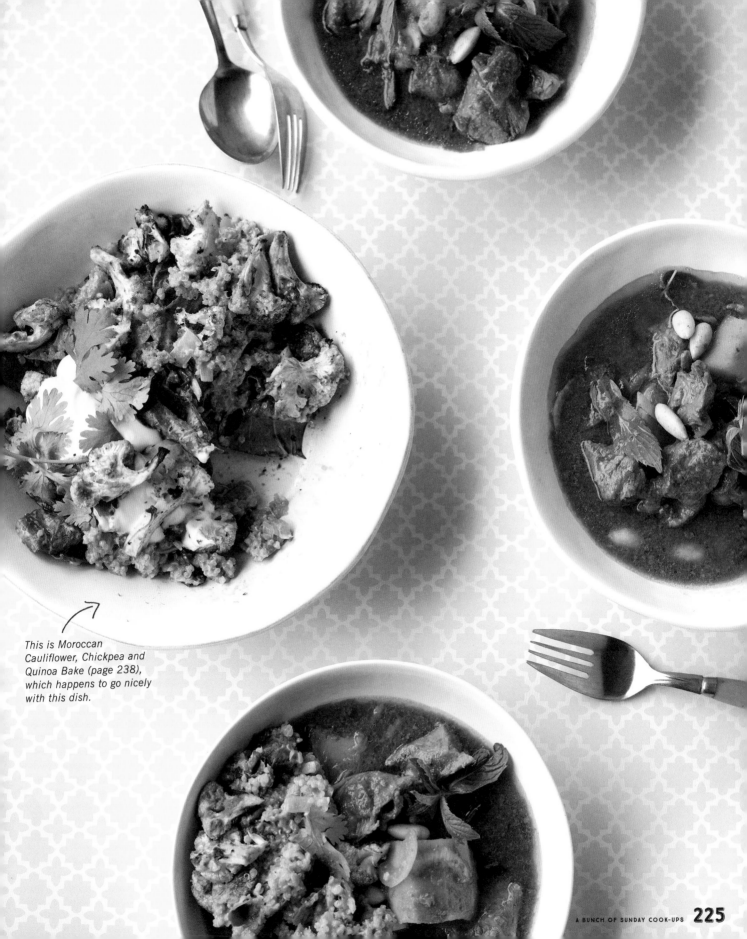

This is Moroccan
Cauliflower, Chickpea and
Quinoa Bake (page 238),
which happens to go nicely
with this dish.

MIDWEEK
ONE-PAN
WONDERS

Very fun, complete meals made using [one] pot,
Dinner done.
[one] baking sheet, or [one] skillet.

TRAY-DINNER-FOR-TWO AUBERGINE PARMIGIANA

SERVES 2

2 aubergines, each cut into 5 rounds

¼ teaspoon sea salt

200 g ball fresh buffalo mozzarella, sliced

1½ cups (350 ml) Nomato Sauce (page 51) or sugar-free tomato passata

½ cup (50 g) grated parmesan

1 bunch tenderstem broccoli (or 1 small head broccoli, cut into florets)

Preheat the oven to 200ºC (gas 6) and line a baking tray with baking paper.

Lightly season the aubergine with salt and place on the tray in a single layer. Bake for 15 minutes or until the aubergine is beginning to turn golden brown. Remove from the oven. Select the two largest aubergine slices and turn them over. Layer with some mozzarella, Nomato Sauce and parmesan. Take the two next-largest slices and repeat the layering, finishing with the sauce and a sprinkle of parmesan. Arrange the broccoli around the stacks. Return to the oven and bake for 20 minutes or until the cheese is melted and golden.

MAKE IT MEATY:
Add a cooked Basic Meatball or two (page 144), squashed, between the layers.

4 SERVES VEG + FRUIT PER SERVE

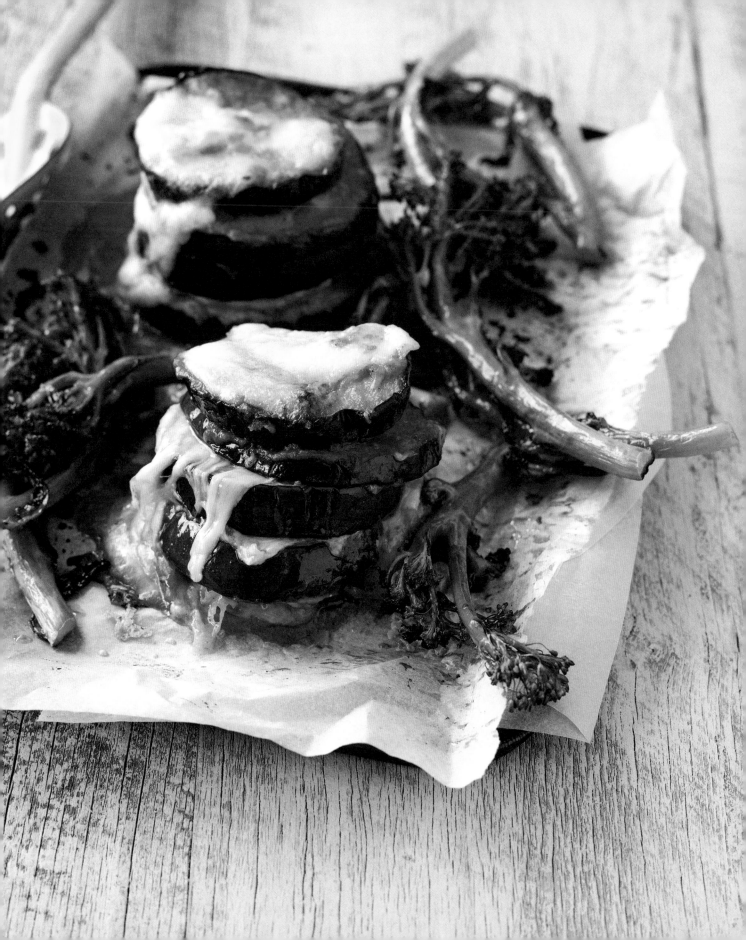

SWEET POTATO NACHOS

1 large sweet potato or 2 small
(about 250 g), halved lengthways

1 cup (130 g) Pulled Pork (page 222), or
Shredded Chicken (page 214)
or (250 ml) Cooked Beans (page 28)

¼ teaspoon sweet paprika

¼ teaspoon ground cumin

½ avocado, chopped

1 lime, halved

1 long red chilli, sliced

50 g cheddar, grated

1 small red onion, thinly sliced

1 corn cob, cut into 6 pieces

6 cherry tomatoes

250 g packet coleslaw mix
or ¼ red cabbage, grated
(or a handful of green beans)

olive oil, for drizzling

sour cream or yoghurt, to serve

coriander leaves, to serve

corn chips or Sweet Potato Skins
(page 23), to serve

Preheat the oven to 200°C (gas 6). Line a baking tray with baking paper. Place the sweet spuds cut-side up on the tray and bake for 1 hour or until soft.

Meanwhile, in a small bowl combine the meat or beans, spices and avocado with a squeeze of lime juice. Mix well.

Remove the spuds from the oven and crank the heat up to 220°C (gas 7). Scoop out some of the flesh from the centre of the potato (reserve for Sweet Potato Purée; page 23) and fill with the avocado mixture. Sprinkle over the chilli and top with the cheddar. Arrange the onion, corn, tomatoes and coleslaw (or cabbage or beans) on the tray and drizzle over plenty of olive oil. Return the tray to the oven and bake for 10–15 minutes until everything is golden.

To serve, dollop with sour cream or yoghurt, sprinkle over the coriander and toss over the corn chips or Sweet Potato Skins.

4 SERVES VEG + FRUIT PER SERVE

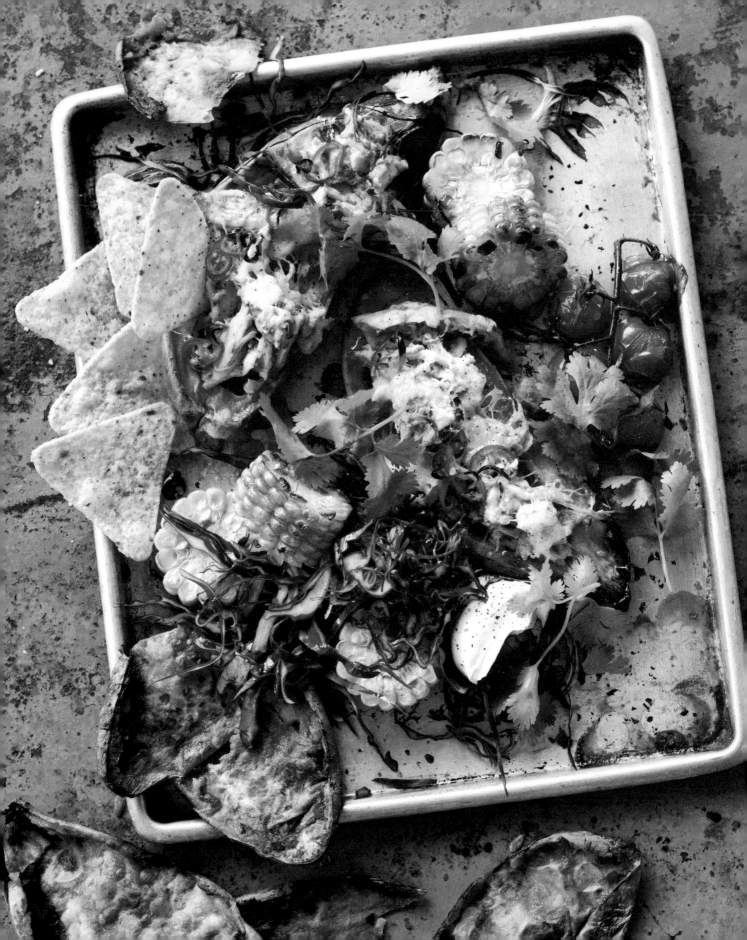

CRUNCHY CHICKEN
SATAY IN A PAN

½ cup (115 g) crunchy natural peanut butter

1 tablespoon coconut oil, melted

3 tablespoons tamari

1 teaspoon chilli flakes

1 clove garlic, finely chopped

2 cm knob of ginger, finely chopped

6 chicken thighs or drumsticks (or a combo)

300 g sugar snap peas, trimmed

1 bunch asparagus, ends snapped, spears halved

2 spring onions, thinly sliced

4 tablespoons peanuts

1 lime, cut into wedges

3 tablespoons white sesame seeds

Preheat the oven to 200°C (gas 6). Combine the peanut butter, coconut oil, tamari, chilli, garlic and ginger in a baking dish and mix well. Add the chicken and chuck around to coat. Place in the oven and bake for 15 minutes.

Remove from the oven and artfully arrange the green veggies, spring onions, peanuts, lime wedges and sesame seeds around and over the chook. Return to the oven and cook for a further 10 minutes, or until the chicken is brown and lush.

1 SERVE VEG + FRUIT PER SERVE

£2 PER SERVE

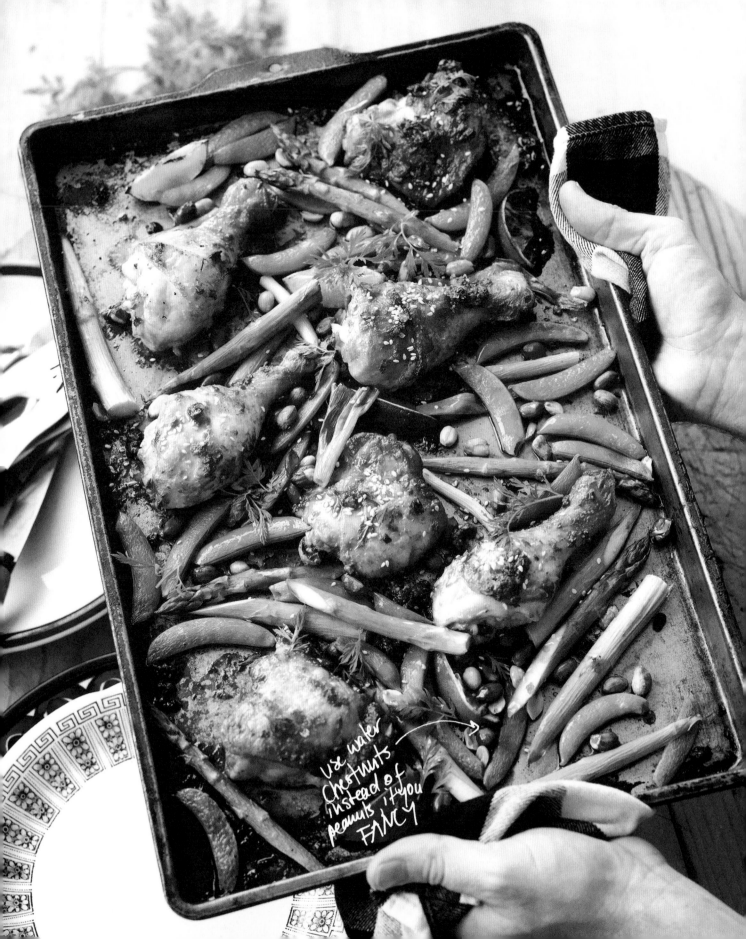

use water chestnuts instead of peanuts if you FANCY

MY RECALIBRATING
PORK MEAL

SERVES 2

When I've been travelling or eating a little too much sugar (you heard right) or I'm just a breathing picture of average-ness (autoimmune inflammation and the like), this is the meal I turn to, generally with a dignified glass of preservative-free red wine.

Go for free-range (outdoor-reared) organic pork to ensure they're not fed recycled food waste (which risks bacterial contamination).

Why get pork on your fork?

My work with *National Geographic*'s Blue Zones longevity team revealed that pork is one of the foods common to all of the Blue Zones (regions and countries boasting the most centenarians). One Japanese study has suggested that the link between eating pork and longevity may have something to do with the fact that pigs are genetically similar to humans and that there may be something in pork protein that helps repair arterial damage. An interesting hypothesis only.

Sustainable cheap cuts:

Where possible, choose pork shoulder chops (also known as blade chops, blade steak, pork shoulder steaks, pork shoulder blade steaks).

2 bone-in pork chops, each about 2 cm thick (about 400 g in total)

1 sweet potato, cut in half lengthways and sliced into rounds (8 mm thick)

sea salt and freshly ground black pepper

2 teaspoons coconut oil

1 fennel, sliced lengthways into 8 wedges (the whole lot including stems and fronds)

1 bunch asparagus, ends snapped, spears halved

1 firm peach or apple, cut into eighths

1 teaspoon chopped sage, rosemary or thyme

3 tablespoons apple cider vinegar or sauerkraut brine (page 337)

big splash of Homemade Chicken Stock (page 42) or 2–3 frozen stock cubes (page 25)

1 teaspoon Dijon mustard

Preheat the oven to 210°C (gas 6). Season the pork and sweet potato with salt and pepper. Heat the coconut oil in an ovenproof skillet over a medium–high heat. Brown the chops and sweet potato, turning once (about 3 minutes each side). Lift the chops out briefly, adding the fennel, asparagus, peach or apple, and herbs to the pan. Stir to combine, then return the chops to the pan, placing them on top of the veggies, fruit and herbs. Mix the vinegar, stock and mustard together and pour over the lot. Place in the oven and cook for 15 minutes.

MAKE IT SERVE 6:

After sealing 6 chops in the skillet, transfer to a large baking dish with triple the amount of each of the remaining ingredients and cook the lot for 20 minutes.

MAKE IT IN A FRYING PAN:

Alternatively, you can cook the lot in your pan – simply cover with a lid or plate and simmer for 10 minutes.

2½ SERVES VEG + FRUIT PER SERVE

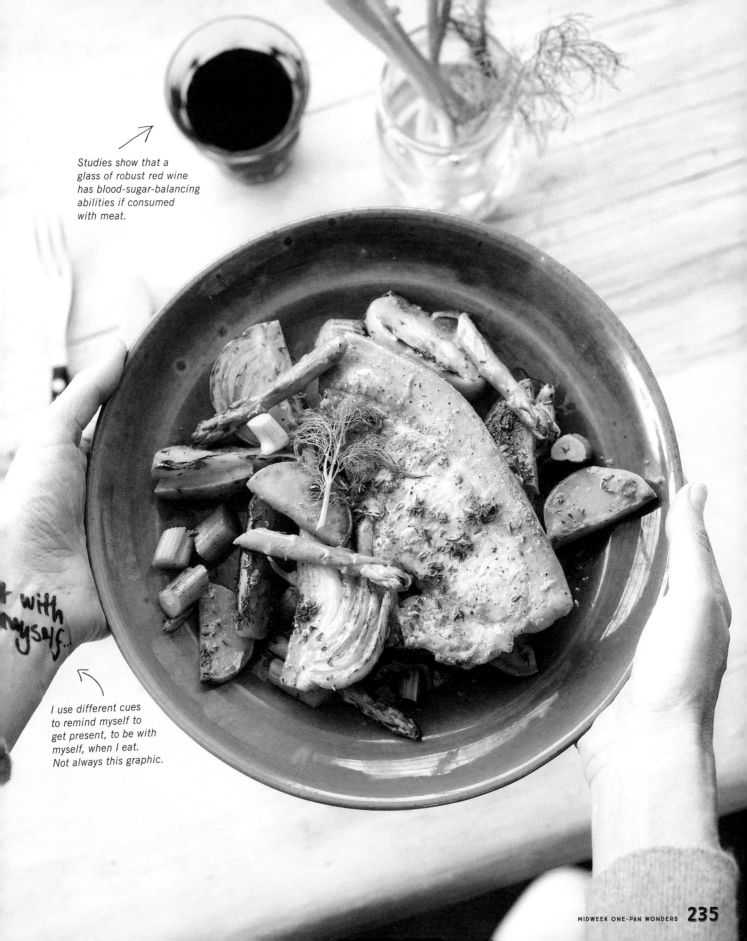

Studies show that a glass of robust red wine has blood-sugar-balancing abilities if consumed with meat.

I use different cues to remind myself to get present, to be with myself, when I eat. Not always this graphic.

SLOW-COOKER APPLE CIDER CHICKEN

SERVES 6

1 kg chicken thighs
(skin left on, bones intact)

2–3 cloves garlic, crushed

2 spring onions, thinly sliced

2 bay leaves

4 tablespoons tamari or soy sauce

4 tablespoons apple cider vinegar

juice of ½ lemon

1 cup (225 g) quinoa, rinsed twice

1½ cups (350 ml) Homemade Chicken Stock (page 42)

2–3 bunches baby pak choi
(or 4 cups (400 g) any Oriental greens)

If the chicken has started to fall off the bone (nice!) feel free to shred it, discarding the bones, before returning it to the slow cooker. →

Place the chicken in the base of a slow-cooker insert. Add the garlic, spring onions, bay leaves, tamari or soy sauce, vinegar and lemon juice, and toss to coat the chicken. Cover and cook on low for 5½ hours or high for 2½ hours. Remove the chicken from the slow cooker and set aside.

Add the quinoa and stock to the slow-cooker insert and stir. Cover and cook on high for 40 minutes, or until the quinoa is cooked (it should have 'tails' sprouting). Return the chicken to the slow cooker. Add the greens, then cover and cook for a further 20 minutes or until tender. To serve, arrange the greens on serving plates. Stir the quinoa and chicken, and spoon over the greens.

1 SERVE VEG + FRUIT PER SERVE

£1.76 PER SERVE

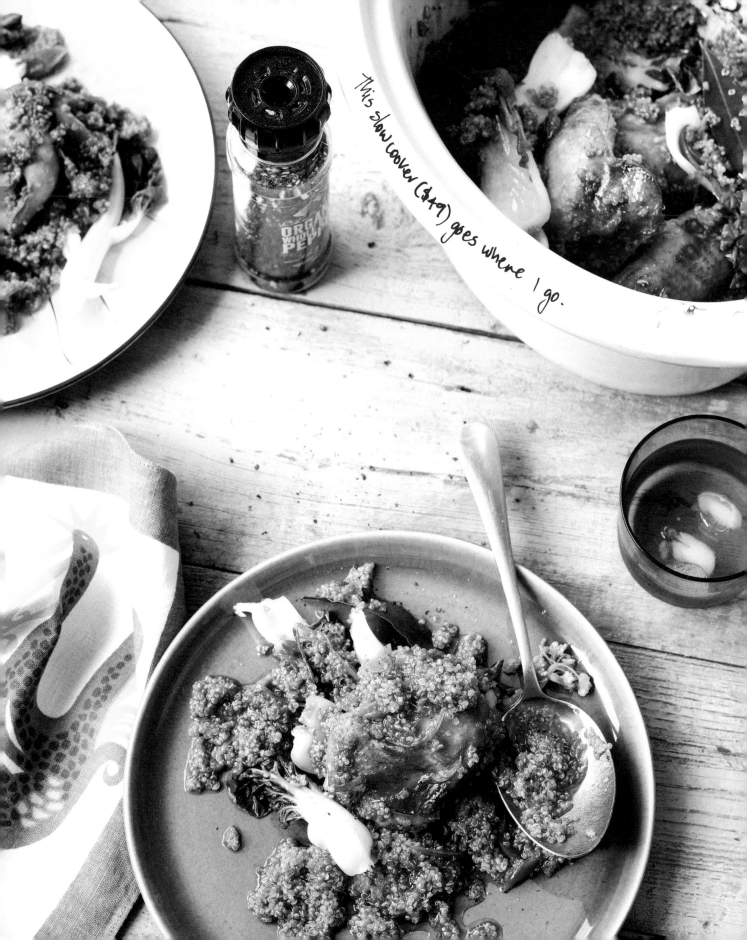

This slow cooker ($49) goes where I go.

MOROCCAN CAULIFLOWER, CHICKPEA AND QUINOA BAKE

SERVES 6

This one is pictured on page 225.

1 head cauliflower, chopped into florets

1 onion, finely diced

2 cups (270 g) Cooked Quinoa (page 26)

2 cups (325 g) cooked chickpeas (page 28) or 400 g can chickpeas, drained and rinsed

½ cup (75 g) almonds, chopped (optional)

2 teaspoons curry powder

1 teaspoon ground turmeric

2 teaspoons ground cumin

sea salt and freshly ground black pepper

juice of 2 lemons

¼ cup (50 g) coconut oil, melted

⅔ cup (130 g) full-fat organic plain yoghurt, mixed with a big pinch of ground cumin

coriander or flat-leaf parsley leaves, to serve

Preheat the oven to 180°C (gas 4). Combine all of the ingredients except the yoghurt in a large baking dish and toss well until the cauliflower is evenly coated in spices and coconut oil. Roast for 20 minutes or until the cauliflower is crispy and brown on top.

Remove from the oven and serve with a dollop of cumin yoghurt and a sprinkle of coriander or parsley leaves.

MAKE IT A MOROCCAN CHICKEN AND CAULIFLOWER BAKE:
Omit the chickpeas and replace with 2 cups (250 g) of Shredded Chicken (page 214).

 1½ SERVES VEG + FRUIT PER SERVE

 £0.92 PER SERVE

STEAK 'N' FIVE VEG

SERVES 2

This recipe works equally well with lamb chops, pork chops or even sausages.

If brussels sprouts aren't in season, use 1 cup (150 g) coarsely chopped broccoli or cauliflower florets.

Know your sustainable steak

Inside skirt steak (called hanger steak in the US or butcher's steak 'cos butchers liked to keep it for themselves) is from the diaphragm and is a relatively tender piece of meat on its own. (None of these muscles get much of a workout!) It is best cooked in a cast-iron skillet or grilled until medium–rare.

Oyster blade or butler's steak (called flat iron steak in the US) is a flat muscle off the shoulder blade. It's super-tender considering it's so close to a joint. Also best cooked in a cast-iron skillet or grilled.

1 sweet potato

1 parsnip

40 g coconut oil, melted

sea salt and freshly ground black pepper

2 × 150 g sustainable beef steaks

1 small red onion, thinly sliced

1 small clove garlic, crushed

8 brussels sprouts, trimmed and thinly sliced

1 cup (100 g) thinly sliced red cabbage

1 cup (100 g) thinly sliced kale or Swiss chard

juice of 1 lemon

pinch of chilli flakes

Preheat the grill to medium–high and place the rack about 15 cm below the element. Using a vegetable peeler, slice the sweet potato and parsnip lengthways into ribbons and place on a baking tray. Toss with half the coconut oil and a sprinkle of salt. Season the steak and place on top.

In a separate bowl, toss the onion, garlic, brussels sprouts, cabbage and kale or chard in the rest of the coconut oil, the lemon juice and chilli until well coated. Add to the baking tray, around the steaks, and grill for 1–2 minutes. Remove from the heat, turn the steaks and veggies and grill for a further 1–2 minutes, or until the steaks are browned.

Remove the meat and let it sit, covered, for 5–10 minutes. Meanwhile, continue to grill the veggies until they are cooked through. Serve immediately.

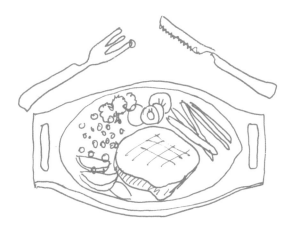

4½ SERVES VEG + FRUIT PER SERVE

LAMB ROAST
FOR TWO

WITH MINTED PEA PISTOU

SERVES 2

Which lamb chops are best?
From a planetary and hip-pocket perspective, go for leg/forequarter (chump chops) over loin chops. Lamb breast can also be used.

1 tablespoon olive oil, plus extra for drizzling

2 teaspoons chopped oregano or ½ teaspoon dried oregano

juice of ½ lemon (use the other half for the Minted Pea Pistou, below)

2 small cloves garlic, crushed

4 lamb chops

2 small onions, skin left on, sliced into wedges (not quite right down to the root, waterlily-like) or 1 small red onion, cut into wedges

1 red pepper, cut into chunks

2 small courgettes, sliced into rounds

sea salt and freshly ground black pepper

6 cherry tomatoes

¼ cup (40 g) olives

¼ cup (60 g) cubed feta

TO SERVE

Minted Pea Pistou (optional; see below)

mint or oregano leaves

Preheat the oven to 200°C (gas 6).

Combine the oil, oregano, lemon juice, garlic and lamb in a bowl. Cover and refrigerate for at least 25 minutes (all day is fab).

Place the onion, pepper and courgette in a large baking dish with a good drizzle of olive oil and season with salt and pepper. Bake for 25 minutes.

Add the lamb, cherry tomatoes, olives and feta to the baking dish and cook for another 20 minutes, turning the chops after 10 minutes. Serve with Minted Pea Pistou (if using) and a sprinkling of mint or oregano leaves.

MINTED PEA PISTOU

½ cup (75 g) frozen peas, blanched in some boiling water and cooled

½ cup (20 g) mint leaves

zest and juice of ½ lemon

4 tablespoons extra-virgin olive oil

Combine all the ingredients in a blender or food processor and whizz until smooth.

Or simply blend ½ cup (125 ml) Leftovers Pesto (page 55) with the peas.

2 SERVES VEG + FRUIT PER SERVE

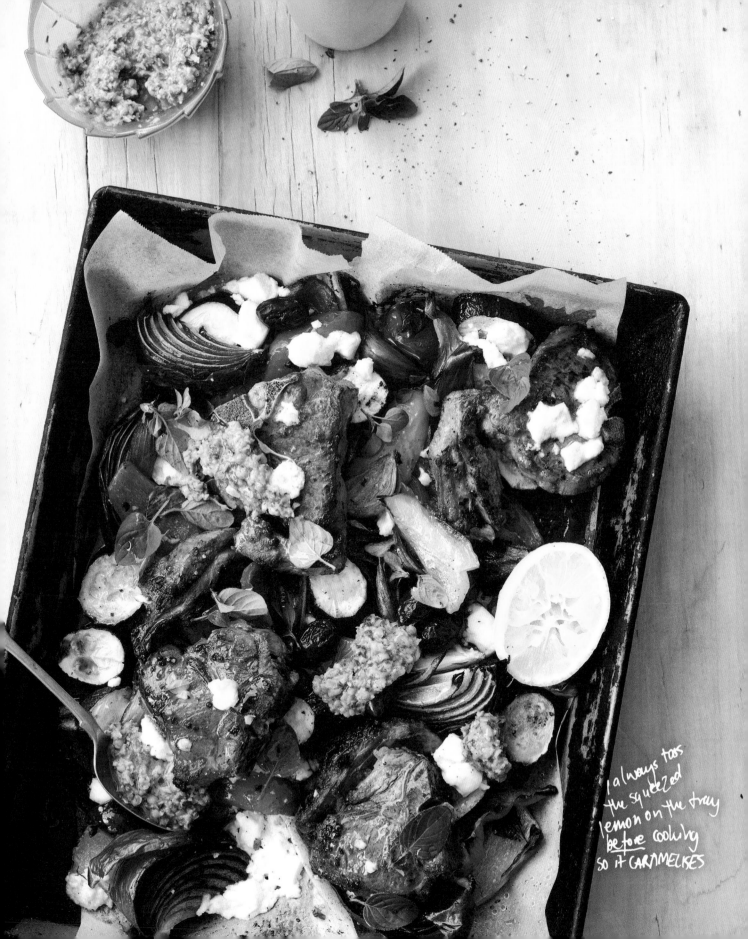

I always toss
the squeezed
lemon on the tray
before cooking
so it CARAMELISES

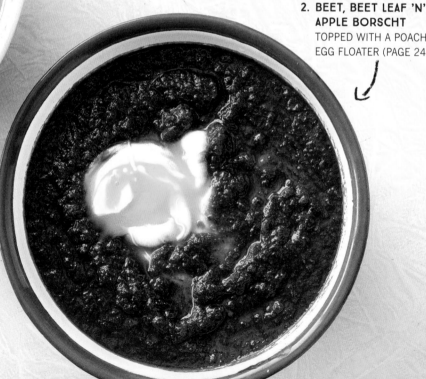

1. **PARSNIP, PEAR 'N' THYME SOUP**
   TOPPED WITH HALOUMI CRISPS (PAGE 245)

A "ROOT 'N' A SHRUB" SOUPS

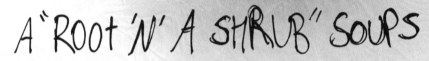

In which I pimp my 'Grounding Roots Soup',
three ways, using a root veggie + blending
it with some lovely herbaciousness

2. **BEET, BEET LEAF 'N' APPLE BORSCHT**
   TOPPED WITH A POACHED EGG FLOATER (PAGE 245)

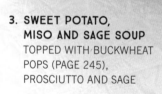

3. **SWEET POTATO, MISO AND SAGE SOUP**
   TOPPED WITH BUCKWHEAT POPS (PAGE 245), PROSCIUTTO AND SAGE

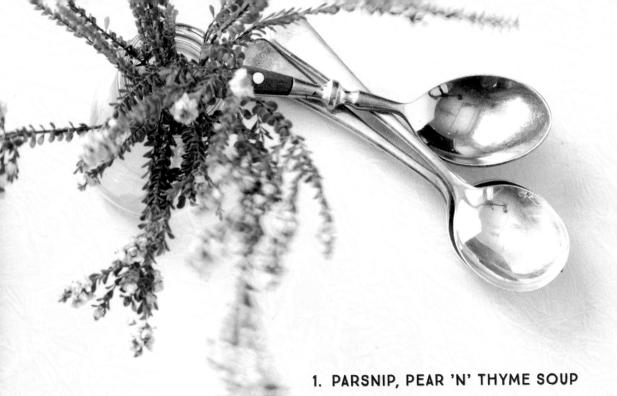

1. PARSNIP, PEAR 'N' THYME SOUP

SERVES 6

3 tablespoons coconut oil, olive oil, butter or ghee

2 onions, diced

4 large parsnips, roughly chopped

2 small pears, peeled, cored and roughly chopped

1 teaspoon sea salt

freshly ground black pepper

1.5 litres Homemade Stock (a veggie variation; page 42)

4 sprigs thyme, leaves picked, plus extra sprigs to serve

cream or full-fat organic plain yoghurt, to serve

Heat the oil, butter or ghee in a large saucepan over a medium–high heat. Add the onion and cook gently for 8–10 minutes, until soft and translucent. Add the remaining ingredients and bring to the boil. Reduce the heat and simmer for about 20 minutes or until all of the vegetables are cooked through. Pour the soup into a blender and blitz to a purée. Serve with extra thyme sprigs and a dollop of cream or yoghurt.

1 SERVE VEG + FRUIT PER SERVE

£0.83 PER SERVE

recipes continue ....

2. BEET, BEET LEAF 'N' APPLE BORSCHT

SERVES 6

1 tablespoon butter or ghee

3 cloves garlic, finely chopped

1 large onion, roughly chopped

1 celery stalk, roughly chopped

1 carrot, roughly chopped

1 bunch beetroot (about 800 g), trimmed, scrubbed and cubed, leaves finely chopped

2 apples, peeled, cored and cut into large cubes

1.5 litres Homemade Stock (a veggie variation; page 42)

sea salt and freshly ground black pepper

full-fat organic plain yoghurt or Homemade Cream Cheese (page 46), to serve

Heat the butter or ghee in a flameproof casserole dish or large saucepan over a low heat. Add the garlic, onion, celery and carrot and cook for 15 minutes or until the vegetables have softened. Add the beetroot, chopped beet leaves and apple to the pan and cook for 5 minutes more, stirring to soften slightly. Add the stock and season to taste with salt and pepper. Cover and simmer for 45 minutes or until everything is tender. Serve the soup chunky, or cool it slightly and purée it in a blender. Spoon into bowls and top with a swirl of yoghurt or a dollop of cream cheese.

MAKE IT SUMMER PROBIOTIC BEET SOUP:

Use 1 cup (250 ml) stock only. Once cooked, allow to cool and add 2 peeled and chopped cucumbers, ½ cup (125 ml) sauerkraut brine (page 337) or Grounding Crimson Tonic (page 347) and ½ cup (100 g) yoghurt. Stir or purée and chill for 4 hours or overnight.

3. SWEET POTATO, MISO AND SAGE SOUP

SERVES 6

1 tablespoon coconut oil

2 onions, roughly chopped

2 cloves garlic, finely chopped

3 medium–large sweet potatoes, peeled and roughly chopped

3 tablespoons red miso paste

1.5 litres Homemade Stock (a veggie variation; page 42)

3 tablespoons chopped sage leaves

sea salt and freshly ground pepper

Caesar Salad Boats (opposite), to serve

Feel free to throw in any orange or white–hued roast veggies you have lying around to fill out the soup.

Heat the coconut oil in a flameproof casserole dish or large saucepan over a low heat. Add the onion and garlic and sauté for 5 minutes. Add the sweet potato and continue cooking until slightly softened, then add the miso paste. Pour over the stock and bring to the boil. Cover, then reduce the heat and cook for 20 minutes or until the sweet potato is cooked through. Season to taste. Allow the soup to cool slightly, then blend in batches to your desired consistency. Serve with Caesar Salad Boats.

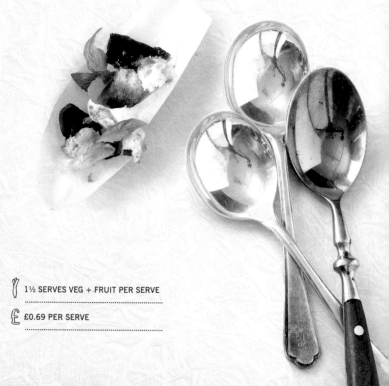

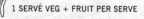 1 SERVÉ VEG + FRUIT PER SERVE

£0.46 PER SERVE

1½ SERVES VEG + FRUIT PER SERVE

£0.69 PER SERVE

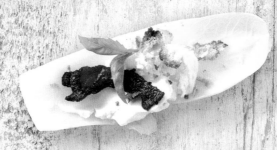
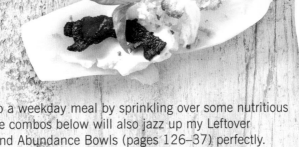
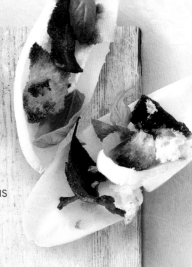

A PAGE OF SOUP TOPPERS

A soup can easily be turned into a weekday meal by sprinkling over some nutritious and filling fairy dust. Most of the combos below will also jazz up my Leftover Mishmashes (pages 246–65) and Abundance Bowls (pages 126–37) perfectly.

BUCKWHEAT POPS

Toast 1 cup (170 g) of Activated Groaties (page 27) in 1 teaspoon of coconut or olive oil over a medium heat. Sprinkle with salt, pepper, chilli flakes, garam masala or ground cumin, to taste.

BONE MARROW BOMBS

This idea comes directly from my mate Matt Preston. (I asked first!)

12 × 5 cm lengths of bone marrow, removed from the bone (ask your butcher to do this)

lots of cornflour or plain flour, for dusting

40 g butter

To prep the marrow, you'll need to soak it in cold, slightly salty water for 24 hours. Next day, remove the soaked marrow and pat dry. Pour the cornflour or plain flour into a cereal bowl and roll each length of marrow in the flour, coating the whole lot. Melt the butter in a frying pan over a medium heat. When the butter is starting to get foamy, slip four bone marrow 'bombs' into the pan and fry until all sides are crunchy. Repeat with the remaining marrow pieces.

HALOUMI CRISPS

Pan-fry strips of haloumi in a frying pan, or grill them in a sandwich press. Allow to cool, then crumble or break into chunks.

BACON GRANOLA

See page 108.

SWEET POTATO CROUTONS

Cut a scrubbed (not peeled) sweet potato into 1.5 cm cubes and pan-fry in coconut oil in a skillet. Sprinkle with sea salt (this will speed up the cooking time) and a little ground cumin and cinnamon. Cook until dark golden.

POACHED EGG FLOATER

Break an egg or two into a teacup. Bring your soup to a gentle boil in a small saucepan over a medium heat (you'll need the soup to be at least 5 cm deep). Gently tip the egg(s) into the soup, turn off the heat immediately and cover the pan tightly. Leave for 3–4 minutes, or until the eggs are cooked.

HARISSA CREAM CHEESE BOMBS

Swirl 1 tablespoon of harissa paste through 1 cup (225 g) of Homemade Cream Cheese (page 46).

CAESAR SALAD BOATS

Pull apart a head of chicory and line individual leaves with Homemade Cream Cheese (page 46). Top with Bacon Bits (page 44), an anchovy fillet and/or leftover Shredded Chicken (page 214).

MY LEFTOVER
MISHMASHES

Officially my favourite chapter where EVERYTHING I stand for comes ⊳ together⊸ and you find yourself using up all your SCRAPS and dregs and bobs + bits... and dregs and bobs + bits...

and ! He makes a lot more flow-y SENSE.

(Generally with an egg chucked in the middle)

Or with a flurry of carrot tops

GREEN SCRAPS SHAKSHOUKA

LEFTOVER GREENS + LEFTOVERS PESTO + SOME EGGS

SERVES 2

A hipster (kale-ified) version of the classic Israeli bubble 'n' squeak.

1 tablespoon butter

½ onion or leek (or use 3 spring onions), thinly sliced

3 cups (450 g) whatever green vegetables you have (sliced fennel (reserve the fronds), grated courgettes, thinly sliced mangetout and asparagus are all great)

Use a few frozen cubes of courgette (page 24) if you like.

¼ teaspoon ground cumin

¼ teaspoon chilli flakes (or a few drops of Tabasco)

juice of ½ lemon

2 handfuls of leafy greens and herbs (kale, beetroot leaves, spinach, flat-leaf parsley, basil, coriander, fennel fronds etc)

sea salt and freshly ground black pepper

3 tablespoons Leftovers Pesto (page 55)

2–3 eggs

4 tablespoons whatever cheese you have, crumbled or grated

sliced olives, to serve (optional)

Melt the butter in a frying pan over a medium–high heat. Add the onion, leek or spring onions, green vegetables and cumin. Sauté for 5–7 minutes. Add the chilli, lemon juice and leafy greens and herbs and cook until wilted. Season with salt and pepper and blob in the pesto.

Create two or three divots in your mixture and break the eggs in one by one. Reduce the heat to low. Sprinkle with cheese. Cover (with a plate or lid) and cook for about 5–7 minutes, or until the eggs are set. To serve, toss in a few black olives and their brine, if you like.

4 SERVES VEG + FRUIT PER SERVE

£0.58 PER SERVE

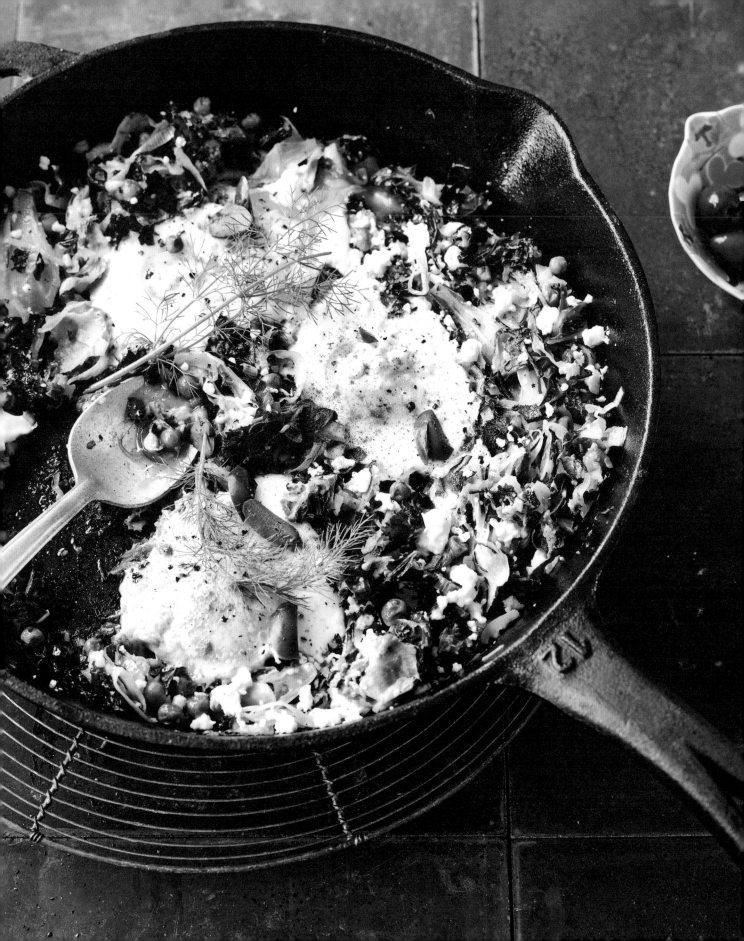

CRISP BIBIMBAP SKILLET PANCAKE

KIMCHI + LEFTOVER SHREDDED MEAT + COOKED QUINOA

SERVES 2

I love this Korean version of bubble 'n' squeak. It's regarded as a winter healing food in Korea and it's all about using leftovers. I've given it a simplicious spin by combining a few steps and abandoning a few pots. Oh, and refashioning the whole lot as a crisp pancake. You're welcome.

If you have a big paella pan, you can triple the recipe to feed the family.

1 tablespoon sesame oil or coconut oil

1 cup (135 g) Cooked Quinoa (page 26)

1 cup (250 ml) 'But the Kitchen Sink' Kimchi (page 337), including a little brine, plus extra to serve (or use 2 cups/200 g shredded leafy greens or cabbage tossed with a big splash of tamari)

3 spring onions, finely chopped

1 tablespoon tamari, soy or fish sauce

2–3 eggs

½ cup (65 g) leftover cooked meat (see any recipe in the Sunday Cook-Ups chapter)

2–3 separate mounds of different coloured cooked or raw vegetables, grated or thinly sliced (carrots, red cabbage, brussels sprouts, squash, courgettes, beans, peas, spinach, bean sprouts etc)

TO SERVE

a generous sprinkle of a crunchy, tasty thing (sesame seeds, dulse flakes, Seaweed Dukkah (page 45) etc)

Simple 'Gochujang' Sauce (see below; optional)

Heat the oil in a frying pan over a medium–high heat. Add the quinoa, kimchi (or greens), spring onions and tamari, soy or fish sauce to the pan, stirring to combine, then press flat with a wooden spoon. Reduce the heat and cook for 5 minutes or until the mixture begins to crisp and caramelise on the base. Crack the eggs on top and swirl to cover. Reduce the heat to low, cover (with a plate or lid) and cook for 4–5 minutes until the eggs are just set. Arrange the meat and coloured veggies on top and heat through.

Remove from the heat and serve with the extra kimchi (or greens, if using), a sprinkling of something crunchy and tasty and some 'gochujang' sauce, if you like.

You can flip the pancake onto a plate before adding the toppings if you want a crunchy vibe.

The egg will spread through the pancake and crisp everything up even further.

SIMPLE 'GOCHUJANG' SAUCE

4 tablespoons Nomato Sauce (page 51)

pinch of chilli flakes or a few drops of Tabasco

½ teaspoon rice malt syrup

Mix in a teacup. Done.

3 SERVES VEG + FRUIT PER SERVE

£0.88 PER SERVE

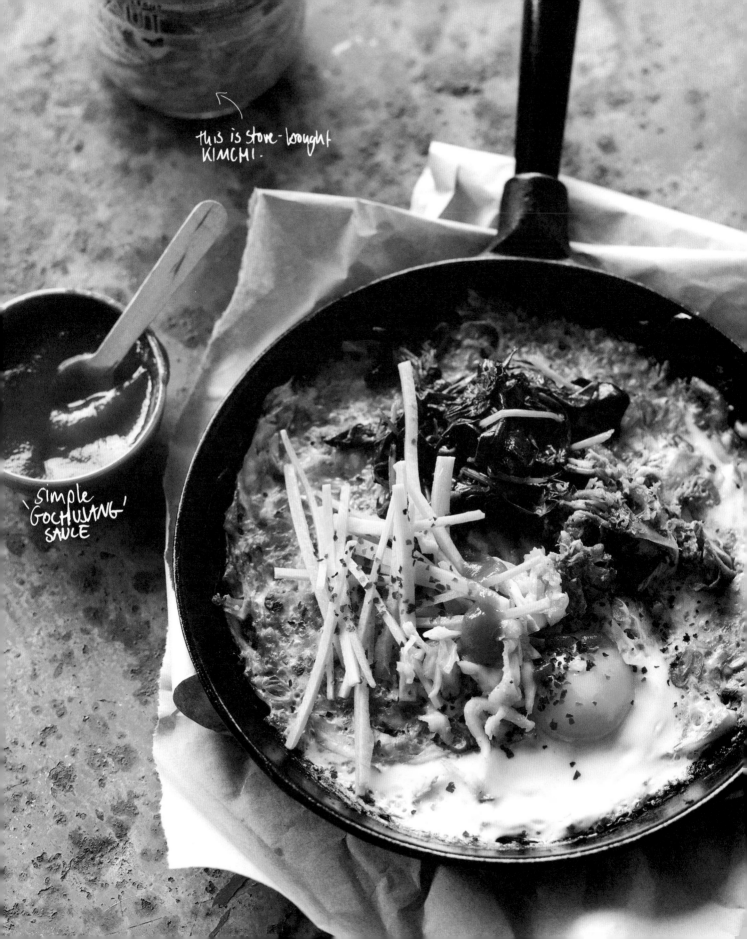

this is store-bought
KIMCHI.

'simple
'GOCHUJANG'
SAUCE

MY SALAD of the SCOUNDREL

SERVES 2

Translated from the French *salade canaille*, this meal is made up of a 'rabble' of bits and pieces, which are given some perk with the addition of fridge-door flavour bombs. Perfectly designed for Sunday-night floor picnics.

PICKLED ROAST VEGGIES

Combine 1–2 cups (150–300 g) of leftover Roasted Roots (page 23) with ½ red onion that's been sliced and soaked in apple cider vinegar for 10 minutes. Sprinkle with celery leaves (optional), a pinch of sea salt and a drizzle of extra-virgin olive oil. Toss.

2 SERVES VEG + FRUIT PER SERVE

GRIBICHE SAUCE PLATE

Finely chop ¼ red onion and mix with 1–2 tablespoons of Whey-Good Mayo (page 50) and 1 teaspoon each of Dijon mustard and chopped capers. Dollop over 1 cup (130 g) of leftover cooked meat (any kind; see Sunday Cook-ups chapter), or 2–3 hard-boiled eggs, diced. Garnish with celery leaves.

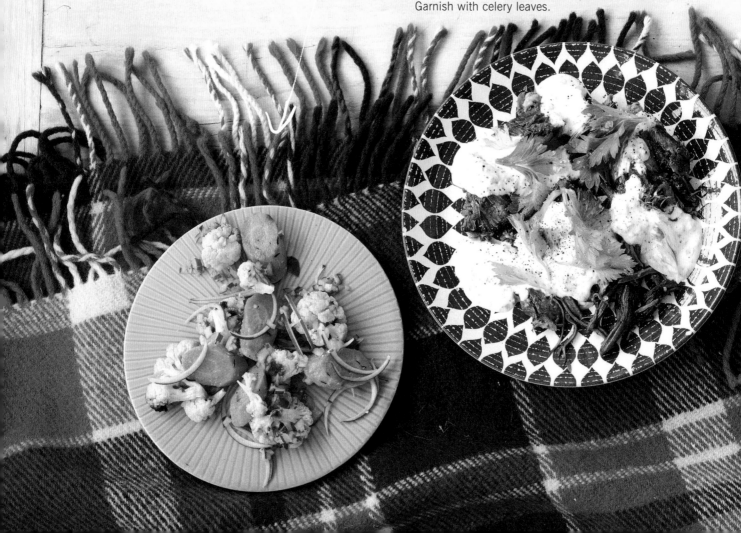

GOLDEN PORRIDGE WEDGES

Combine 2 cups (about 250 g) of leftover porridge, rice, lentils or Cooked Quinoa (page 26) with ⅓ cup (35 g) grated parmesan and 1 tablespoon of chopped thyme, chives or other fresh herbs. If your mixture is a bit soggy, add 1 teaspoon of chia seeds. Line a plate with baking paper. Scoop the porridge onto the plate and press it into a 'pancake' the size of your frying pan. Transfer it to the fridge for 30 minutes to firm. Heat 2 tablespoons of butter in your pan and fry the porridge cake on both sides until golden.

PINK DEVILISH GOOGIE EGGS

Marinate 12 peeled, hard-boiled eggs in 1½ cups (350 ml) of leftover pink ferment brine (page 337) for at least 2 hours (or overnight) in the fridge. Pat the eggs dry and slice in half lengthways. If you like, remove the yolks and mash with 1 tablespoon of Whey-Good Mayo (page 50), then spoon the mixture back in and sprinkle with curry powder.

If you don't have pink brine, slice 1 old beetroot and boil it in 1 cup (250 ml) water and ½ cup (125 ml) white vinegar for 20 minutes. Strain and cool.

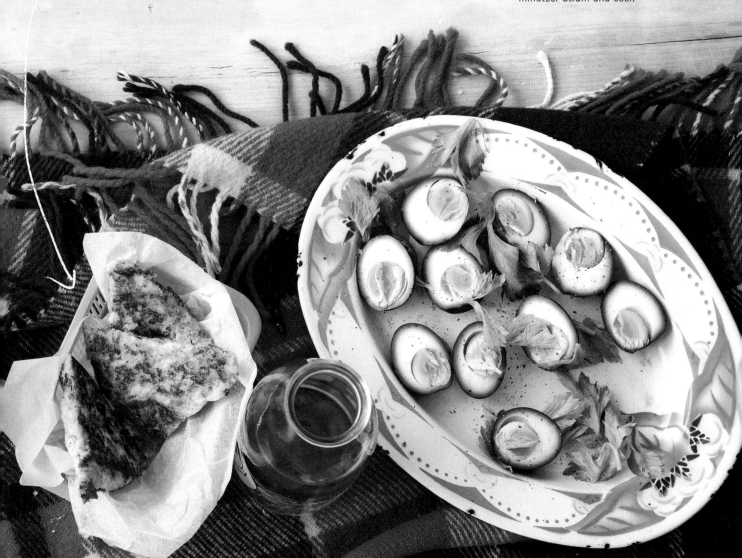

FRIDGE-DOOR TONNATO

MAKES 1½ CUPS (350 ML)

FIVE WAYS TO USE FRIDGE-DOOR TONNATO:

1. Pour over Shredded Lamb (page 220) and steamed beans and sprinkle with celery leaves to make Cheat's Vitello Tonnato (pictured).

2. Dollop on a grilled lamb chop with a side salad.

3. Toss through pasta and broccoli (cooked in the one pot).

4. Drizzle over a plate of boiled eggs.

5. Spoon over a wedge of iceberg lettuce.

1 × 425 g can pole-and-line-caught tuna, drained (reserve liquid; see below)

1 tablespoon capers

1 tablespoon chopped anchovies, or a splash of fish sauce

½ cup (125 ml) Whey-Good Mayo (page 50)

juice of ½ lemon

Combine all of the ingredients in a blender and purée. Store in the fridge and use within 2–3 days.

USE THE LEFTOVER TUNA BRINE OR OIL:
Use it to make a dressing, for sautéing or drizzling or freeze it in an ice-cube tray with herbs (page 25).

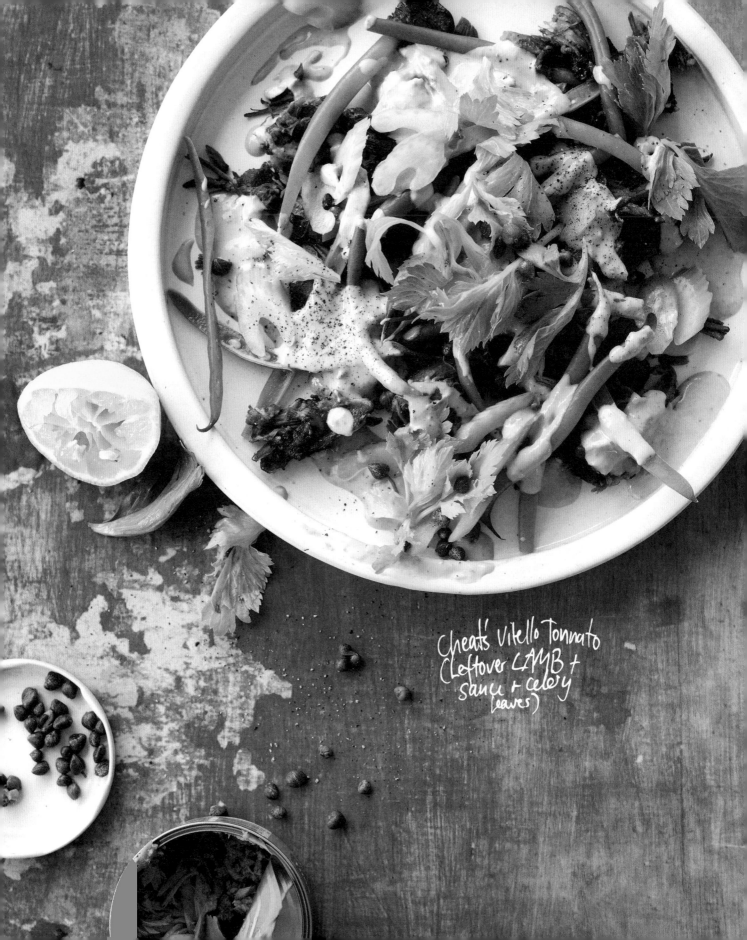

Cheat's Vitello Tonnato
(Leftover LAMB +
sauce + celery
leaves)

LAST NIGHT'S DINNER
WITH AN EGG STUCK IN IT

LEFTOVER DINNER + HOMEMADE STOCK + EGG

SERVES 1

I call it 'Doggie Bag Dinner the Next Day' or 'Repurposed Stew'. The French call it *oeufs en restes*, which lends things a little *élan*. Whatever. The idea entails putting a leftover meal in a pan – it can be a whole meal (chopped up), a soup, a pasta or a stew – adding a dash of broth and sticking an egg in the middle of it.

If you need to thicken a stew or soup, add 5 tablespoons of grated potato or 1–2 teaspoons of chia seeds.

The 2:4 Doggie-Bag Rule
Don't be scared of food poisoning: simply get the meal to a fridge within 2 hours, and keep it there for no more than 4 days before eating. Oh, and reheat it in the microwave for at least 2 minutes until it's steaming hot (above 75°C).

3 cups (about 450 g) leftover dinner (chop up anything that doesn't have a goopy consistency)

4 tablespoons Homemade Stock (page 42) or 2–3 frozen stock cubes (page 25)

1 egg

a good glug of olive oil

sea salt

Heat the leftovers in a skillet or a small saucepan with a little stock. Once hot and bubbling, create a divot in the middle of the mixture and crack in your egg. Cover (with a plate or lid), then reduce the heat and cook until the egg is set. Remove from the heat, pour over the olive oil and season with salt.

I add a small handful of peas: I believe a pea can improve most things.

3 SERVES VEG + FRUIT PER SERVE

£0.23 PER SERVE

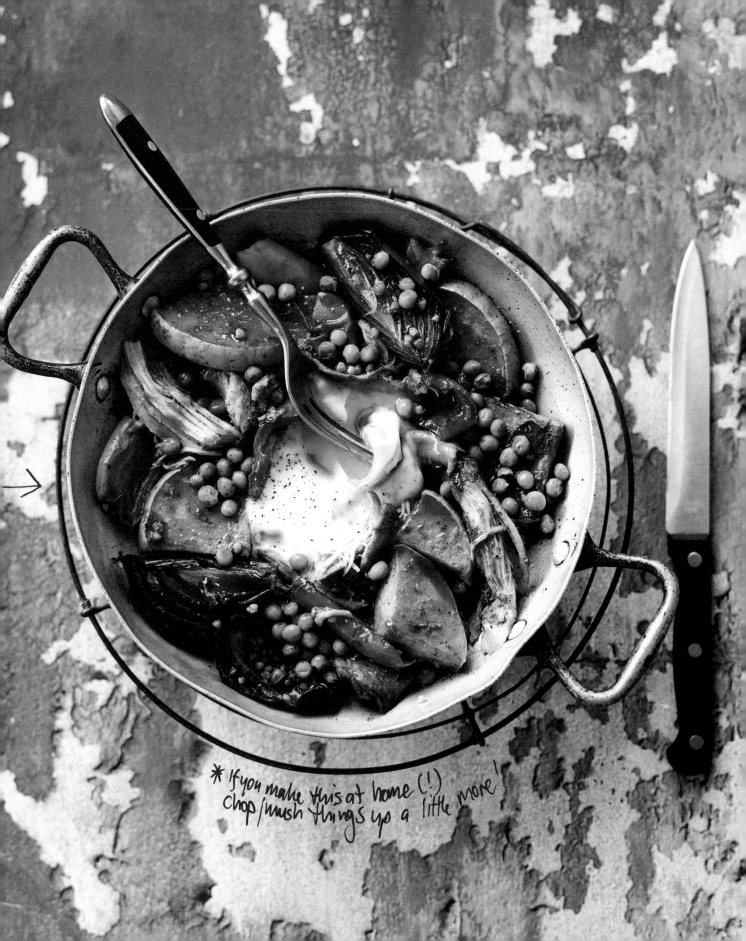

* If you make this at home (!)
chop / mush things up a little more!

SHORTCUT CHOUCROUTE

LEFTOVER MEAT + CABBAGE + OLD SAUERKRAUT

SERVES 2

A great trick for using up 'kraut that's about to turn.

4 good-quality pork sausages
or 8 Basic Meatballs (page 144)

1 onion, cut into wedges

½ apple, cut into wedges

250 g packet coleslaw mix
or 3 cups (300 g) shredded cabbage

1 cup (250 ml) excess Simplicious
Sauerkraut (page 337), including juices

Preheat the oven to 200°C (gas 6).

Place the sausages or meatballs and onion in a baking dish and roast for
10 minutes. Add the apple, coleslaw or cabbage and sauerkraut and cook
for a further 20 minutes, or until the sausages are plump and golden.

**MAKE IT KIMCHI CHICKEN
CHOUCROUTE:**
Use chicken sausages or meatballs
instead of pork and 'But the Kitchen Sink'
Kimchi (page 337) instead of sauerkraut.

*You can also finish the
cooking under the grill if
things aren't browned to
your liking.*

3 SERVES VEG + FRUIT PER SERVE

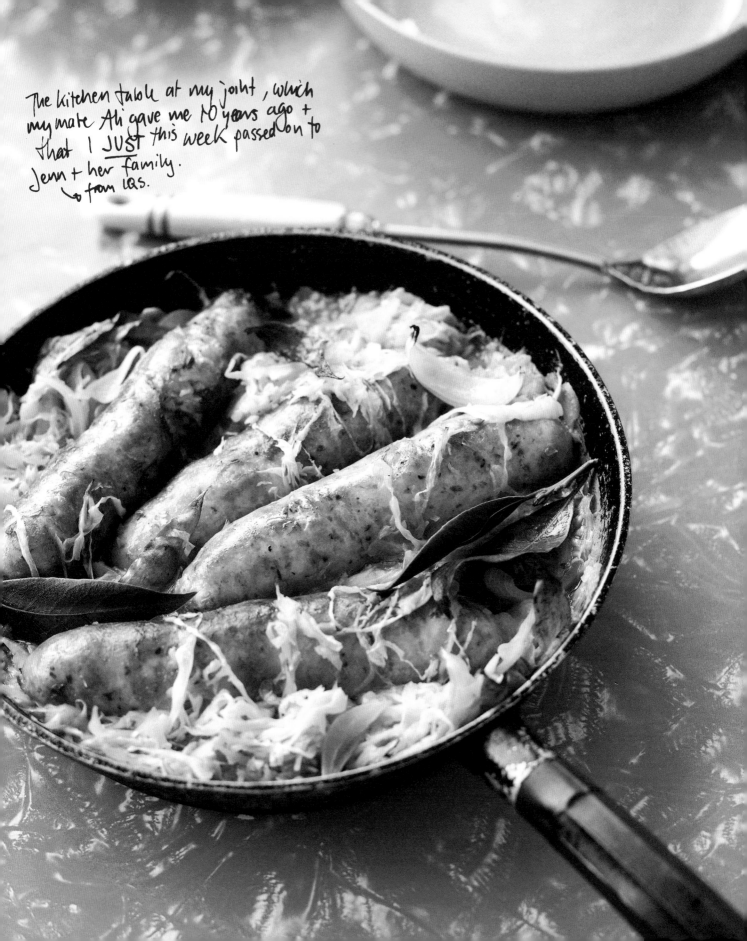

The kitchen table at my joint, which my mate Ali gave me 10 years ago + that I JUST this week passed on to Jenn + her family.
↳ from LQS.

VEGAN WHATCHAGOT QUICHE

LEFTOVER VEGGIES + MORE LEFTOVER VEGGIES + CHIA

SERVES 6

You might not be vegan, but you might run out of eggs sometimes . . .

No leftover cooked cauli? Throw 4 cups (600 g) chopped raw florets (and the red onion) into a baking dish with some coconut oil and roast for 20 minutes in an oven preheated to 190°C (gas 5).

coconut oil, for greasing

3 cups (450 g) leftover roasted cauliflower, chopped

1 red onion, finely chopped

3 cups (450 g) grated veggies (e.g. a mix of 1 large courgette, 1 sweet potato or swede and 1 parsnip or carrot)

½ cup (75 g) pitted black olives, chopped

4 tablespoons chia seeds, stirred into 1 cup (250 ml) cold water

2 teaspoons chopped thyme, sage or rosemary, plus extra whole sprigs and leaves to serve

4 tablespoons gluten-free flour (buckwheat flour or chickpea flour are great)

mixed seeds (e.g. linseeds, pumpkin seeds, sunflower seeds), to serve

lemon zest, to serve

Sweet Paprika Stem Chips, to serve (optional)

Grease a large quiche dish or spring-form cake tin with coconut oil. Combine all the ingredients in a large bowl and mix well. Pour into the dish or tin. Cover and refrigerate for at least 2 hours (or overnight) to allow the ingredients to bind.

Preheat the oven to 190°C (gas 5). Bake the quiche for 40–45 minutes, or until the top is nicely browned. To serve, sprinkle over the seeds, lemon zest and extra herbs.

SWEET PAPRIKA STEM CHIPS
LEFTOVER BROCCOLI AND CAULIFLOWER STALKS

Whenever I cook with broccoli and cauli, I cut the stalks into sticks and store them in the freezer ready for this cause.

This is a great way to use up the stalks of your broccoli and cauliflower.

stalks of 3–4 heads broccoli or cauliflower

1 tablespoon coconut oil

½ teaspoon salt

½ cup (50 g) grated parmesan

pinch of sweet paprika

Cut the broccoli and cauli stalks into chips 1.5 cm wide and toss with the oil and salt. Line a baking tray with baking paper and lay the chips out evenly. Bake for 10 minutes, then turn, sprinkle with parmesan and paprika and bake for a further 10–15 minutes. Serve as a side or with The Whole Brassicus Hummus (page 187).

MAKE IT VEGAN:
Use 4 tablespoons of nutritional yeast powder instead of parmesan.

 2 SERVES VEG + FRUIT PER SERVE

£0.39 PER SERVE

THE FISH THAT GOT AWAY PIE

LEFTOVER FISH + LEFTOVER VEGGIES + EGGS

SERVES 6

Sometimes I realise I have some white fish in the freezer or in the fridge that's been there a touch too long. When this is the case, I make this pie or my Sustainable Sweet Fish Curry (page 164). You can also use leftover Shredded Chicken (page 214).

50 g butter

1 onion-y thing (1 onion, 1 leek or 6 spring onions), thinly sliced

3 tablespoons flour

1½ cups (350 ml) milk

600 g leftover fish or offcuts, cut into bite-sized pieces

2–3 hard-boiled eggs, quartered (optional)

3 cups (450 g) chopped veggies (use any frozen or leftover veggies, such as cauliflower, courgette or carrot – I always include frozen peas)

1 tablespoon Dijon mustard

½ cup (20 g) finely chopped flat-leaf parsley

GREEN NUTTY CRUST

3–4 cups (about 500 g) raw broccoli or cauliflower, grated or blitzed

⅓ cup (35 g) finely grated parmesan

4 tablespoons sunflower seeds

Preheat the oven to 180°C (gas 4). Melt the butter in a saucepan over a medium heat. Add the onion-y thing and cook for 1 minute or until softened. Add the flour and cook, stirring, for 1–2 minutes. Gradually add the milk, whisking to remove any lumps. Bring the mixture to the boil and simmer, stirring constantly, for 3–4 minutes. Reduce the heat to low–medium and stir through the fish, eggs (if using), veggies, mustard and parsley. Dump the lot into a large baking dish.

To make the crust, combine the ingredients in a bowl and mix well. Spoon the crust mixture over the fish and veggies and bake for 20–25 minutes until golden and bubbling at the edges.

MAKE IT AN ORANGE NUTTY CRUST:
Use grated root veggies (sweet potato, carrot etc) instead of the broccoli or cauliflower and 2 tablespoons of butter instead of the parmesan.

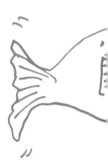

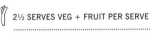 2½ SERVES VEG + FRUIT PER SERVE

 £0.80 PER SERVE

'PIZZA' BREAD AND BUTTER CRUMBLE

LEFTOVER MEAT + LEFTOVER VEGGIES + NOMATO SAUCE

SERVES 2

2–3 cups (about 250 g) Par-Cooked 'n' Frozen kale or Swiss chard (page 22)

1 cup (130 g) leftover meat (any kind; see Sunday Cook-ups chapter)

1–2 frozen stock cubes with herbs (page 25) or ¼ teaspoon dried herbs

½ cup (120 ml) Nomato Sauce (page 51) or sugar-free passata

BREAD AND BUTTER CRUMBLE

1 tablespoon butter, melted

1 cup (150 g) Cooked Quinoa (page 26) or Cooked Buckwheat (page 27)

3 tablespoons grated cheese (any hard cheese is fine)

Preheat the oven to 200°C (gas 6). Combine the kale or chard, meat, stock or herbs, and Nomato Sauce or passata in a small baking tray or skillet.

To make the crumble, combine the ingredients in a small bowl and mix well. Spoon the crumble over the meat and vegetable mixture and bake for 15–20 minutes until golden and bubbling.

MAKE IT A CREAMY GRATIN:
Use cream instead of Nomato Sauce.

I actually prefer this "white" version. but it meant ditching the catchy "pizza" title.

🍴 2 SERVES VEG + FRUIT PER SERVE

£ £1.27 PER SERVE

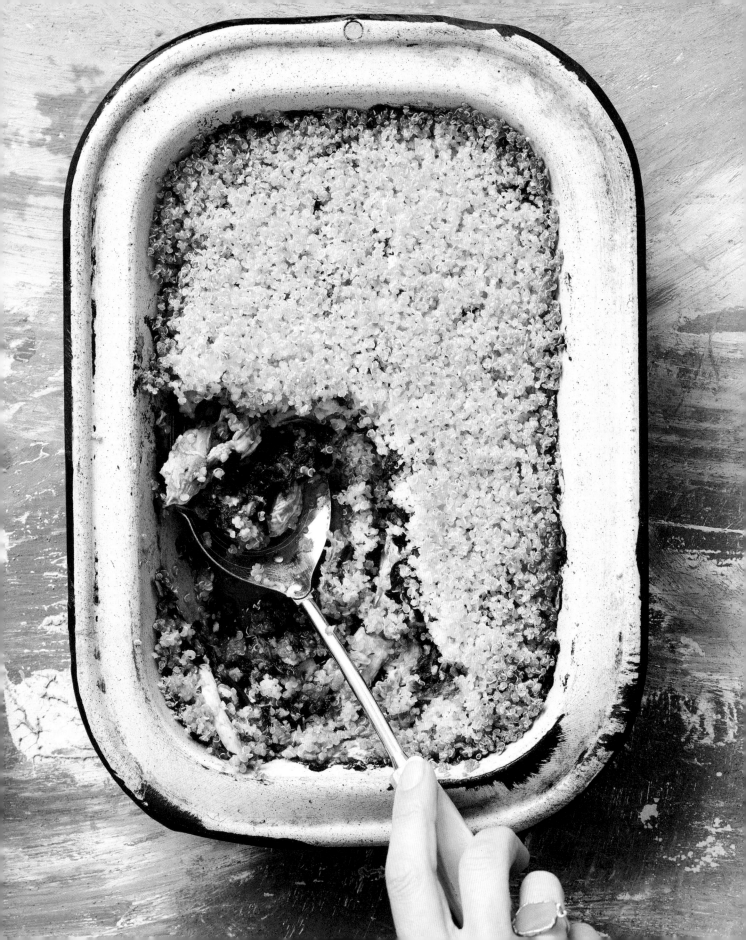

FOUR HEALING THINGS TO DO WITH A CUP OF HOMEMADE STOCK

I pride myself on finding better and simpler ways to maketh some bone broth/stock into a quick, gut-lining meal. (See page 42 for beef, chicken and fish stock recipes.)

You can use any for these recipes, but beef and chicken are best.

EGG-DROP SOUP

Whisk 1 egg and pour slowly into a small saucepan of simmering stock, stirring with a spoon. Cook for half a minute and serve with a sprinkle of chopped flat-leaf parsley, if you like.

LEFTOVERS KIMCHI SOUP

Combine equal quantities of stock (preferably chicken; page 42), Shredded Chicken (page 214), water and 'But the Kitchen Sink' Kimchi (page 337) in a saucepan. Bring to the boil and simmer for 5 minutes, tossing in some spring onions and frozen peas towards the end.

EASIEST EVER KOREAN BREAKFAST CUSTARD

Whisk 2 eggs with ¼ teaspoon of sea salt and ½ cup (125 ml) of stock in a ramekin or mug until foamy. Place the ramekin in a saucepan of simmering water (the water should come halfway up the sides of the ramekin). Cover the saucepan and gently simmer for 10–15 minutes until the eggs are set but still a bit wobbly. Serve with Indian Kimchi (page 338), sliced spring onions and Seaweed Dukkah (page 45).

MY GUT-HEALING BREW

(see page 87)

Face + head beyond the fold

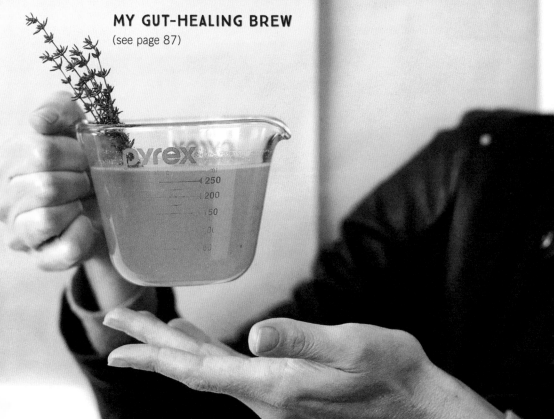

GREEN GUMBO

LEFTOVER SOUP + LEFTOVER HAM

SERVES 2

Use any greens you like: kale, Swiss chard, cavolo nero, parsley etc.

6 cups (600 g) chopped leafy greens

2 portions of Slow-Cooked Green Peas and Ham (the soup variation; page 217)

2 teaspoons apple cider vinegar

2 portions of Ham Hock Chunks (page 217)

Celery Leaf Salt, to serve (optional)

Bring a saucepan of salted water to the boil over a medium heat. Add the greens and blanch, uncovered, for about 5 minutes, or until quite soft. Drain most of the water out. Add the soup portions and vinegar and simmer for another 5 minutes. Sprinkle over the ham and serve with Celery Leaf Salt, if you like.

CELERY LEAF SALT
LEFTOVER CELERY LEAVES

MAKES ½–1 CUP (125–250 ML)

Grandad Tim put celery salt on everything. With white pepper. I think I've inherited his taste for it. Or perhaps it's the taste of smugness from knowing I've found another way to use stuff that's mostly turfed. Lovely on eggs, salads and on top of soups.

1 bunch celery, leaves only

sea salt flakes (not ground salt or crystals – Maldon sea flakes are good)

Preheat the oven to 180°C (gas 4). Place the dry celery leaves on a baking tray in a single layer. Bake in the oven for 5–8 minutes until dried out and crunchy, but not browned. Remove from the oven, cool and either crumble in your hands into small flakes or process briefly in a food processor. Place in a jar and add salt in a 1:1 ratio if you like lots of salt, or 2:1 ratio if you want a stronger celery flavour. Shake to combine.

3½ SERVES VEG + FRUIT PER SERVE

£0.88 PER SERVE

A SMALL CHAPTER OF SHOW-STOPPING TREATS

Frankly, I've scaled everything back for this chapter. Originally, my plan was to shrink the whole chapter. Literally. But it was going to make it hard for you to read. And my publisher Ingrid gave me her "Are you serious, Sarah?!" look. So I just concentrated on making sure the amount of sugar sweetener used was small. Ditto portion sizes. You won't notice, of course. But I wanted to MAXIMISE my minimising point. Now. Please enjoy.

LAMINGTON ICE CREAMS

400 ml can coconut cream, shaken lightly before opening

1/3 cup (75 g) cashew butter

1 teaspoon pure vanilla extract (or make your own; page 45)

1 tablespoon rice malt syrup

200 g dark (85–90% cocoa) chocolate, chopped into small pieces

1½ cups (115 g) desiccated or shredded coconut

5 tablespoons Raspberry Chia Jam (page 57)

Line a 22 cm square brownie tin with baking paper. Pour the coconut cream into the prepared tin and place in the freezer for 2–3 hours until frozen.

Remove the coconut cream slab and break into shards using a masher or the end of a rolling pin. Pulse the shards in a food processor until they resemble a fine powder. Add the cashew butter, vanilla extract and rice malt syrup and process until smooth and fluffy like ice cream. Pour the mixture back into the tin and smooth the top with a spatula or palette knife. Freeze for 1–2 hours until the mixture is firm to the touch but not rock solid.

Melt the chocolate in a bowl in the microwave (or in a heatproof bowl over a saucepan of boiling water, making sure the base of the bowl doesn't touch the water). Put the coconut into another bowl.

Remove the ice cream from the freezer and slice into 36 small squares. (You may want to trim the outer edges for a neater result.) Spread 18 squares with a thin layer of jam. Place the remaining squares on top to make 'sandwiches'.

Using two forks, or a cocktail stick, gently dip the squares into the melted chocolate, coating all sides, then dip in the coconut until covered, placing them on a lined tray as you go. Store in the freezer in a sealed container for up to 3 months.

If you're serving these straight from the freezer, let them sit out for 2–3 minutes to thaw slightly and they'll be crunchy on the outside and soft and smooth on the inside.

¼ TSP ADDED SUGAR PER SERVE

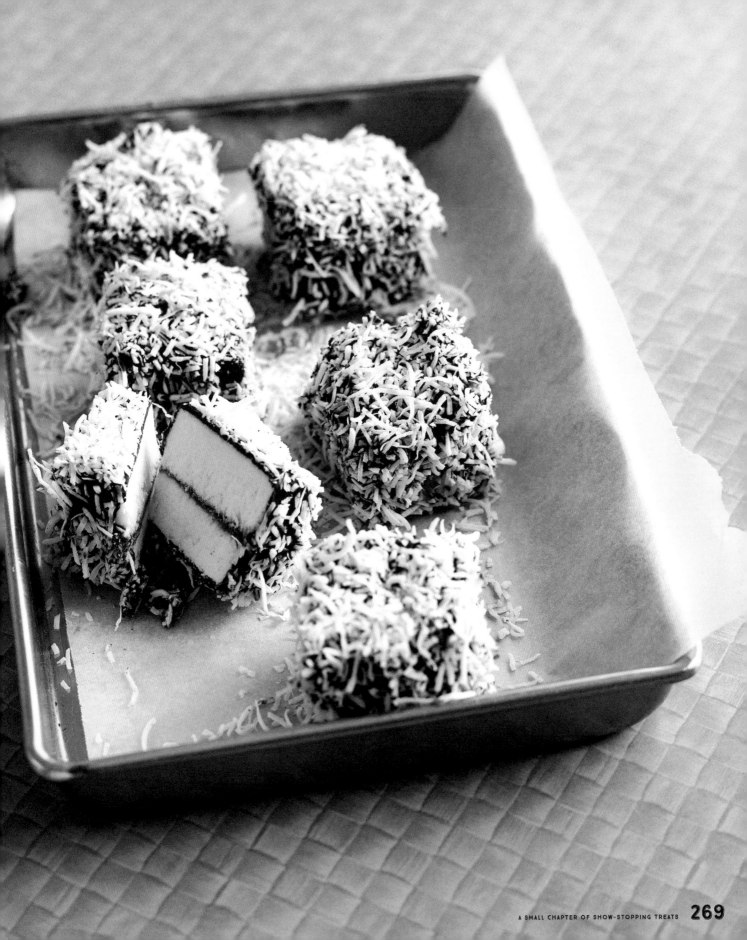

CHOC-BEET
ALLSPICE TRUFFLES

½ cup (75 g) Cooked 'n' Frozen Beetroot (page 23) or 1 large beetroot, trimmed, peeled, chopped and steamed

½ cup (125 ml) double cream

1 teaspoon ground allspice (or a big pinch of ground cumin for something quite wild)

50 g dark (85–90% cocoa) chocolate, roughly chopped

raw cacao powder, for rolling

Purée the beetroot, then simmer in a small saucepan for 5 minutes, stirring frequently, to remove the excess liquid. In another saucepan, heat the cream and spice until it's at simmering point. Add the beet purée and chocolate, stirring until the chocolate is melted. Leave in the fridge for a few hours.

Once cold, roll teaspoonfuls of the truffle mix into balls with your hands (refrigerate for an extra 10 minutes if your balls are a little too moist) and then roll in the cacao powder to coat. Store in the fridge for 3–4 days or freeze for up to 3 months.

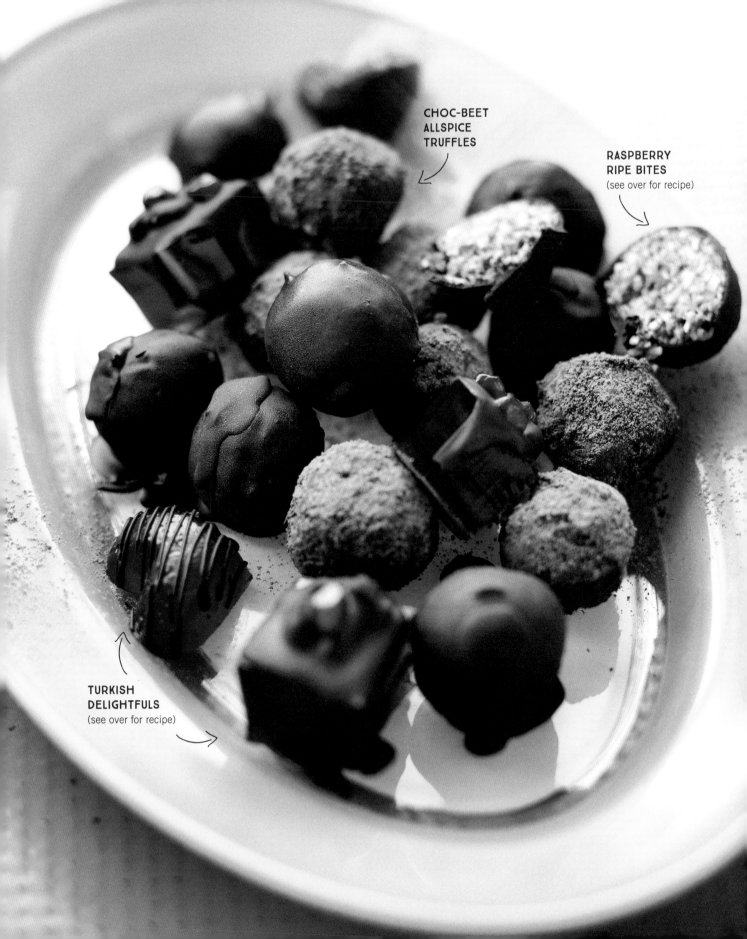

CHOC-BEET
ALLSPICE
TRUFFLES

RASPBERRY
RIPE BITES
(see over for recipe)

TURKISH
DELIGHTFULS
(see over for recipe)

TURKISH DELIGHTFULS

If you can't find a pomegranate, use 1 cup (120 g) raspberries or an extra ½ cup (125 ml) water and a tablespoon of beetroot powder.

You might need up to 1 tablespoon – it depends on the strength of your rosewater.

A note on pomegranates
Pomegranate is probably best viewed as a treat food. It's not a low-fructose fruit (although the amount you eat means it's not something to be too concerned about).

4 tablespoons gelatine powder

when to buy gelatine?
(see page 348)

1 pomegranate (reserve 1 tablespoon seeds for decorating, smash the rest a little to release the juice)

3 tablespoons lemon juice

3 tablespoons rice malt syrup or 4 drops liquid stevia

1–2 teaspoons rosewater

3 cubes frozen Basic Raw Chocolate (page 56) or 4 tablespoons chopped dark (85–90% cocoa) chocolate (optional)

chopped pistachios, to decorate

'Bloom' the gelatine by stirring it into ⅓ cup (75 ml) of cold water and letting it sit for 5 minutes. Meanwhile, combine the pomegranate pulp and lemon juice in a small saucepan with 1½ cups (350 ml) water and bring to the boil. Remove from the heat and strain out the pomegranate seeds. Return the pan to the heat and add the rice malt syrup or stevia and the gelatine and stir to dissolve. Remove from the heat and stir in the rosewater. Allow to cool slightly, then pour into silicone moulds or a glass or plastic dish and set in the fridge for at least 2 hours.

Remove the jelly from the moulds (or cut into squares if using a dish). Melt the chocolate in a cup in the microwave (slowly on a low heat, checking frequently). Dunk the jelly shapes into the chocolate or drizzle the chocolate over them. Decorate with the reserved pomegranate seeds and chopped pistachios, using an extra drizzle of chocolate to keep them in place. These will keep in the fridge for up to 1 week.

½ TSP ADDED SUGAR PER SERVE

RASPBERRY RIPE BITES

1¼ cups (100 g) shredded coconut

1 tablespoon rice malt syrup

1 tablespoon coconut oil, melted

2 tablespoons coconut milk

1 teaspoon pure vanilla extract (or make your own; page 45), optional

½ cup (60 g) raspberries or cherries (fresh or frozen)

1 cup (240 ml) Basic Raw Chocolate (page 56) or 1 cup (225 ml) chopped dark (85–90% cocoa) chocolate

Line a baking tray with baking paper. Place all of the ingredients (except the chocolate) in a food processor. Pulse until the mixture comes together but still has texture. Roll tablespoons of the mixture into balls, place on the baking tray and freeze for at least 1 hour.

Meanwhile, make your own raw chocolate, or melt store-bought chocolate in a microwave on low (or in a heatproof bowl over a saucepan of boiling water, making sure the base of the bowl doesn't touch the water).

Remove the coconut balls from the freezer and roll them in the melted chocolate so they are completely coated (stabbing the balls with a skewer and dunking works well). Return the balls to the lined tray and allow to set in the fridge for 30 minutes before serving. These will keep in the fridge for up to 1 week or in the freezer for up to 3 months.

½ TSP ADDED SUGAR PER SERVE

TAM TIMS

You know, a clearly bastardised version of the Aussie Big Food one, renamed to avoid being sued. And, yes, you can still drink your tea through one.

1 cup (125 g) gluten-free plain flour, plus extra for dusting

2 teaspoons granulated stevia

$^1/_3$ cup (40 g) raw cacao powder

75 g cold unsalted butter, diced

4 tablespoons milk (any kind, though full-fat dairy is best)

GANACHE

40 g unsalted butter, at room temperature

3 tablespoons rice malt syrup

3 tablespoons raw cacao powder

CHOCOLATE COATING

100 g dark (85–90% cocoa) chocolate, chopped into small, even-sized pieces

Preheat the oven to 180°C (gas 4) and line a baking tray with baking paper.

Place the flour, stevia, cacao powder, butter and milk in a food processor bowl and process to make a firm dough. Transfer the dough to a lightly floured work surface and knead until smooth. Roll the dough out between two sheets of baking paper to make a rectangle (about 5 mm thick). Cut into 16 smaller rectangles. Transfer to the baking tray and bake in the oven for 10 minutes.

For a firmer frosting, set the ganache mixture in the fridge for 15 minutes.

Meanwhile, to make the ganache, place all the ingredients in a small bowl and beat until fluffy.

Remove the biscuits from the oven and allow to cool. Once cooled, spread a thin layer of ganache over eight of the biscuits and top each one with another biscuit, sandwiching them together. Place in the fridge while you make the chocolate coating.

Melt the chocolate slowly in a microwave (or in a heatproof bowl over a saucepan of boiling water, making sure the base of the bowl doesn't touch the water). Dip each biscuit sandwich in the melted chocolate and place on the baking paper. Return to the fridge to set before serving. Store in a sealed container in the fridge for up to 1 week or in the freezer for up to 3 months.

1 TSP ADDED SUGAR PER SERVE

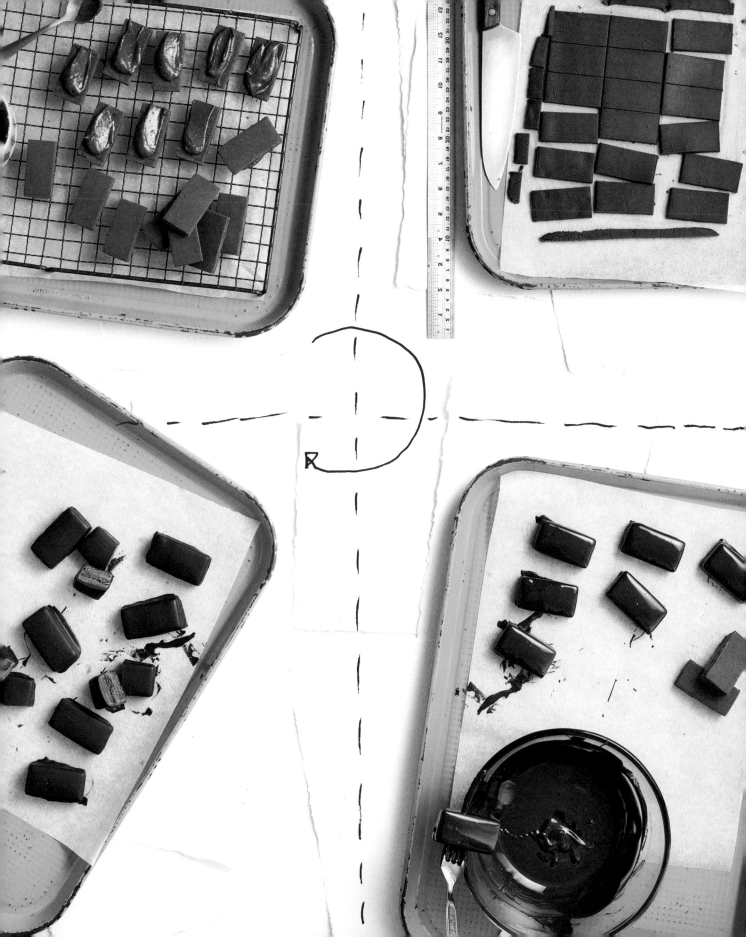

THREE COOKIE DOUGH SLICES
Happily use the BAKED or RAW bases interchangeably, if you like.

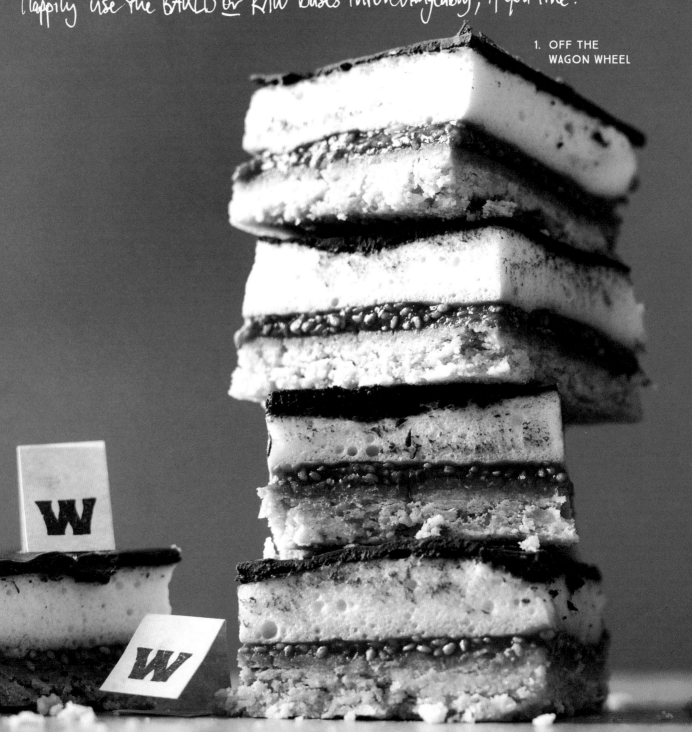

1. OFF THE
   WAGON WHEEL

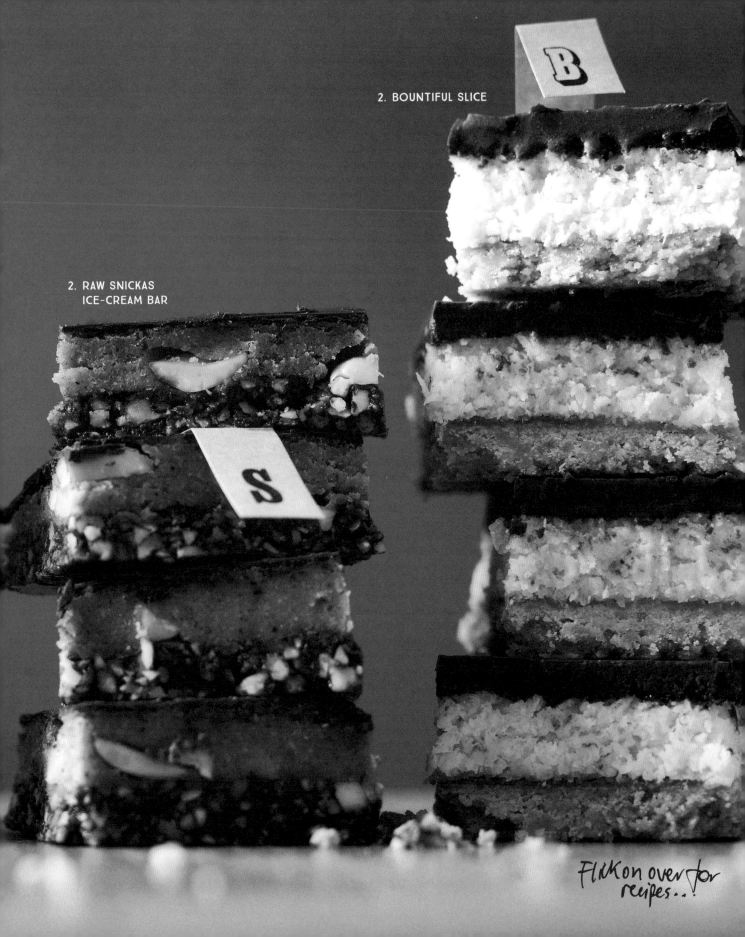

2. BOUNTIFUL SLICE

2. RAW SNICKAS
ICE-CREAM BAR

Flik on over for recipes..!

1. OFF THE WAGON WHEEL

MAKES 28 SMALL SQUARES

1 cup (250 ml) Raspberry Chia
Jam (page 57)

BAKED COOKIE DOUGH BASE

150 g unsalted butter

3 tablespoons rice malt syrup

¾ cup (90 g) buckwheat flour

¾ cup (90 g) gluten-free plain
flour

½ cup (40 g) desiccated coconut

pinch of sea salt

MARSHMALLOW FILLING

2 tablespoons gelatine powder

4 tablespoons rice malt syrup

1 teaspoon pure vanilla extract
(or make your own; page 45)

¼ teaspoon sea salt

CHOC COATING

100 g dark (85–90% cocoa)
chocolate or Basic Raw Chocolate
(page 56)

yes!!

Preheat the oven to 180°C (gas 4). Grease and line a 28 cm ×
18 cm baking tin with baking paper.

To make the Baked Cookie Dough Base, melt the butter and
rice malt syrup in a small saucepan (or in a mixing bowl in the
microwave). Combine with the remaining ingredients and mix well.
Press the mixture into the prepared tin and bake for 15–20 minutes
until light golden. Remove from the oven and allow to cool.

When cool, spread the jam over the base and refrigerate.

Meanwhile, to make the marshmallow filling, 'bloom' the gelatine
by stirring it into ⅓ cup (75 ml) water until it dissolves. Allow to sit
for 5 minutes – it will become firm like a rubber ball. Meanwhile,
combine the rice malt syrup, vanilla and salt in a saucepan with
1 cup (250 ml) water and bring to the boil. Reduce the heat and
simmer, stirring constantly, for 8 minutes. Turn off the heat, add
the gelatine blob to the mixture and stir to dissolve. Using a stick
blender, blitz until it forms a thick cream (or transfer to a high-
powered blender to cut time).

*Flick to page 348 to
nerd up on gelatine.*

Pour the marshmallow over the cooled jam layer. Now rub your
hands in coconut oil and use your fingers to smooth the surface.
Refrigerate for at least 1 hour or until set.

Melt the chocolate slowly in a microwave (or in a heatproof bowl
over a saucepan of boiling water, making sure the base of the bowl
doesn't touch the water) and pour over the marshmallow layer,
spreading it evenly. Return the tray to the fridge for at least 1 hour
or until the chocolate is set. Cut into squares to serve. Store in the
fridge in a sealed container for up to 5 days.

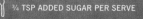

¾ TSP ADDED SUGAR PER SERVE

2. RAW SNICKAS ICE-CREAM BAR

MAKES 28 SMALL SQUARES

Pecans have a good flavour, but almonds, pistachios or hazelnuts are great too.

RAW COOKIE DOUGH BASE

2 cups (250 g) nuts (preferably activated; page 28)

4 tablespoons raw cacao powder

4 tablespoons rice malt syrup

40 g coconut oil, melted

pinch of sea salt

'NOUGAT'

¾ cup (175 ml) coconut cream

⅓ cup (75 ml) rice malt syrup

good pinch of sea salt

½ cup (50 g) coconut flour, plus extra if needed

⅔ cup (150 g) natural peanut butter

4 tablespoons raw unsalted peanuts

CHOCOLATE TOPPING

100 g dark (85–90% cocoa) chocolate, diced

Line a 28 cm × 18 cm baking tin with baking paper.

To make the Raw Cookie Dough Base, process the nuts in a food processor to a fine crumb. Add the remaining ingredients and process until just combined. Add more coconut oil (if needed) to achieve a dough-like consistency. Alternatively, keep blitzing until the nuts give up their oil. Press the mixture evenly into the base of the prepared tin. Place in the freezer to set.

Meanwhile, to make the 'nougat', place all of the ingredients except the peanuts in a bowl and mix until smooth. (Add extra coconut flour if the mixture is too runny. It should be the consistency of cookie dough.) Fold through the peanuts. Spread the mixture over the chilled cookie dough base and whack it back in the freezer.

Melt the chocolate slowly in a microwave (or in a heatproof bowl over a saucepan of boiling water, making sure the base of the bowl doesn't touch the water), stirring until melted. Pour the chocolate over the chilled nougat and return to the freezer until ready to serve. Store in the freezer for up to 3 months.

MAKE IT PEANUT-FREE:
Swap the peanut butter and peanuts for cashew butter and cashews.

3. BOUNTIFUL SLICE

MAKES 28 SMALL SQUARES

The taste of paradise . . . with the nutritional profile to match.

1 portion of Baked Cookie Dough Base (opposite)

You can also use the Raw Cookie Dough Base from the Snickas recipe if you prefer. Both work.

1 cup (250 ml) coconut milk

⅓ cup (75 ml) rice malt syrup

¼ cup (50 g) coconut oil

2 cups (150 g) desiccated coconut

pinch of sea salt

CHOC COATING

1 batch (325 ml) of Basic Raw Chocolate (page 56)

Make the Baked Cookie Dough Base (opposite) and allow to cool.

Heat the coconut milk, rice malt syrup and coconut oil in a saucepan over a low heat. Stir until well combined. Remove from the heat and stir in the desiccated coconut and salt. Spoon over the cookie dough base and press evenly so that it is about 1.5 cm thick. Freeze until the coconut filling is set (about 1 hour).

Melt the chocolate slowly in a microwave (or in a heatproof bowl over a saucepan of boiling water, making sure the base of the bowl doesn't touch the water). Spread the melted chocolate over the coconut layer and return to the fridge for at least 1 hour before cutting into squares. Store in a sealed container in the fridge for up to 1 week or in the freezer for up to 3 months.

MAKE IT A CHERRY RIPE SLICE:
Add ½ cup (60 g) of raspberries to the coconut filling.

1 TSP ADDED SUGAR PER SERVE

½ TSP ADDED SUGAR PER SERVE

CHOCOLATE PEANUT BUTTER CRACKLES

Seven ingredients, one pot, 4½ minutes, some time in the fridge, and you're done.

¾ cup (175 g) coconut oil

3 tablespoons rice malt syrup

4 tablespoons raw cacao powder

½ cup (115 g) crunchy natural peanut butter

½ cup (40 g) desiccated coconut

½ cup (70 g) Activated Groaties (page 27)

1½ cups (25 g) puffed quinoa or puffed rice

Remember you can use store-bought 'buckinis' if you like.

Line two cupcake trays or muffin tins with 18 paper cases.

Gently heat the coconut oil in a saucepan over a low–medium heat. Remove from the heat and stir in the rice malt syrup. Add the cacao powder and peanut butter and stir to combine. Add the coconut, groaties and puffed quinoa or rice and mix well. Spoon the mixture into the prepared trays. Refrigerate for 2 hours to completely set, then serve. Store leftovers in a sealed container in the fridge for up to 2 weeks.

¼ TSP ADDED SUGAR PER SERVE

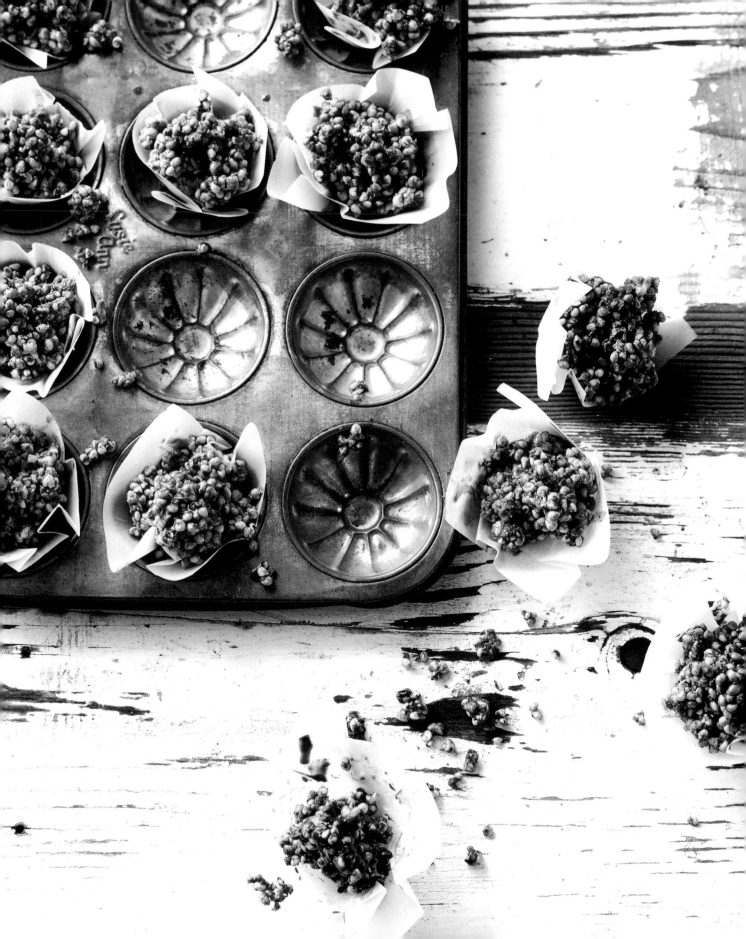

MISO AND WALNUT SLOW BROS

SERVES 16

A slow-cooker brownie . . . yeah! This masterpiece is seriously disaster-proof. And no matter how hard you try to mess it up, it will still come out with a lovely glazed top, crunchy outer bits and a gooey volcano-like centre. Serve with yoghurt or cream. If your slow cooker is larger than a 4.5 litre version, you'll need to double the batch quantity.

coconut oil, butter or ghee, for greasing

1½ cups (150 g) almond meal

½ cup (60 g) raw cacao powder

1 teaspoon gluten-free baking powder

½ teaspoon sea salt

½ cup (115 g) unsalted butter or coconut oil, melted

⅓ cup (75 ml) rice malt syrup

3 tablespoons red miso paste

3 eggs

½ cup (75 g) chopped walnuts

80 g dark (85–90% cocoa) chocolate, chopped into small, even chunks

full-fat organic plain yoghurt or cream, to serve

Grease the slow-cooker insert and line it with baking paper so it reaches halfway up the side.

In a large bowl combine the almond meal, cacao powder, baking powder and salt.

In a separate bowl whisk together the melted butter or oil, rice malt syrup and miso paste. Add the eggs and continue whisking until the mixture is well combined.

The centre will always be moister than the perimeter of the brownie; don't burn the outside waiting for the centre to firm up.

Pour the butter and syrup mixture into the dry ingredients and mix thoroughly. Stir through the walnuts and the chocolate chunks. Pour the batter into the lined slow-cooker insert. Cover and cook on low for 2½ hours or 1½ hours on high, or until the outside of the mixture is firm and the centre is no longer liquid. Remove the lid and continue cooking for a further 30 minutes or until the centre cooks through.

Once cooked, switch off the slow cooker and leave the cooked mixture to rest for 10–15 minutes. Carefully remove from the slow cooker by grabbing the edges of the baking paper and gently lifting out. Allow to cool completely before slicing. Store the brownies on the baking paper in a sealed container for 3–4 days or freeze for up to 4 months.

MAKE IT PEANUT BUTTER SLOW BRO FUDGE:
Follow the recipe above, replacing the walnuts with 4 heaped tablespoons of softened crunchy natural peanut butter. Cook for 3 hours on low or 1½ hours on high.

1½ TSP ADDED SUGAR PER SERVE

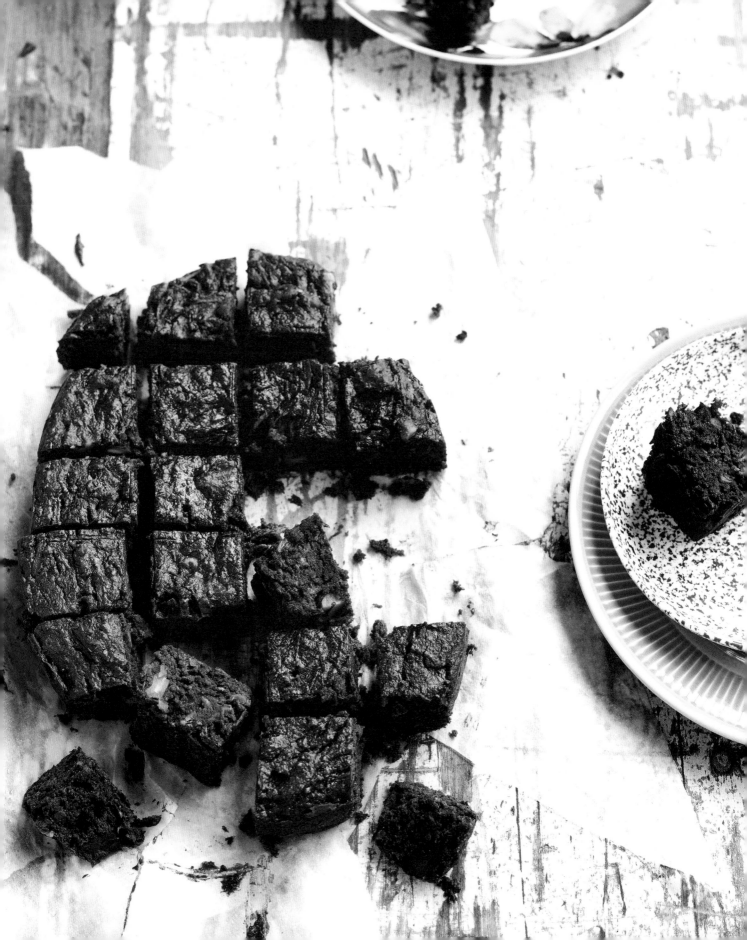

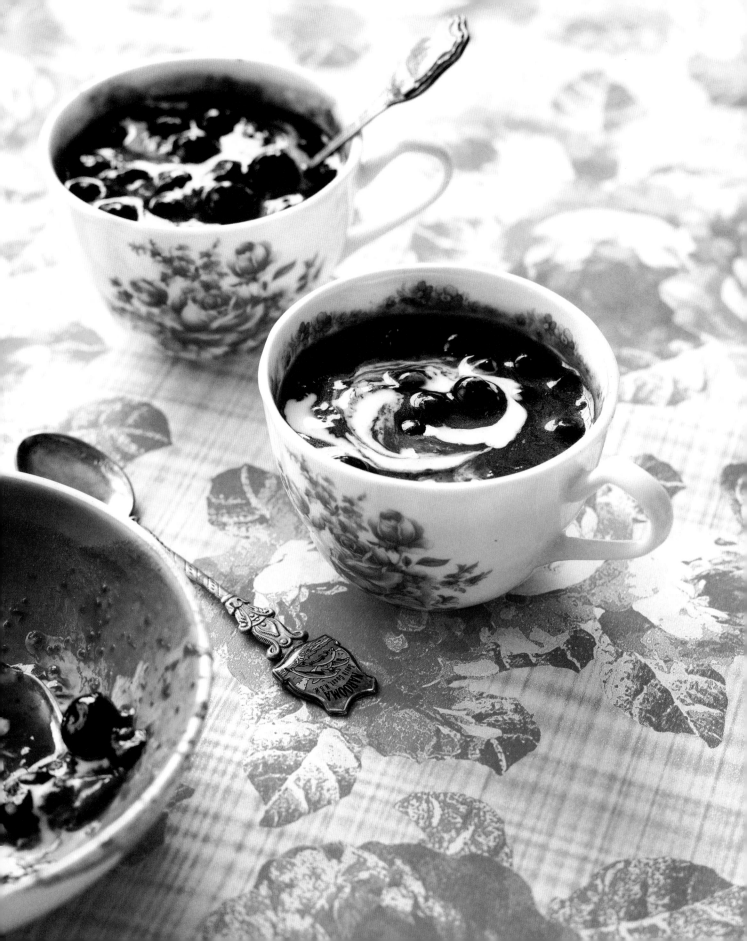

BUTTERED BLUEBERRY AND BLOOD ORANGE SOUP

So severely simple I feel embarrassed calling it a recipe.

1 tablespoon unsalted butter

4 cm knob of ginger, finely chopped

3 cups (350 g) blueberries (fresh or frozen)

juice of 2 small blood oranges
or mandarins (or 1 large orange)

zest of 1 orange or mandarin

1 tablespoon rice malt syrup

Whipped Coconut Frosting (page 56)
or whipped cream, to serve (optional)

pinch of ground nutmeg
or cinnamon, to serve (optional)

Heat the butter in a small frying pan over a medium heat and sauté the ginger for 2–3 minutes. Add the berries, juice, zest and rice malt syrup and sauté for 5 minutes.

Serve in small bowls (or teacups) with a swirl of cream and a sprinkle of nutmeg or cinnamon, if you like. Eat with a spoon!

½ TSP ADDED SUGAR PER SERVE

1 SERVE VEG + FRUIT PER SERVE

FRIDAY NIGHT
CHOCKITO
ON A STICK

MAKES 15–30

When I was a kid, Dad would come home with a Friday Night Surprise each week. Mostly it was the one Chokito bar – a caramel fudge, rice crispy, chocolate log thing – divided between all five of us kids (as we were back then). Perhaps you've not encountered a Chokito. That's because it periodically gets discontinued. I think the Big Food Giant responsible for this might like to reformulate its next incarnation without sugar. Here's a recipe for them now. On a stick.

½ cup (85 g) Activated Groaties (page 27) or crushed peanuts

30 lollipop sticks (or use bamboo skewers cut in half)

100 g dark (85–90% cocoa) chocolate

CARAMEL FILLING

⅓ cup (75 g) coconut oil, slightly softened

3 tablespoons hulled tahini

3 tablespoons rice malt syrup

½ cup (50 g) almond meal

To make the caramel filling, place the coconut oil, tahini and rice malt syrup in a bowl and mix until smooth. Stir in the almond meal. Refrigerate the mixture for 1 hour to firm.

or just do stickless truffles instead

Roll teaspoons of the mixture into balls and coat each one in groaties or peanuts. Insert a lollipop stick or skewer into the centre of each ball and place upside down on a baking tray or plate lined with baking paper. Pop in the freezer for at least 10 minutes.

Melt the chocolate in a heatproof bowl over a saucepan of boiling water, making sure the base of the bowl doesn't touch the water. Dip the balls in the chocolate and coat well. Refrigerate for at least 1 hour or until the chocolate is set. These will keep in the fridge in a sealed container for up to 2 weeks, or in the freezer for 3–4 months.

¼ TSP ADDED SUGAR PER SERVE

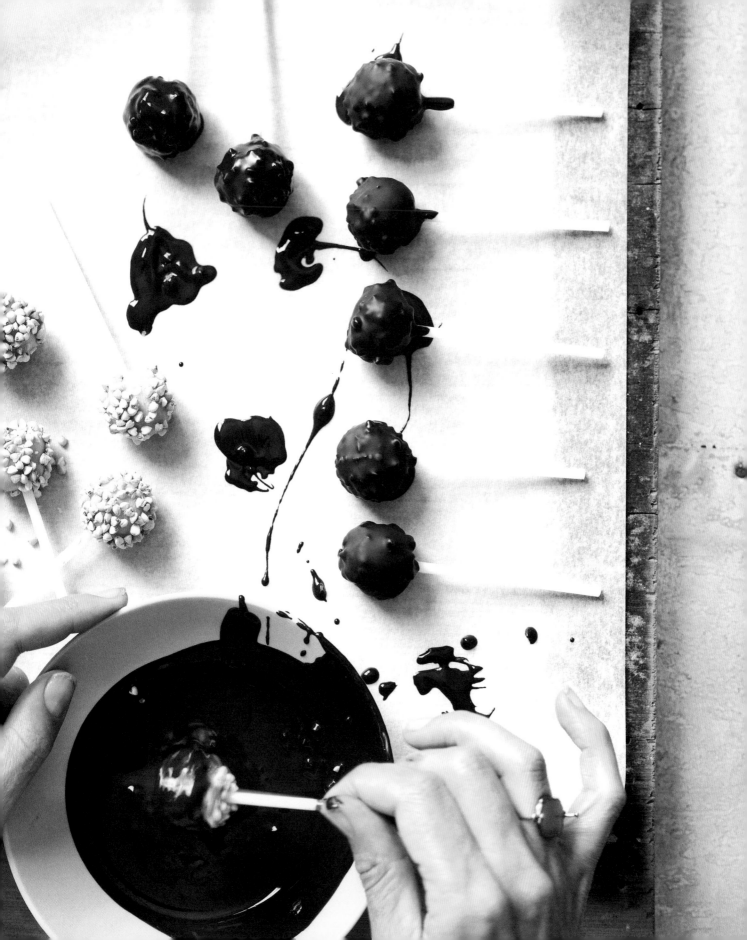

FOUR VERY LUSH MUG CAKES

Treats for one made in the microwave in two.

1. GINGER BREAD MUGGIN

4 tablespoons almond meal or gluten-free self-raising flour

3 tablespoons desiccated coconut

¼ teaspoon baking powder

¼ teaspoon ground ginger

½ teaspoon Pumpkin Spice Mix (page 45) or ground cinnamon

1 tablespoon crushed pecans, plus extra to serve

½ teaspoon rice malt syrup

1 cube frozen Sweet Potato Purée (page 23) or 4 tablespoons grated sweet potato

4 tablespoons milk (any kind)

full-fat organic plain yoghurt, to serve

Place all of the ingredients in a microwave-safe porcelain mug and mix with a spoon. Microwave on high for 2 minutes. Serve with yoghurt and pecans.

½ TSP ADDED SUGAR PER SERVE

½ SERVE VEG + FRUIT PER SERVE

2. CHOC GINGER AND PEAR MUGGIN

4 tablespoons almond meal or gluten-free plain flour

3 tablespoons desiccated coconut

¼ teaspoon baking powder

1 teaspoon raw cacao powder

½ teaspoon ground ginger

¼ pear, cored and chopped

4 tablespoons milk (any kind)

1 cube frozen Basic Raw Chocolate (page 56)

pear wedges, to serve

Place all of the ingredients, except the cube of frozen chocolate, in a microwave-safe porcelain mug and mix with a spoon. Place the chocolate cube in the centre of the mixture and push down. Microwave on high for 2 minutes. Serve with pear wedges.

4. LEMON SYRUP AND POPPY SEED MUGGIN

4 tablespoons almond meal or gluten-free plain flour

3 tablespoons desiccated coconut

¼ teaspoon baking powder

zest of ½ lemon

1 tablespoon lemon juice

1 teaspoon poppy seeds, plus extra to serve

½ teaspoon rice malt syrup

4 tablespoons milk (any kind)

Homemade Cream Cheese (page 46), to serve

Place all of the ingredients in a microwave-safe porcelain mug and mix with a spoon. Microwave on high for 2 minutes. Serve with a dollop of cream cheese and a sprinkle of poppy seeds.

½ TSP ADDED SUGAR PER SERVE

3. STRAWBERRY CHEESECAKE MUGGIN

4 tablespoons almond meal or gluten-free plain flour

3 tablespoons desiccated coconut

¼ teaspoon baking powder

1 tablespoon pistachios, chopped, plus extra to serve

1 tablespoon Strawberry Chia Jam (page 57) or 2–3 strawberries, chopped, plus extra to serve

4 tablespoons milk (any kind)

1 tablespoon full-fat ricotta, plus extra to serve (or use Homemade Cream Cheese; page 46)

Place all of the ingredients in a microwave-safe porcelain mug and mix with a spoon. Microwave on high for 2 minutes. Serve with a dollop of ricotta, and the extra pistachios and jam or strawberries.

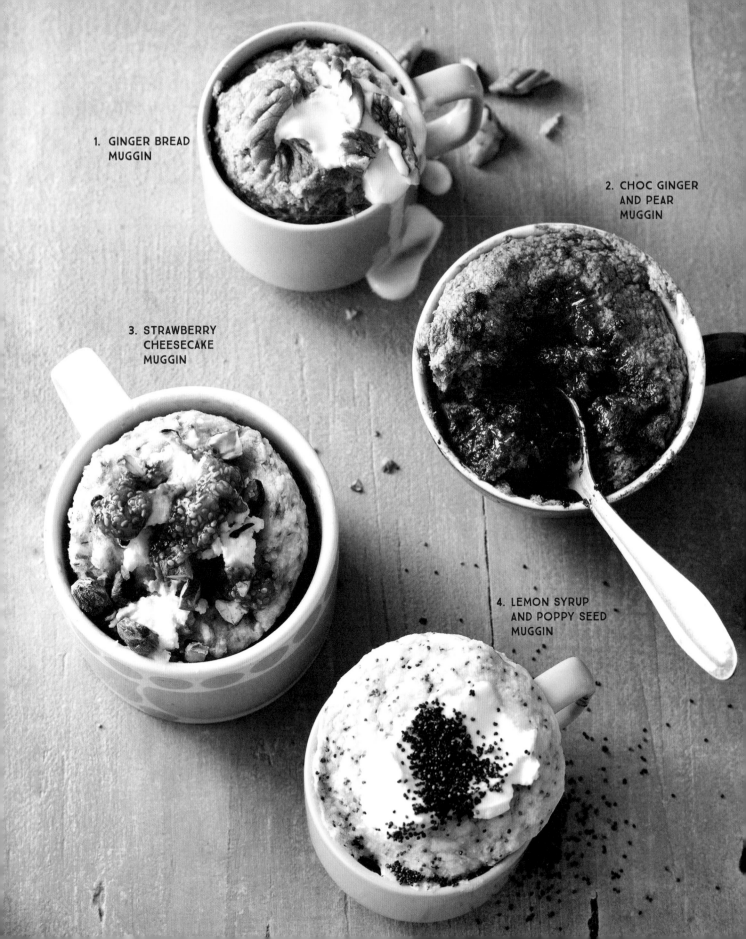

1. GINGER BREAD MUGGIN

2. CHOC GINGER AND PEAR MUGGIN

3. STRAWBERRY CHEESECAKE MUGGIN

4. LEMON SYRUP AND POPPY SEED MUGGIN

PULL-APART CATERPILLAR BIRTHDAY CAKE

SERVES 13 ——

A cupcake pull-apart cake is the best way to manage portion control with kids.

Double the recipe if you've been roped into making a cake for the whole class and make him a fat, hungry caterpillar with two cupcakes per 'segment'.

400 g can black beans, rinsed and drained

1 cup (250 ml) Sweet Potato Purée (page 23)

125 g coconut oil

1/3 cup (75 ml) rice malt syrup

1½ teaspoons ground cinnamon

1½ teaspoons baking powder

1 teaspoon bicarbonate of soda

5 eggs

½ cup (60 g) raw cacao powder

ICING

2 tablespoons frozen raspberries, thawed and mushed through a sieve to extract the juice

several pinches of pure vanilla powder (optional)

1 quantity Cream Cheese Frosting (page 56) or Supercharged Coconut Frosting (page 56)

1 cup (50 g) baby spinach leaves, puréed with 1 tablespoon water and pressed through a sieve

Preheat the oven to 160°C (gas 3). Line one or two muffin or cupcake trays with 13 paper cases.

Place the beans, sweet potato, coconut oil, rice malt syrup, cinnamon, baking powder, bicarbonate of soda and 1 of the eggs in a food processor. Process until smooth. Add the remaining eggs and the cacao powder and process until combined. Divide the mixture between the cases, overfilling one of the paper cases (with an extra 1–2 tablespoons of mixture) to make the head. Bake for 25 minutes, leaving the larger cupcake for another 3 minutes. Leave in the trays for 5 minutes then transfer to a wire rack to cool.

Assemble the caterpillar on a baking tray or serving tray lined with baking paper (or other paper).

To make the icing for the head, mix the raspberry juice with 1 teaspoon of frosting in a cup. Mix in a pinch of vanilla powder (if using) and spread evenly over the largest cupcake.

To make the icing for the body, add the spinach juice to the remaining frosting (reserve a tiny amount of cream-coloured frosting for the eyes, if you like), a little at a time. Add a few pinches of vanilla powder and mix until thick. Spread over the remaining cupcakes and decorate as desired. I use half a blueberry to make each pupil, a blueberry sliver for the mouth and tiny spinach leaves for the antennae.

To reduce the sugar load, I suggest making the frosting with no added sweetener

1 TSP ADDED SUGAR PER SERVE

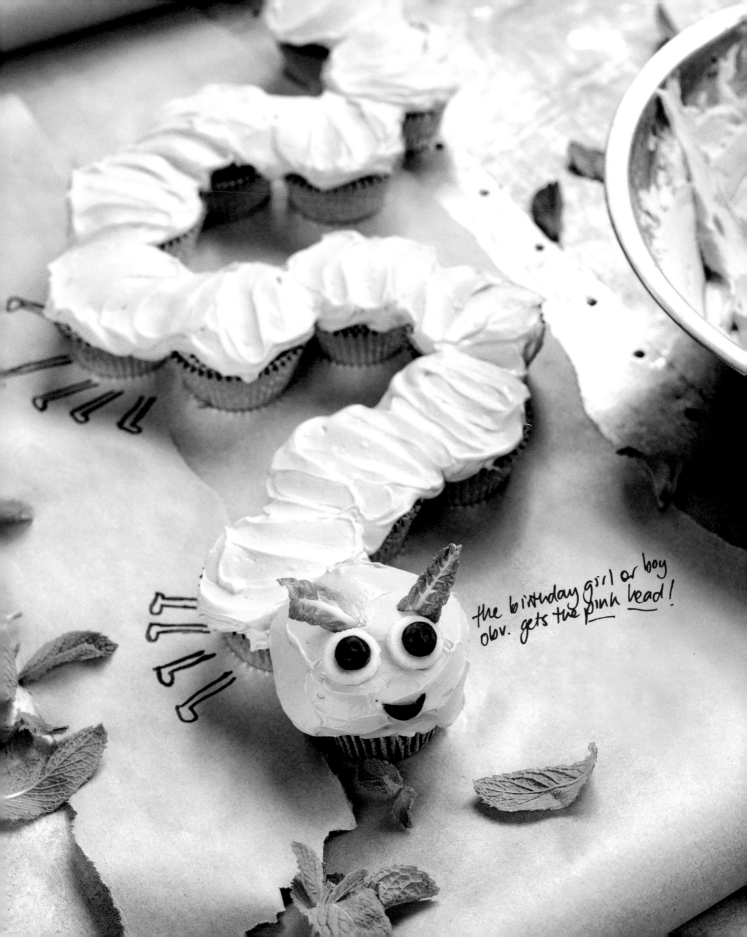

the birthday girl or boy
obv. gets the pink head!

PARTY POLENTA CAKES WITH POPPING TOPPING

MAKES 12

175 g unsalted butter, cubed and at room temperature, plus extra for greasing

½ cup (125 ml) rice malt syrup

3 eggs

220 g almond meal

100 g coarse polenta

1 teaspoon baking powder

1 teaspoon pure vanilla extract (or make your own; page 45)

½ teaspoon ground turmeric

zest of 2 oranges

juice of ½ orange

1 cup (250 g) Cream Cheese Frosting (page 56)

TOPPING

⅓ cup (75 g) popcorn kernels

1 tablespoon unsalted butter

1 tablespoon rice malt syrup

big pinch of sea salt

Preheat the oven to 180°C (gas 4) and grease a 12-hole muffin tray with butter or line with paper cases.

Beat the butter until pale. Add the rice malt syrup and beat until light and creamy. Beat in the eggs one at a time. Fold in the almond meal, polenta, baking powder, vanilla, turmeric and the orange zest and juice and mix until just combined. Spoon the mixture into the muffin tray or paper cases and bake for 45 minutes or until just golden and the sides are coming away from the tin (or cases). Set aside to cool.

Meanwhile, for the topping, place the popcorn kernels in a large bowl with the butter. Cover with a plate and heat in the microwave on high for 2½–3 minutes until the popping eases off. While the popcorn is still hot, drizzle over the rice malt syrup and sprinkle with salt. Toss to combine.

Smooth the frosting over the cooled cakes and top with the popcorn. Store in a sealed container in the fridge for 3–4 days.

2 TSP ADDED SUGAR PER SERVE

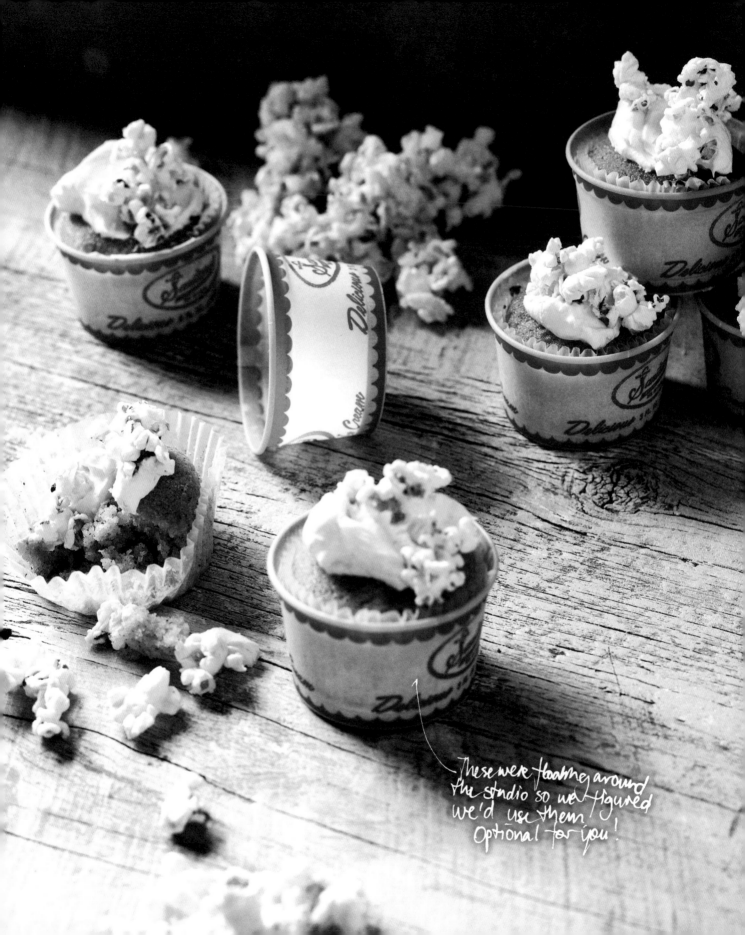

These were floating around the studio so we figured we'd use them. Optional for you!

CHEESECAKE-STUFFED PEACHES WITH BASIL

SERVES 12

6 peaches, halved and stones removed

¼ cup (50 g) unsalted butter, melted

2 teaspoons ground cinnamon

1 cup (225 g) Homemade Cream Cheese (page 46)

3 tablespoons rice malt syrup

1 egg

1½ teaspoons pure vanilla extract (or make your own; page 45)

basil leaves, to serve

Preheat the oven to 180°C (gas 4) and line a baking tray with baking paper.

Trim a very thin slice from the round side of each peach half (so the halves don't topple in transit). Coat each peach half in melted butter and place, cut-side up, on the lined baking tray. Sprinkle with cinnamon.

Beat the cream cheese in a bowl with a stick blender until smooth. Add the rice malt syrup, egg and vanilla and mix together until creamy. Spoon the mixture into the peach centres. Bake for 35 minutes, until everything is crispy and golden.

Serve with a sprinkle of basil leaves.

½ TSP ADDED SUGAR PER SERVE

½ SERVE VEG + FRUIT PER SERVE

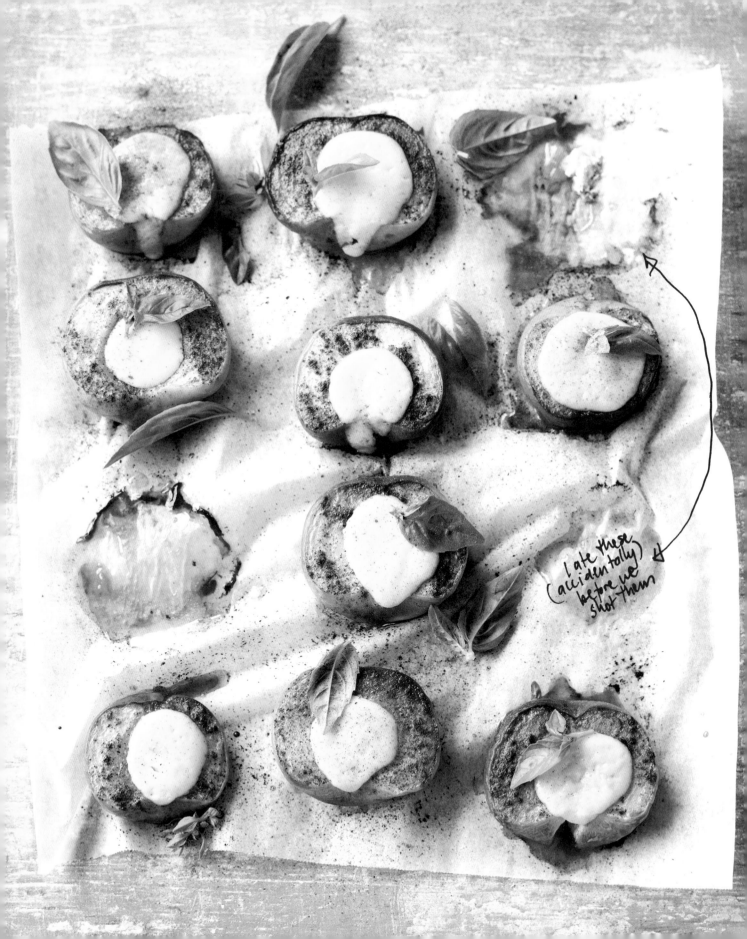

I ate these
(accidentally)
before we
shot them

GOLDEN
HAPPY TIMES

MAKES 6–8

Here's my version of one of Australia's favourite ice creams – made healthy enough to actually feed to kids (though note that they do contain nuts).

400 ml can coconut cream

1/3 cup (75 g) almond butter or cashew butter

1 tablespoon pure vanilla extract (or make your own; page 45)

1/4 teaspoon sea salt

2 tablespoons rice malt syrup

1 teaspoon each coconut oil and rice malt syrup, melted

1/2 cup (85 g) Activated Groaties (page 27)

1/2 cup (125 ml) Basic Raw Chocolate (page 56)

In a small saucepan, combine 1/2 cup (125 ml) of the coconut cream with the nut butter, vanilla, salt and rice malt syrup and whisk continuously over a very low heat until a thick caramel forms (about 10 minutes). Remove from the heat and stir through the rest of the coconut cream until the mixture is creamy. Pour into ice-block moulds and freeze for 4 hours or until set.

Preheat the oven to 180°C (gas 4) and line a baking tray with baking paper.

Since you have the oven on, you might like to make a big batch of these and keep as toppers for yoghurt, porridge, cakes or smoothies. Store in a container for up to 2 months.

Mix the melted coconut oil and rice malt syrup with the groaties and spread them out on the baking tray. Bake in the oven for 10 minutes or until browned. Use your fingers to break up any clusters and set aside.

When the ice creams are set, melt the chocolate in a cup in the microwave (do it gradually on low). Remove the ice creams from their moulds by running the moulds under warm water. Dip each ice cream into the melted chocolate (you might like to do a few coats) and then sprinkle the groaties over the top. You will need to work quickly, as the chocolate will set fast. Place the ice creams on a lined baking tray and freeze for another 5 minutes before serving. Store these in the freezer for 3–4 months.

3/4 TSP ADDED SUGAR PER SERVE

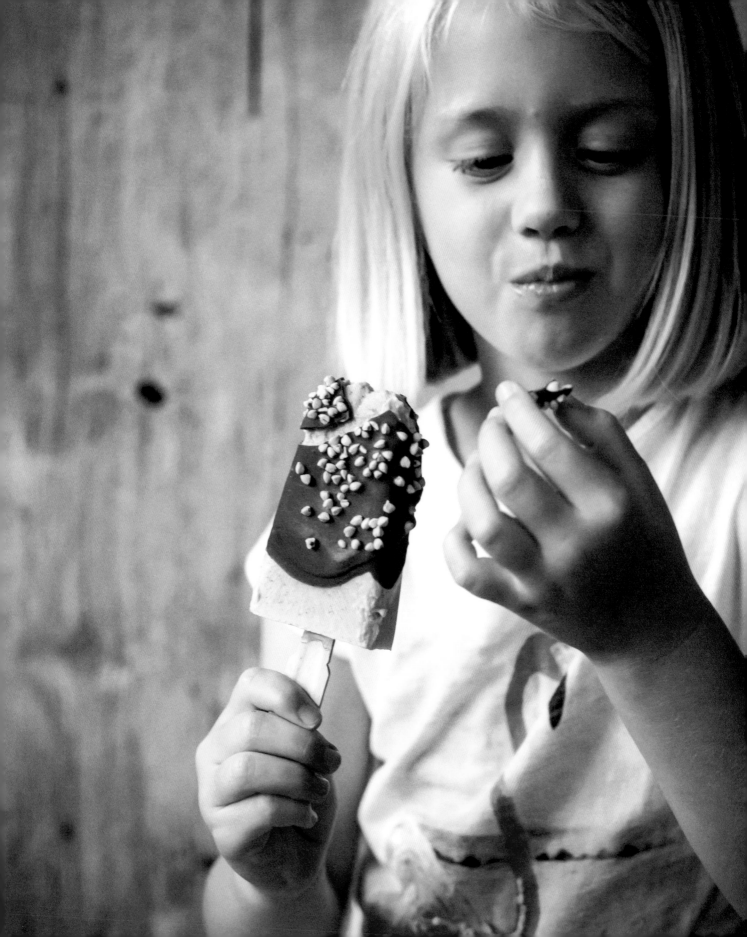

SUNFLOWER STRAWBERRY THUMBLES

MAKES ABOUT 16

These are usually called thimbles, after the sewing thingummyjig you're supposed to use to make the little jam indents. No one I know owns a thimble. Thumbs can be used instead.

1½ cups (200 g) sunflower seeds

½ cup (60 g) buckwheat flour

2 tablespoons arrowroot

1 teaspoon baking powder

pinch of sea salt

¼ cup (50 g) butter or coconut oil, melted

3 tablespoons rice malt syrup

1 egg, separated

1 teaspoon pure vanilla extract (or make your own; page 45)

3 tablespoons Strawberry Chia Jam (page 57)

Preheat the oven to 180°C (gas 4) and line a baking tray with baking paper.

Spread the sunflower seeds on the baking tray and roast in the oven for 10 minutes, tossing them around after 5 minutes, until lightly browned. Put three-quarters of the sunflower seeds into a high-speed blender or food processor and blitz until a coarse meal forms. Transfer to a large mixing bowl and stir in the buckwheat flour, arrowroot, baking powder and salt.

In a small bowl, combine the butter, rice malt syrup, egg yolk and vanilla and whisk with a fork. Fold into the dry ingredients and stir until a dough forms.

Whisk the egg white in a small, clean bowl until foamy. Coarsely chop the remaining sunflower seeds and place in another small bowl.

Roll dessertspoons of the dough into balls. Roll each ball in the foamy egg white and then coat it in the sunflower seeds. Arrange on the baking tray and push down with your thumb (or use a thimble!) to create a well in the centre. Repeat with the remaining dough. Fill each well with ½ teaspoon of jam. Bake for 10–15 minutes, until lightly golden. Transfer to a wire rack and leave to cool; they will firm up once they cool. Store these in an airtight container in the fridge for 4–5 days or freeze for up to 1 month.

Handy for lunchboxes if you pop in a couple of frozen ones.

¼ TSP ADDED SUGAR PER SERVE

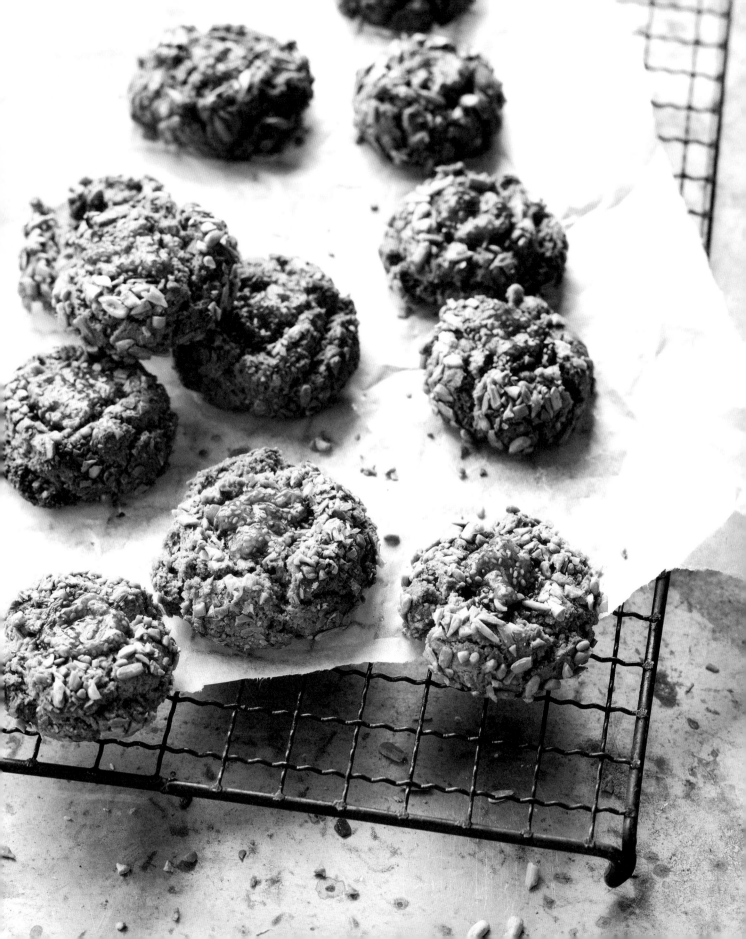

A CELEBRATION MENU

kids' birthdays

CHRISTMAS

Easter

special afternoon teas

weddings.

dinner parties

all of which are
STILL rather healthy

(and LOOK MORE FANCY
than they really are!)

(but don't look too earnest
either!!!)

TOTALLY GAUDY CHRISTMAS TREE CHEESE BALL

500 g cream cheese, preferably homemade (see page 46), at room temperature

250 g cheddar, finely grated (or use 125 g cheddar and 125 g feta or gorgonzola)

1 tablespoon Dijon mustard

3 spring onions, thinly sliced

sea salt and freshly ground black pepper

½ cup (20 g) finely chopped flat-leaf parsley

TO GARNISH

Bacon Bits (page 44)

almond flakes

pomegranate seeds

Blend the cream cheese, cheddar and mustard in a bowl with a stick blender. Stir through the spring onions and season with salt and pepper. Cover and refrigerate for at least 2 hours or overnight (heaps better) to firm.

Get organised! You can make your tree ball to this stage and freeze for up to 2 months.

Before serving, form into a ball and then into a tree shape. Roll the tree-shaped cheese mixture in the parsley, reshaping it with your hands as necessary. Decorate with bacon bits, almond flakes and pomegranate seeds.

Serve with crackers or crudités.

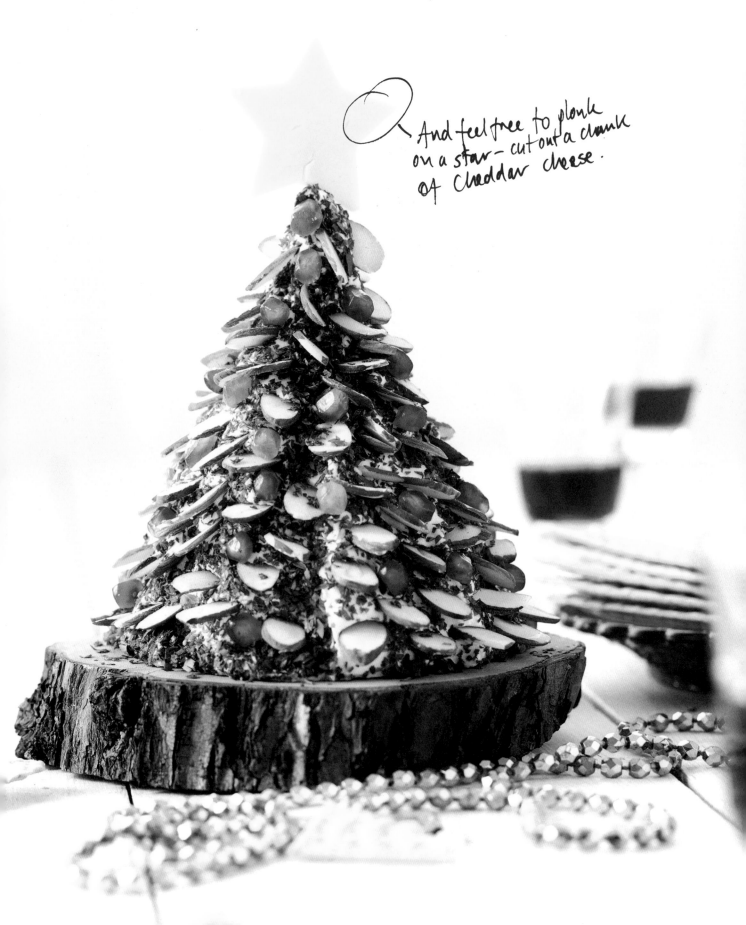

And feel free to plonk
on a star — cut out a chunk
of Cheddar cheese.

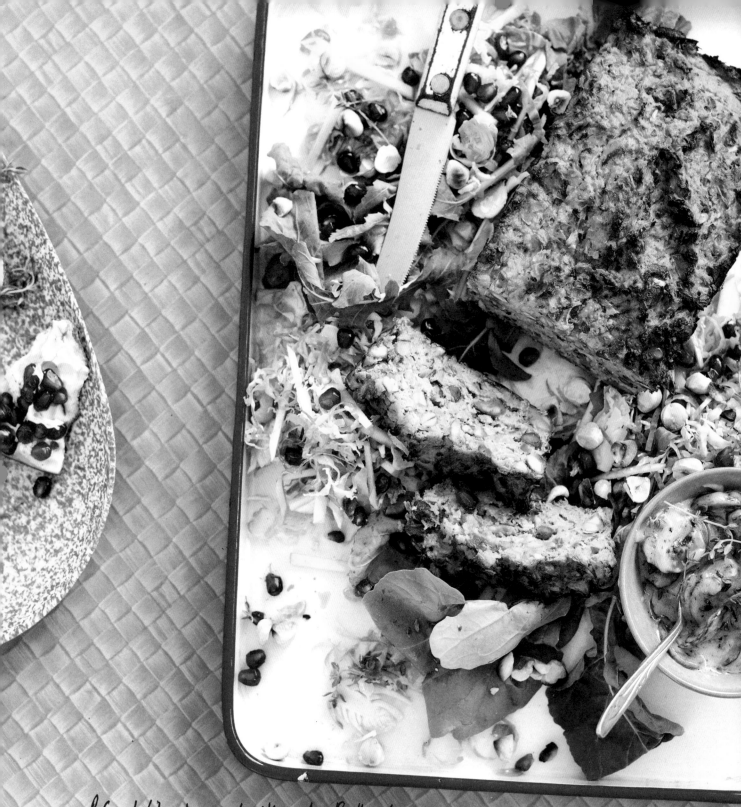

P.S. I like to make this loaf the day
after making a big roast (the Jerk Pork)
I cook extra veg + reserve some of the
juices + add to the mushroom sauce. →

BAKED STUFFING LOAF

WITH MUSHROOM SAUCE AND SHAVED SPROUTS AND PECORINO SALAD

SERVES 6–8

Yep, a vegetarian baked dinner in a loaf with added bits
to make it a dish worthy of a celebration.

*A combo of cauliflower, sweet
potato and celery is great; or
a combo of parsnip, pumpkin
and carrot also works well.*

5 cups (750 g) chopped raw veggies

1 onion, chopped

4 cloves garlic, skin on

3 eggs

1 teaspoon chopped rosemary

1 tablespoon chopped thyme
plus extra sprigs to garnish (optional)

good pinch of sea salt

3 tablespoons flour (any kind)

40 g coconut oil, melted

1 cup (150 g) chopped pistachios

MUSHROOM SAUCE

3 knobs of butter

pinch each of sea salt and
freshly ground black pepper

150 g button mushrooms, sliced

½ cup (125 ml) cream

Preheat the oven to 200°C (gas 6) and line a baking tray and a loaf tin (23 cm ×
13 cm) with baking paper.

*To make it with leftover
veggies, use 4 cups
(600 g) of Roasted
Roots (page 23), skip
the roasting step and
follow the rest of the
recipe (oh, and use just
1 tablespoon of melted
coconut oil).*

Place the vegetables and garlic on the baking tray and roast for 30 minutes. Transfer
to a food processor (squeeze the garlic out of its skin first) and pulse until the
vegetables resemble breadcrumbs. Add the eggs, herbs and salt and blend until
combined, leaving some chunks. Stir through the flour, coconut oil and pistachios.

Pour the mixture into the lined loaf tin and bake for 40–50 minutes until a skewer
inserted into the centre of the loaf comes out clean. (Remove from the oven after
25 minutes and press the extra thyme sprigs into the top of the loaf, if you like.) Set
aside to cool a little.

To make the mushroom sauce, place the butter, salt, pepper and mushrooms in a
small frying pan over a low heat. Cook the mushrooms for 10 minutes until softened,
then stir in cream. Reduce the sauce until the desired consistency is reached.

Lift the loaf from the tin and slice into thick slices. Serve with the Shaved Sprouts
and Pecorino Salad (see below) and the mushroom sauce.

SHAVED SPROUTS AND PECORINO SALAD

SERVES 6–8 AS A SIDE

1 green apple, cut into matchsticks

400 g brussels sprouts, shaved
or grated

½ cup (125 ml) Powerhouse Dressing
(page 53)

2 big handfuls of rocket or watercress leaves

1 cup (100 g) grated pecorino or parmesan

chopped hazelnuts and pomegranate seeds,
to garnish (optional)

Toss the apple, sprouts and dressing in a large bowl and leave to sit for
20 minutes. Serve with the leaves and grated cheese, and sprinkle over the
hazelnuts and pomegranate seeds, if using.

3 SERVES VEG + FRUIT PER SERVE

£1.29 PER SERVE

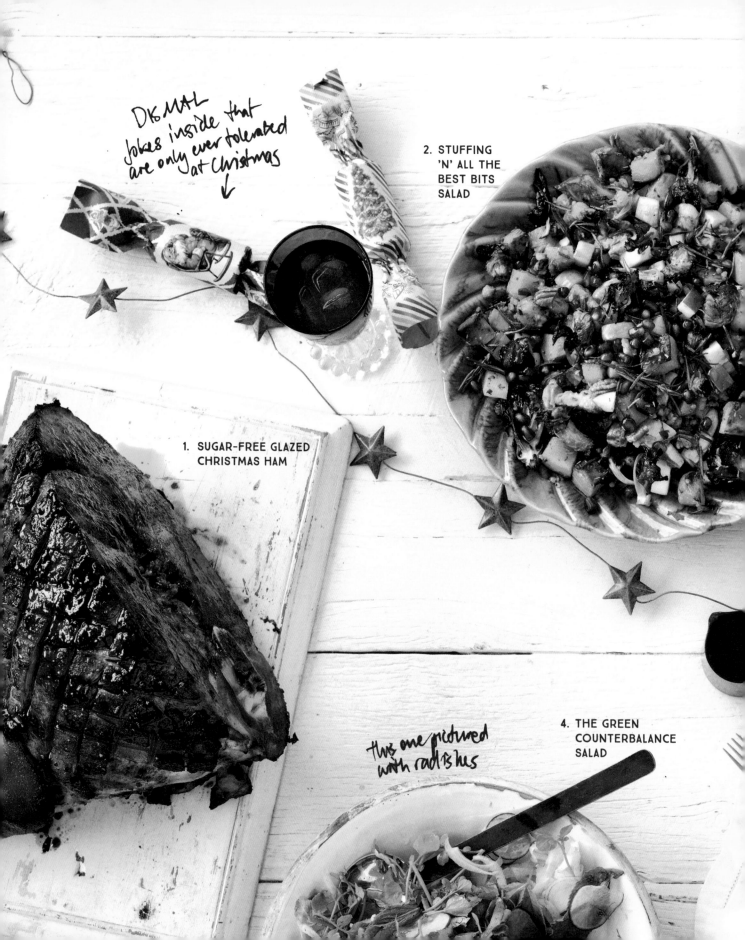

DISMAL jokes inside that are only ever tolerated at Christmas ↓

2. STUFFING 'N' ALL THE BEST BITS SALAD

1. SUGAR-FREE GLAZED CHRISTMAS HAM

this one pictured with radishes

4. THE GREEN COUNTERBALANCE SALAD

A HEALTHY CHRISTMAS DAY SPREAD

Designed to save time, pans, effort + family conflict!

SERVES 12

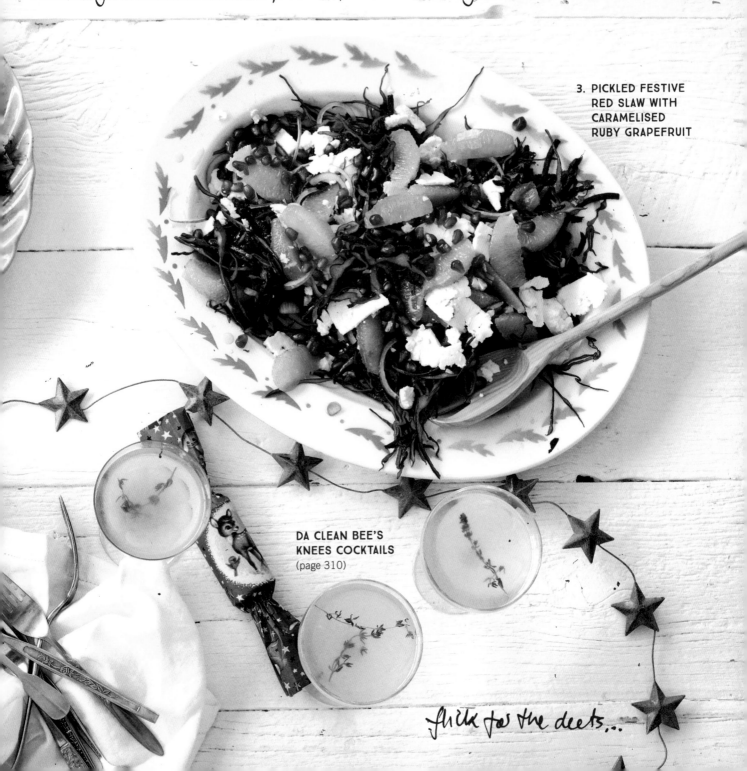

3. PICKLED FESTIVE
RED SLAW WITH
CARAMELISED
RUBY GRAPEFRUIT

DA CLEAN BEE'S
KNEES COCKTAILS
(page 310)

flick for the deets...

1. SUGAR-FREE GLAZED CHRISTMAS HAM

SERVES 8, PLUS LOTS OF LEFTOVERS

Pork neck is an economical cut and pork leg (leg of ham) is, too, surprisingly. Because so few people buy them fresh (everyone buys them pre-smoked as ham), you can get them for a good price.

1.8 kg pork neck
or 2 kg pork leg

½ cup (125 ml) rice malt syrup

4 tablespoons olive oil

1 tablespoon paprika

2 teaspoons ground cloves

1 teaspoon ground cinnamon

1 teaspoon each sea salt
and freshly ground black pepper

zest of 1 orange

3 tablespoons orange juice

Christmas Eve: Line a baking dish with baking paper. Wash the meat under cold running water and pat dry with kitchen paper.

Place the rice malt syrup and olive oil in a jug with 4 tablespoons water. Stir in the spices, salt, pepper and orange zest and juice. Pour over the pork, using your hands to rub the marinade well into the meat. Place in the prepared baking dish. Cover and marinate in the fridge for at least 8 hours or overnight.

Christmas Day: Preheat the oven to 200ºC (gas 6). Remove the ham from the fridge and allow it to stand for 10 minutes. Add a cup of water to the base of the dish and pop the lot in the oven. Bake for 30 minutes, then turn the baking dish around and bake for a further 30 minutes, adding another ½ cup (125 ml) water if necessary. Bake for a further 30 minutes, turning the dish around after 15 minutes. Serve warm with the salads opposite.

2. STUFFING 'N' ALL THE BEST BITS SALAD

SERVES 8

500 g brussels sprouts

800 g butternut squash

2 large parsnips

Cut 'em all into 2.5 cm chunks.

3 sprigs rosemary or thyme, leaves picked and roughly chopped, plus extra to garnish

200 g pancetta, cut into 1 cm cubes

½ cup (125 ml) olive oil or 115 g coconut oil

sea salt and freshly ground black pepper

2 cups (300 g) Cooked Buckwheat (page 27)

1 cup (115 g) pecans, roughly chopped

1 pink lady apple, cut into 1 cm cubes

dash of apple cider vinegar

pomegranate seeds, to garnish

Christmas Eve: Preheat the oven to 200ºC (gas 6). Spread the vegetables, herbs and pancetta on one or two baking trays. Coat with oil and season to taste with salt and pepper. Roast for 45 minutes, turning halfway.

Spread the buckwheat and pecans on another tray and place in the oven. Roast everything (including the veggies) for another 10 minutes or until the pecans are golden. Remove from the oven and allow to cool. Once cooled, transfer each tray of goodies to separate containers and keep them somewhere cool (the laundry perhaps . . . no need to take up fridge space).

Root vegetables improve with cooling – both in texture and flavour – and also provide great resistant starch . . . which will help with post-Christmas digestion.

Christmas Day: In a large serving bowl, toss the vegetables with the roasted buckwheat and pecans. Add the cubed apple and drizzle with a dash of apple cider vinegar. Garnish with pomegranate seeds and the extra rosemary or thyme.

some of this drains away

1½ TSP ADDED SUGAR PER SERVE

£1.39 PER SERVE

2 SERVES VEG + FRUIT PER SERVE

3. PICKLED FESTIVE RED SLAW WITH CARAMELISED RUBY GRAPEFRUIT

SERVES 8

½ red cabbage, shredded

2 beetroots, trimmed, scrubbed and grated

2 purple (or orange) carrots, grated

1 red onion, thinly sliced

½ cup (125 ml) Powerhouse Dressing (page 53)

sea salt and freshly ground black pepper

2 ruby grapefruit or 3 blood oranges or 2 oranges, segmented

a few dobs of butter

½ cup (70 g) crumbled feta, to serve

Christmas Eve/morning: Toss the red cabbage, beetroot, carrot and onion in a bowl with the dressing. Season with salt and pepper. Cover and leave in the fridge overnight (or for a few hours if you want to prepare it on the day).

Christmas Day: Place the grapefruit or orange segments on a tray lined with baking paper. Dot with butter and a sprinkle of salt. Place under the grill (or in a hot oven – with the ham!) and cook for 5–8 minutes. Allow to cool.

To serve, add the caramelised grapefruit or orange to the slaw and sprinkle over the crumbled feta.

4. THE GREEN COUNTERBALANCE SALAD

SERVES 6–8

1 large bunch watercress, leaves picked (or rocket leaves and/or chicory leaves, halved)

2 small fennel bulbs, stalks removed, cored, halved and thinly sliced (reserve the fronds)

2 handfuls of mint leaves

½ red onion, halved and thinly sliced

1 green apple, halved and thinly sliced or 6 radishes, thinly sliced

⅓ cup (75 ml) Powerhouse Dressing (page 53)

Place the leaves, fennel, mint, onion and apple or radish in a large bowl (or on a serving plate). Pour over the dressing and mix. Toss the fennel fronds on top.

MAKE IT BULKIER:
Add 2 cups (270 g) Cooked Quinoa (page 26) or a 400 g can of brown lentils, rinsed and drained, along with 1 cup (150 g) frozen peas, cooked in hot water for 2 minutes, and ½ cup (60 g) toasted pumpkin seeds.

something bitter + green to get gastric juices fired up

1 SERVE VEG + FRUIT PER SERVE

1 SERVE VEG + FRUIT PER SERVE

THREE CLEAN DIGESTIVE COCKTAILS

I called on my mates the Trolley'd boys – two guys who serve cocktails from an old airline trolley at events – to help fine-tune these boozy treats. All three cocktails serve as refreshing aperitifs, with gut-boosting properties.

1. THE BRIGHT SIDE

MAKES 8

4 cm knob of turmeric, peeled and sliced

1 teaspoon fennel seeds

3 tablespoons rice malt syrup

1 cup (250 ml) boiled water

160 ml grapefruit juice

240 ml vodka

fennel flowers, to serve

Muddle the turmeric in a bowl (smash around a little with a spoon to release the juices). Add the fennel seeds, rice malt syrup and boiled water and allow to brew for 20 minutes. Strain and cool.

Make two cocktails at a time by shaking one-quarter of the fennel and turmeric liquid with one-quarter of the remaining ingredients. Strain into chilled cocktail glasses and garnish with fennel flowers.

2. THE CULTURED MULE

MAKES 8

360 ml vodka

1/3 cup (75 ml) lime juice

3 tablespoons rice malt syrup (mixed with 1–2 teaspoons hot water)

650 ml Kombucha (page 344) or use store-bought kombucha

ice and lime wedges, to serve

Combine all of the ingredients in a large jug. Pour into tall glasses over ice and lime wedges.

3. DA CLEAN BEE'S KNEES

MAKES 8

1 cup (250 ml) boiled water

3 tablespoons rice malt syrup

12 sprigs thyme, plus extra to serve

360 ml vodka or gin

120 ml lemon juice

120 ml apple cider vinegar

You may want to add more syrup if you like

Combine the boiled water, rice malt syrup and thyme in a jug and allow to brew for 20 minutes. Strain and cool.

Make two cocktails at a time by shaking one-quarter of the thyme liquid with one-quarter of each of the remaining ingredients. Strain into chilled cocktail glasses and garnish with a sprig of thyme.

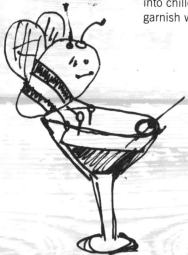

¾ TSP ADDED SUGAR PER SERVE

¾ TSP ADDED SUGAR PER SERVE

¾ TSP ADDED SUGAR PER SERVE

'MAPLE SYRUP' PORK BELLY WITH PECANS

SERVES 6–8

Pork belly is a very fatty, rich piece of meat, but beautifully succulent.
Be sure to eat it with plenty of greenery.

1 kg pork belly, cut into 6–8 thick slices

1/3 cup (75 ml) rice malt syrup

2 cinnamon sticks

1 large red chilli, finely chopped

8 cloves

3 cloves garlic, finely chopped

1/3 cup (75 ml) soy sauce or tamari

1/2 cup (125 ml) Homemade Chicken Stock (page 42)

zest of 1/2 orange, flesh cut into segments (seeds removed)

3 tablespoons apple cider vinegar

TO SERVE

6 cups (600 g) steamed greens (tenderstem broccoli, courgettes and kale is a good combo)

1/2 cup (60 g) pecans, lightly toasted

In the morning: Place the pork slices in the slow-cooker insert, fatty-side up (try to wedge them all in so they fit in one layer). Pour over the rice malt syrup, then add the remaining ingredients. Cover and cook on low for 6–7 hours or high for 4 hours.

If the top of your pork hasn't browned in the slow cooker, place on a foil-lined baking tray and pop under a hot grill for 5 minutes to crisp.

Just before serving: Remove the pork and keep warm. Skim off as much fat from the top of the cooking liquid as you can, place in a jar and refrigerate (lard is great for cooking). Strain the sauce through a fine sieve and return it to the slow-cooker insert. Cook on high with the lid off to thicken while you steam your greens.

Serve the pork with the steamed greens. Sprinkle over the pecans and pour over the sauce.

as I say, this is a rich dish

2 TSP ADDED SUGAR PER SERVE

CACAO CAYENNE PECANS

MAKES 4 CUPS (450 G)

These make a great grown-up Christmas gift. A dad who came to one of my events with his daughter took me aside once and told me I should do more 'chocolate stuff for men'. Hopefully this fits the brief and his daughter finds this recipe.

butter, for greasing

3 egg whites

pinch of sea salt

1/3 cup (75 ml) rice malt syrup

1/3 cup (40 g) raw cacao powder

1/2 teaspoon ground ginger

1/4 teaspoon cayenne pepper (add more if you like a bit of heat)

1 teaspoon ground cinnamon

4 cups (450 g) pecans (preferably activated; page 28)

Preheat the oven to 80°C (for gas ovens, on the pilot light) and grease a stainless-steel baking tray with butter.

Beat the egg whites and salt in a clean bowl. Gradually add the rice malt syrup, then stir in the cacao powder and spices and mix well. Fold in the pecans until well coated. Spread the pecans on the baking tray and place in the oven for 1½ hours, or until the coating hardens. Once cool, store in airtight jars for up to 1 month.

USE THE LEFTOVER EGG YOLKS:
Make an omelette or frittata.
Or freeze them (see page 25).

1 TSP ADDED SUGAR PER SERVE

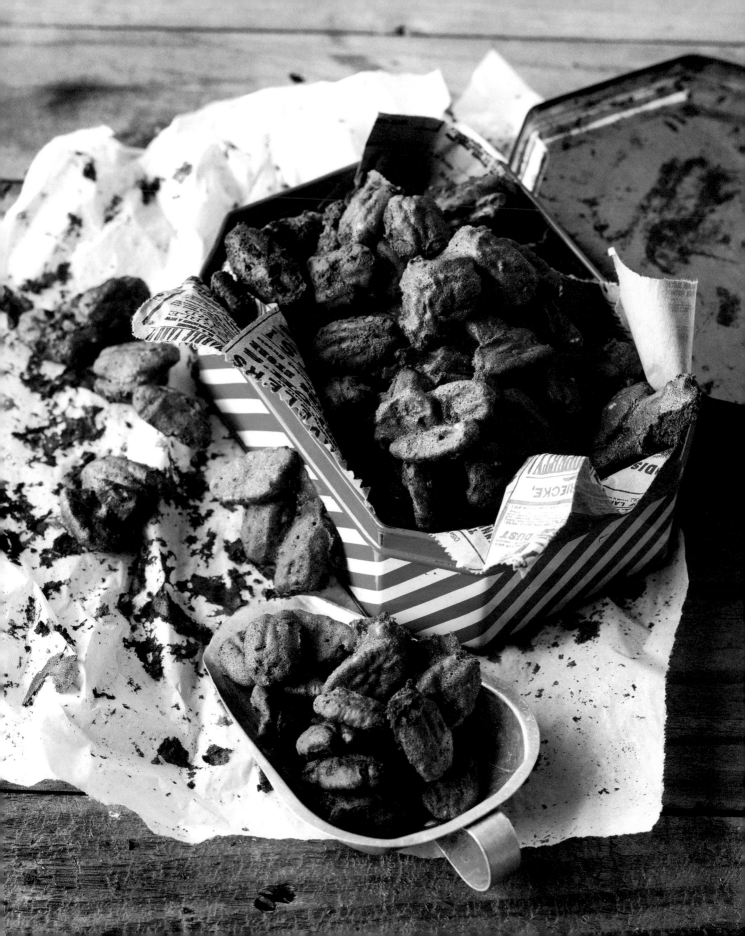

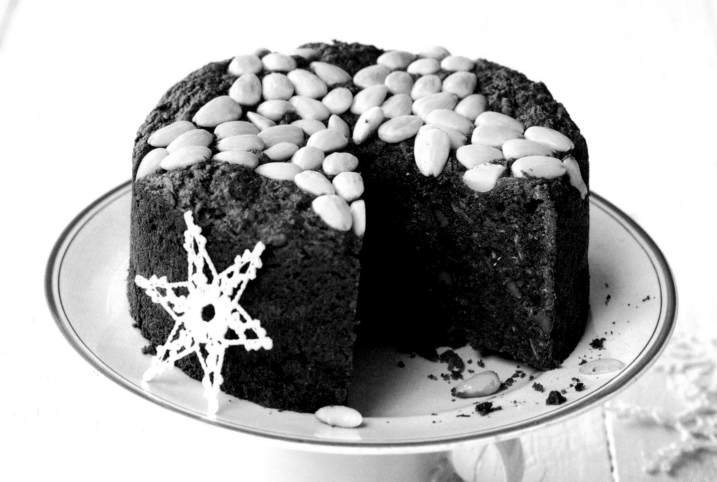

I slice straight from the
freezer, heat in the microwave
+ eat with butter.

MY TOTALLY MESSED-WITH CHRISTMAS CAKE

SERVES 16

I've taken out the dried and glacéed fruit and the gluten, but kept the brandy and almonds, then added dark chocolate, coconut, walnuts and, yeah, beetroot. The result kicks some foolhardy festive goals.

A storage warning
The reason traditional fruit-filled Christmas cakes last for so long is that they're full of sugar and alcohol. Both work as preservatives and in some cases they can keep the cake moist and mould-free for several months. This cake ain't like that. Store it in an airtight container and it should keep for up to a week. Or freeze it for up to 2 months.

2 cups (250 g) gluten-free self-raising flour

1 cup (75 g) shredded coconut

1 cup (100 g) almond meal

4 tablespoons raw cacao powder

1 tablespoon gluten-free baking powder

2 teaspoons ground cinnamon

2 teaspoons ground ginger

2 teaspoons ground cardamom

½ teaspoon ground cloves

1 tablespoon orange zest

1 cup (115 g) walnuts, chopped

100 g dark (85–90% cocoa) chocolate, coarsely chopped

200 g butter, cubed

½ cup (125 ml) rice malt syrup

4 eggs

3 tablespoons brandy

2 cups (300 g) grated beetroot (about 2–3 beetroots)

½ cup (70 g) blanched almonds (optional)

Preheat the oven to 160°C (gas 3) and grease a 20 cm spring-form cake tin.

In a large bowl combine the flour, coconut, almond meal, cacao powder, baking powder, spices and zest. Stir in the walnuts and chocolate.

Melt the butter and rice malt syrup in a small saucepan over a medium heat (or in the microwave). Cool slightly.

Break the eggs into a separate bowl and whisk. Stir in the brandy, then whisk in the melted butter and rice malt syrup.

Pour the wet ingredients into the dry ingredients. Add the beetroot and stir well. Transfer the mixture to the prepared tin and smooth the top. Decorate with blanched almonds (if using). Cover the tin with foil and bake for 1 hour 15 minutes. Remove the foil and cook for a further 15–25 minutes until a skewer inserted into the centre comes out clean. Allow the cake to cool for 20 minutes before removing from the tin.

This cake can be served warm or cold.

1½ TSP ADDED SUGAR PER SERVE

£0.60 PER SERVE   *seriously!*

ISRAELI WHOLE-BAKED CAULIFLOWER

I loved the idea of serving a whole cauli on the table for dinner ('cos I love cauli *that* much) so I did just that, but gave it an Israeli twist. It makes a great dinner-party conversation starter.

1 cup (200 g) full-fat organic plain yoghurt (preferably Greek-style)

1 tablespoon Ras el Hanout Mix (page 45) or 1 teaspoon each sweet paprika, ground cumin and ground coriander

2 teaspoons sumac (optional)

2 teaspoons ground turmeric

1 tablespoon chopped thyme or 1 teaspoon dried thyme

2 cloves garlic, finely chopped

2 cm knob of ginger, finely chopped

1 teaspoon sea salt

zest and juice of 1 lemon

1 head cauliflower, leaves and stalk trimmed

1 tablespoon coconut oil

Green Minx Dressing (page 54), Leftovers Pesto (page 55) or TMT Dressing (page 53), to serve

If your cauli is quite large, feel free to pre-cook it: simmer it in a stockpot with enough water to cover for 20 minutes. Then bake for 40 minutes only.

In a large mixing bowl, combine the yoghurt, spices, thyme, garlic, ginger, salt, zest, and half of the juice. Place the cauliflower headfirst into the yoghurt mixture, moving it around until the entire top is coated. Using your hands, make sure the mixture gets under the florets on the base of the cauliflower. Cover and place in the fridge to marinate for at least 1 hour, preferably overnight.

Preheat the oven to 180°C (gas 4) and line a baking tray with baking paper.

Remove the cauliflower from the bowl, reserving the leftover marinade for serving. Place the cauli on the baking tray and drizzle over the coconut oil. Bake for 1½ hours on the middle shelf of the oven or until the cauli is soft.

Remove from the oven and slice into 6 wedges (do it at the table for effect). Mix the leftover marinade with the remaining lemon juice to make the dressing. Serve the cauli with the marinade dressing and a robust salad – try the Green Counterbalance Salad (page 309) or A Salad of Crushed Olives (page 170).

1 SERVE VEG + FRUIT PER SERVE

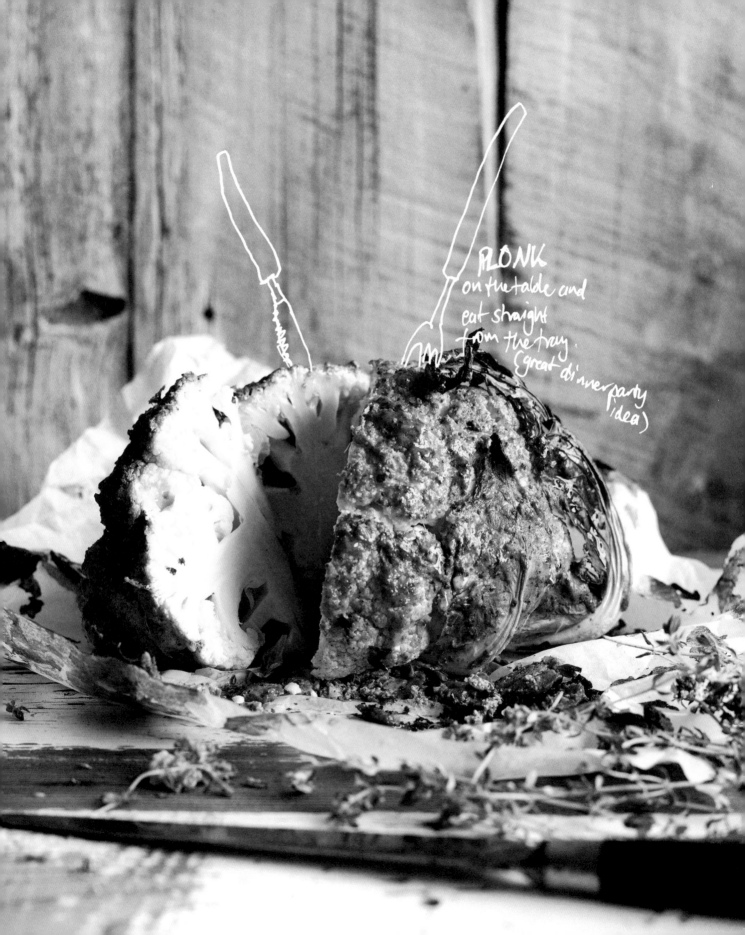

PLONK on the table and eat straight from the tray. (great dinner party idea)

CARDAMOM AND SEA SALT GANACHE TART

SERVES 16

270 ml can coconut cream

2 tablespoons cardamom pods, lightly crushed with a flat blade until the outer husks crack

½ teaspoon pure vanilla powder or 1 teaspoon pure vanilla extract (or make your own; page 45)

100 g dark (85–90% cocoa) chocolate, chopped

pinch of sea salt, plus coarse sea salt, to garnish

berries, edible petals and Activated Groaties (page 27), to garnish (optional)

CRUST

⅓ cup (75 g) coconut oil

4 tablespoons rice malt syrup

2 cups (150 g) shredded coconut

1 tablespoon raw cacao powder

Preheat the oven to 180°C (gas 4).

To make the crust, melt the coconut oil and rice malt syrup in a saucepan. Remove from the heat, add the shredded coconut and cacao powder and mix well. Press the mixture into the base and up the side of a quiche or tart tin – no need to grease it – so that the mixture's approximately 5 mm thick all over. Bake the crust for 15–20 minutes. Remove from the oven and set aside to cool and firm up.

Meanwhile, heat the coconut cream, cardamom pods and vanilla in a saucepan to a simmer, then turn off the heat and cover with a lid. Allow to steep for 10 minutes.

Strain the coconut cream mixture into a bowl, reserving 4 tablespoons in the pan for emergency use later, if needed. Discard the cardamom pods (or save to spice up chai tea). Add the chocolate and salt to the bowl, whisking it through until silky and melted. If the fats separate and your ganache develops a chocolatey cottage-cheese appearance, just add the reserved coconut cream, whisking swiftly to bring it all back together.

Once silky, pour into the tart shell and refrigerate until the ganache sets (at least 2 hours). Garnish with a pinch of coarse sea salt and berries, petals and activated groaties, if desired.

1 TSP ADDED SUGAR PER SERVE

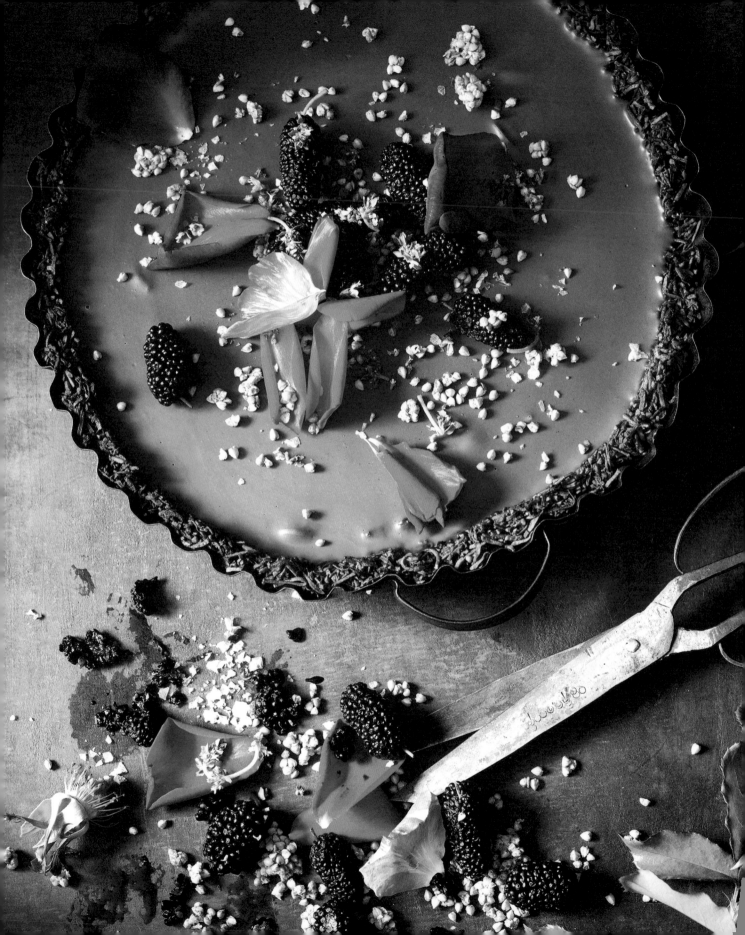

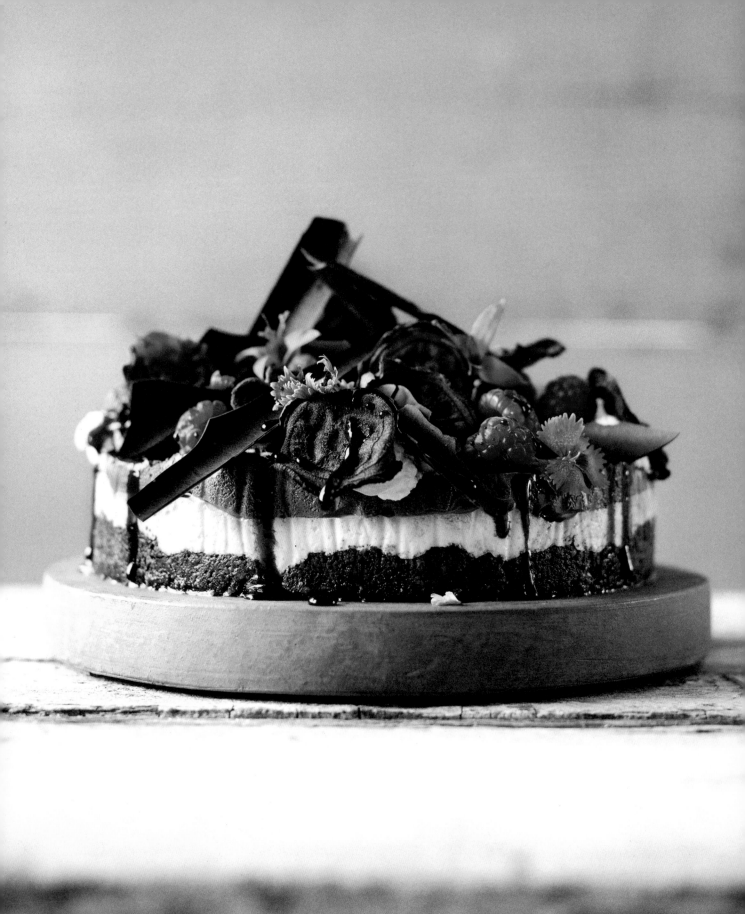

BEETROOT RED VELVET CHEESECAKE

IN WHICH I 'PIMP' TWO FAVOURITE TREATS

SERVES 12

I put out a 'What would you like to see in my next cookbook?' call to action on the interweb. I was overwhelmed with requests to 'pimp' the Crunchynut Cheesecake from my first book as well as the Beetroot Red Velvet Cupcakes from my second book. So I figured I'd do the whole crazy thing in the one spring-form cake tin!

The recipe might look tricky . . . but there is an extraordinary amount of flow to it.

CANDIED BEETROOT

1 beetroot, trimmed and peeled

3 tablespoons rice malt syrup

½ teaspoon pure vanilla powder

BASE

1 cup (125 g) nuts (preferably activated; page 28; skinless hazelnuts are best, but you can use pistachios too)

1 cup (100 g) desiccated coconut

½ cup (50 g) almond meal

½ cup (60 g) raw cacao powder

120 g unsalted butter, softened

CHEESECAKE FILLING

750 g Homemade Cream Cheese (page 46; or use store-bought), at room temperature, plus extra to garnish

3 tablespoons full-fat organic plain yoghurt or sour cream

4 tablespoons coconut cream

4 tablespoons rice malt syrup

1 egg

pinch of pure vanilla powder

4 tablespoons raw cacao powder

GARNISH

50 g dark (85–90% cocoa) chocolate, chopped

edible flowers and raspberries, to garnish

Preheat the oven to 120°C (gas ½) and line a baking tray with baking paper.

To make the candied beetroot, slice the beetroot thinly (about 2 mm) using a sharp knife or mandoline. In a small saucepan, heat the rice malt syrup and vanilla with ½ cup (125 ml) water, stirring until the syrup dissolves. Bring to the boil. Add the beetroot slices and top with more water so that the beetroot is just covered. Return to the boil and simmer for 20 minutes, or until the beetroot slices are tender and translucent. Remove the beetroot, reserving the leftover liquid for making the cheesecake filling. Lay the beetroot slices on the prepared tray and bake for 1 hour, or until crispy. Remove from the oven and allow to cool.

To make the base, increase the oven temperature to 180°C (gas 4) and line a 23 cm spring-form cake tin with baking paper. Grind the nuts in a food processor until semi-fine. Transfer to a mixing bowl with the coconut, almond meal, cacao powder and butter and rub with your fingers to make a dough. (The more you rub, the more you'll release the oils in the nuts and achieve the right consistency.) Add more butter if required. Press the mixture evenly into the base of the tin so the crust is about 1.5 cm thick. Bake for 10 minutes. Remove and allow to cool completely.

1½ TSP ADDED SUGAR PER SERVE

continued over...

BEETROOT RED VELVET CHEESECAKE [... CONT'D]

To make the cheesecake filling, combine the cream cheese, yoghurt or sour cream, coconut cream, rice malt syrup, egg and vanilla in a large bowl. Don't over-mix, and try to keep the aeration to a minimum while stirring (too much air will make the filling puff up and then collapse during cooking). Transfer half of the mixture to another bowl and stir through 2–3 tablespoons of the reserved beetroot liquid and the cacao powder. Spoon the vanilla layer onto the cooled base, then layer the beetroot and cacao mix on top. Return to the oven for 20–30 minutes until the mixture pulls away from the side a little and the centre is custard-like (don't overcook). Place in the fridge for at least 2 hours to firm.

To make chocolate shards for the garnish, melt the chocolate slowly in a microwave (or in a heatproof bowl over a saucepan of boiling water, making sure the base of the bowl doesn't touch the water). Pour onto a sheet of baking paper and spread evenly with a palette knife. Cover with a second sheet of baking paper and smooth out any bubbles. Gently roll up to form a 3.5 cm tube. Place in the fridge for 30 minutes to set. Unroll carefully to reveal instant shards.

Adorn the cold cheesecake with the candied beetroot chips, edible flowers, chocolate shards and raspberries, using the extra cream cheese to keep things in place.

THAI LATTES

1½ tablespoons gelatine powder

3 teaspoons lemongrass and ginger tea leaves (or use 3 teabags)

½ small red chilli, chopped, or 2 kaffir lime leaves, chopped (optional)

3 tablespoons rice malt syrup

1 cup (250 ml) Supercharged Coconut Frosting (page 56)

4 tablespoons roasted peanuts and/or coconut flakes, toasted

shredded kaffir lime leaves or lime zest, to serve

'Bloom' the gelatine by stirring it into ⅓ cup (75 ml) cold water until dissolved. Let it sit for 5 minutes until it becomes rubbery.

Meanwhile, place the tea (in a tea ball if using leaf tea), chilli or kaffir lime leaves (if using) and rice malt syrup in a saucepan with 2 cups (500 ml) boiling water. Leave to steep, then remove the tea and chilli or kaffir lime and strain. Use a whisk or stick blender to blend the gelatine into the mixture until smooth.

Pour into teacups or glasses and chill in the fridge for 4 hours to set.

To serve, top with the coconut frosting, sprinkle with peanuts and/or coconut and garnish with shredded kaffir lime leaves or lime zest.

1½ TSP ADDED SUGAR PER SERVE

MY SPECTACULAR
POPSTICK CAKE

For many, the end of a dinner party is the real test of their no-sugar resolve. So, here you go: dessert, chocolate and wine all combined into one fun, distracting package. I used an old polystyrene ball chopped in half to poke the sticks into. You could use some of your kid's play dough or I guess an orange, halved, would do it. But that would seem a waste of an orange. Source flowers from your garden/neighbourhood to add extra flourish and dig up some sparklers from that drawer where such things get lost.

POMEGRANATE AND COCONUT
VODKA POPSTICKS

MAKES 6

COCONUT LAYER

4 tablespoons gelatine powder

270 ml can coconut cream

½ teaspoon granulated stevia, or to taste

VODKA LAYER

4½ tablespoons gelatine powder

¾ cup (175 ml) boiling water

½ teaspoon granulated stevia, or to taste

¾ cup (175 ml) vodka

1–2 teaspoons rosewater, to taste (you may need to use more, depending on the strength)

seeds of 1 pomegranate

To make the coconut layer, 'bloom' the gelatine by stirring it into ⅓ cup (75 ml) cold water until dissolved. Let it sit for 5 minutes until it becomes 'rubbery'.

Put the coconut cream and stevia in a saucepan and heat until almost boiling. Remove from the heat and add the bloomed gelatine, breaking up the blobby bits and using a stick blender to purée. When cooled a little, pour into ice-block moulds to one-third full and freeze for 1 hour.

To make the vodka layer, make up another batch of jelly, blooming the gelatine as above. Combine the boiling water with the stevia. Allow to cool a little, then stir in the vodka and rosewater. Sprinkle pomegranate seeds over the set coconut layer and pour over the vodka mixture. Insert the ice-block sticks and return to the freezer to set. Serve with a few more pomegranate seeds sprinkled on top, if you like.

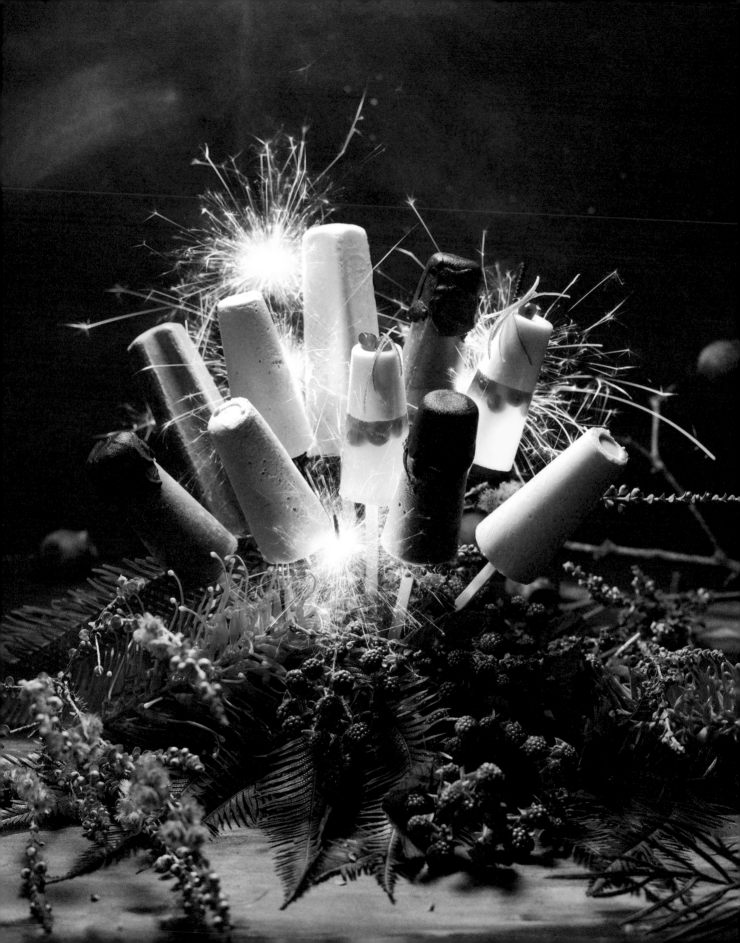

MARGARITA POPSTICKS

MAKES 6

Made specifically for my mate Zoe who's partial to some salt and lime on a rim.

juice of 5 limes, plus 1 lime, peeled and cubed

1½ cups (350 ml) coconut milk

1 large avocado

4 tablespoons tequila, or to taste

1½ tablespoons rice malt syrup or 5 drops liquid stevia

1½ teaspoons sea salt

Place everything except the lime chunks in a blender and whizz until smooth. Pour the margarita mixture into six ice-block moulds. Add chunks of lime and insert ice-block sticks. Freeze for at least 1 hour until slushie-like, and then stir to distribute the lime chunks evenly. Freeze for a further 3 hours.

CHOCOLATE AND RED WINE CREAMSTICKS

MAKES 6

¾ cup (175 ml) leftover red wine

1 cinnamon stick or 1 teaspoon ground cinnamon

1 teaspoon ground allspice

1 teaspoon cloves

1 cup (250 ml) coconut cream

½ avocado

1 tablespoon rice malt syrup or 4 drops liquid stevia

3 tablespoons raw cacao powder

50 g dark (85–90% cocoa) chocolate, or 3 cubes frozen Basic Raw Chocolate (page 56)

Heat the wine and spices in a saucepan over a medium heat. Simmer for 10 minutes (it will reduce quite a bit). Cool slightly, then strain and pour into a blender. Add the coconut cream, avocado, rice malt syrup or stevia and cacao powder. Blend until smooth. Pour into ice-block moulds and insert the sticks. Freeze for at least 4 hours.

Melt the chocolate in a cup in the microwave (do it gradually on low), or in a heatproof bowl over a saucepan of boiling water, making sure the base of the bowl doesn't touch the water. Dip the top of each creamstick into the chocolate and return to the freezer (use your mould to keep them propped vertically) until ready to serve.

½ TSP ADDED SUGAR PER SERVE

½ TSP ADDED SUGAR PER SERVE

PUMPKIN SPICE-A-CHINO

2 tablespoons gelatine powder

2 x 400 ml cans coconut cream

1 cup (250 ml) Pumpkin Purée (page 23)

3 tablespoons rice malt syrup

2 teaspoons Pumpkin Spice Mix

ground cinnamon or grated dark (85–90% cocoa) chocolate, to serve

CHINO FOAM

300 ml coconut cream (reserved from above)

1 tablespoon gelatine powder

2 teaspoons rice malt syrup

'Bloom' the gelatine by stirring it into ⅓ cup (75 ml) cold water until dissolved. Let it sit for 5 minutes until it becomes rubbery.

Place 2 cups (500 ml) of the coconut cream in a saucepan with the Pumpkin Purée and rice malt syrup. (Refrigerate the remaining coconut cream for the Chino Foam.) Heat gently, then remove and stir in the gelatine and Pumpkin Spice Mix. Using a stick blender, blend the mixture until smooth. Pour into cups or glasses and refrigerate for 4 hours or until set.

About 10 minutes before the mixture is set, make the Chino Foam. Remove the reserved coconut cream from the fridge and blend with a stick blender. Slowly pour in the gelatine in a thin stream, followed by the rice malt syrup. Continue mixing until the mixture is fluffy (2–3 minutes).

To serve, top with Chino Foam and sprinkle with cinnamon or chocolate.

MAKE IT AN AUSTRALIANA MANGO FLAT WHITE:
Follow the recipe above, replacing the Pumpkin Purée with 1 cup (170 g) chopped mango and omitting the Pumpkin Spice Mix. Top with Chino Foam and serve with a pinch of lime zest and frozen mango cubes, if you have some.

1½ TSP ADDED SUGAR PER SERVE

HOT CROSS MUFFINS

MAKES 8

I've spent four Easters perfecting a HXB that contains no gluten,
no dried fruit and no gooby additives that no one has in their pantry . . .
but that still tastes like the things Woolies starts selling shortly after
Christmas. Here she is . . .

50 g coconut oil or butter,
melted, plus extra for greasing

1½ cups (150 g) almond meal

4 tablespoons arrowroot

1½ teaspoons baking powder

1 teaspoon ground cinnamon

1 teaspoon ground ginger

1 teaspoon ground nutmeg

1 teaspoon Pumpkin Spice Mix (page 45)
or ¾ teaspoon ground cinnamon and
¼ teaspoon ground nutmeg

¼ teaspoon ground cloves

pinch of sea salt

4 tablespoons chopped pecans

50 g dark (85–90% cocoa)
chocolate, roughly chopped

zest of 1 orange

1 teaspoon pure vanilla extract
(or make your own; page 45)

1 tablespoon rice malt syrup

3 eggs, lightly beaten

4 tablespoons gluten-free plain flour
(regular plain and spelt are fine too)

butter, to serve

Preheat the oven to 180°C (gas 4) and grease an 8-hole muffin tray.

Place the almond meal, arrowroot, baking powder, spices, salt, pecans,
chocolate and orange zest in a mixing bowl and stir until combined.

In a separate bowl, lightly whisk the melted butter or coconut oil, vanilla, rice
malt syrup and eggs. Pour the wet ingredients into the dry ingredients and mix
until smooth. Spoon the mixture evenly into the muffin holes.

Whisk the flour with 2–3 tablespoons of water to make a thick paste.
Spoon the mixture into a piping bag (or a zip-lock bag with one corner snipped),
and squeeze onto each muffin to make a cross. Bake for 15 minutes, or until
brown on the top. Cool for a minute or so, then slice open and serve with
a dollop of butter.

½ TSP ADDED SUGAR PER SERVE

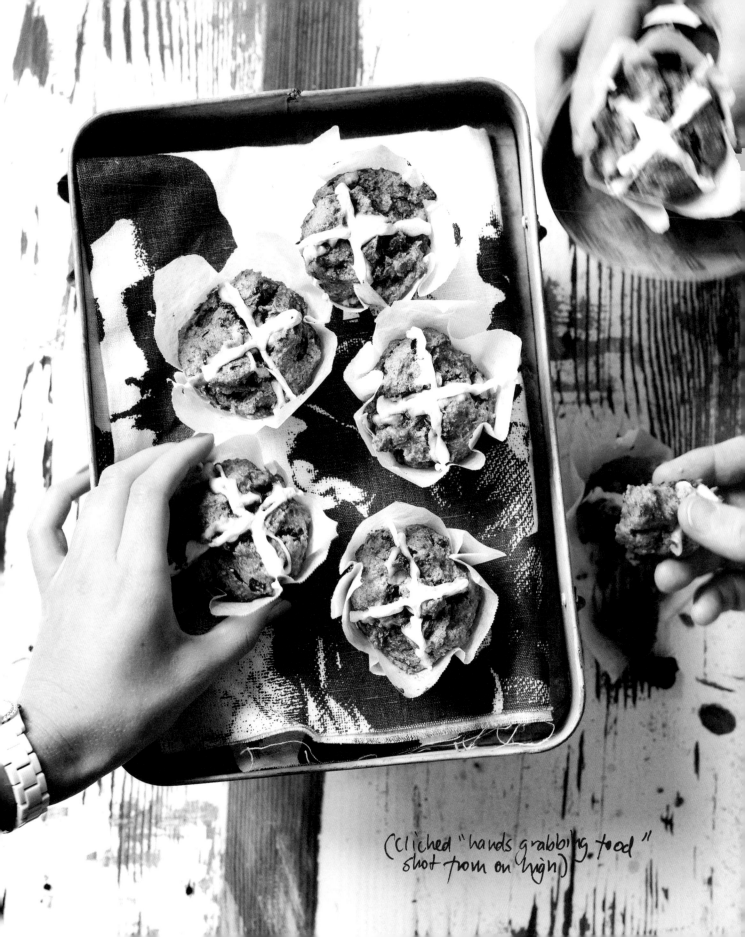

(cliched "hands grabbing food"
shot from on high)

GREEN SMOOTHIE CAKE WITH LEMON CHEESE WHIP

SERVES 14

butter or coconut oil, for greasing

1 bunch spinach (about 300 g), roots trimmed, leaves and stems roughly chopped

zest and juice of 1 lemon

3 eggs

½ cup (125 ml) rice malt syrup

2 teaspoons pure vanilla extract (or make your own; page 45)

1½ cups (250 g) brown rice flour mixed with 2½ teaspoons baking powder

⅓ cup (75 ml) extra-virgin olive oil

1¾ cups (175 g) almond meal

1 courgette, finely grated and squeezed in a clean tea towel to remove moisture

1½ cups (375 g) Cream Cheese Frosting (page 56)

Preheat the oven to 180°C (gas 4). Grease and line a 20 cm square or round cake tin with non-stick baking paper.

Place the spinach in a food processor and process until very finely chopped. Add the lemon juice and process to form a paste.

Beat the eggs and rice malt syrup in a large bowl until thick and glossy – this will take about 4–5 minutes using an electric mixer. (A ribbon should fall from the beaters when lifted.) Beat in the vanilla and lemon zest. Using a large metal spoon, gradually fold in the flour alternately with the oil. Fold in the almond meal and mix until smooth, then stir through the spinach and courgette. Spoon the mixture into the prepared tin and smooth the surface. Bake for 45–50 minutes, or until a skewer inserted into the centre comes out clean. Leave in the tin to cool completely.

When cool, use a small spatula to ice the cake with the frosting. Cut into slices to serve.

This cake is best served fresh but can be stored in an airtight container in the fridge for 3 days. Or you can slice and freeze it for up to 1 month.

1½ TSP ADDED SUGAR PER SERVE

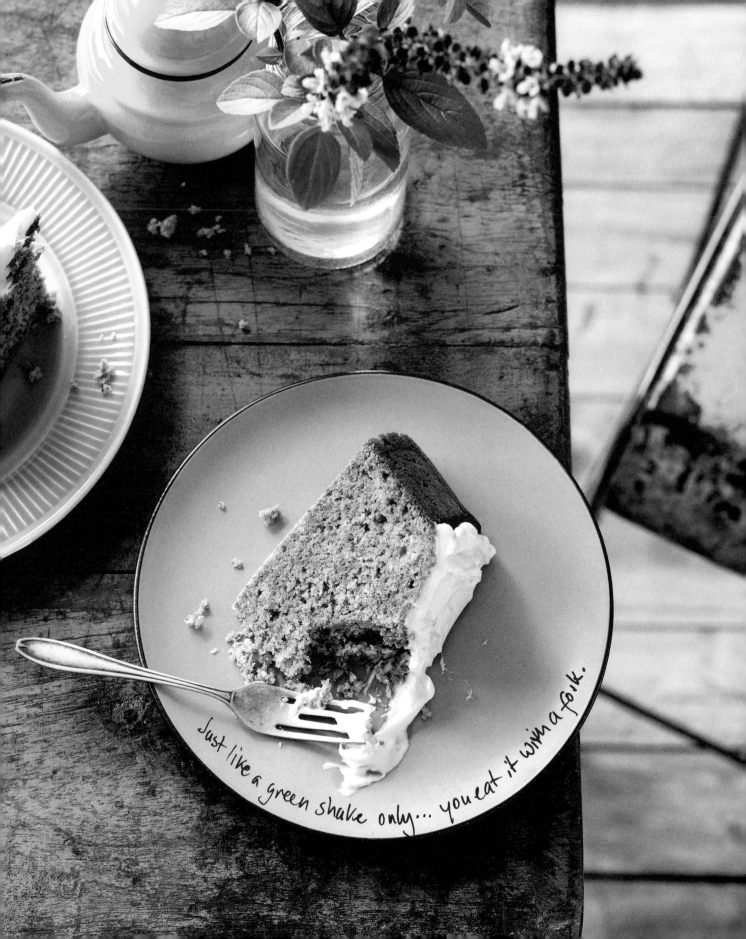

Just like a green shake only... you eat it with a fork.

FERMENTS AND OTHER
GUT-HEALING
FUNCTIONAL FOODS

witchy FERMENTED, sprouted and BACTERIA-blooming stuff

for STUPENDOUSLY healthy, happy, balanced interior health. ☺

FERMENTED VEGETABLES.

New to the concept? Jaded by the multi-step hoopla? I've given the fad a simplicious makeover and streamlined things for us all.

WHY FERMENT?

It saves food
Lacto-fermentation has been around for aeons as a way to preserve food when it's in seasonal abundance. Unlike pickling (which uses heat, vinegar and sugar), lacto-fermentation uses salt (and sometimes whey) to encourage the veggie's natural 'good' (*lactobacillus*) bacteria to flourish, producing lactic acid that staves off dodgy bacteria. Pickling, on the other hand, pretty much kills off everything.

It's a condiment flavour bomb
Ferments are a condiment on their own and ferment juices add kick to sauces, deglazes, dressings and leftovers.

It unlocks extra nutrition
Lactic acid activates enzymes in the vegetable that aid digestion, and unlocks a bunch of vitamins, including vitamin C and vitamin A as well as the much-revered vitamin K2 – a known cancer fighter.

It builds gut health
It promotes the growth of healthy flora in the intestine.

It cuts sugar content
The sugar in the veggie is what ferments; the same process sees red wine end up almost fructose-free.

And reduces sugar cravings
This is the other BIG reason to ferment – it helps you quit the white stuff. Scientists have found that gut bacteria actually secrete special proteins that are similar to hunger-regulating hormones, affecting both our food cravings and mood. In other words, the little buggers try to get us to eat foods that *they* thrive on. So if you eat lots of sugar, you feed the bacteria that love it, locking yourself into the craving cycle. Eating fermented food, however, amps up the healthy bacteria, overpowering the sugar-lovin' microbes and weakening the craving signals.

WHAT DO YOU NEED?

You could follow all the complex methods . . . or you can do as I do and cut steps and ingredients and then to the chase. You just need:

- super-fresh and organic vegetables that are currently abundant

- a few glass jars (about 1 litre is ideal) with tight-fitting lids

- a fair dose of salt and/or whey (see page 46 for how to make your own whey), both of which work as fermenting starters

- some spices to help act as fungicides (fenugreek, fennel, coriander, mustard, caraway or chilli seeds, or just peppercorns)

- something to act as a weight (see 'Always submerge your ferments', opposite)

Which salt?
Himalayan rock salt is best. It's a very dry salt and contains no harmful moulds (which can be found in some sea salt). Don't use bog-standard table salt – for anything! – as the iodine will kill the ferment.

WHAT TO KEEP IN MIND

Follow these tips to make your ferments fabulous.

Always submerge your ferments
Your veg will ferment instead of rot *only* if they're fully covered in liquid – either brine or salt-released veggie juices. If you ever come up short, add some brine.

The best way to keep the vegetables from floating above the liquid is to cut a cabbage-leaf circle slightly larger than the mouth of the jar and fit it over the vegetables. Or use a small glass jar that fits snugly into the mouth of your jar, filled with water. Or a clean stone!

Temperature matters
Around 16–22°C is ideal and will ensure a nicely paced ferment. In colder climates, stick your ferment on top of the fridge and perhaps use a little whey. In warmer places, you'll just have to put up with a faster ferment that's not quite as tangy.

Always add spices and herbs
Chilli, garlic, peppercorns, caraway, fenugreek, fennel, coriander and mustard seeds are chucked in for a reason – they act as mould inhibitors.

Keep the lid loose
This stops the jar exploding. You might like to place a bowl underneath in case it does bubble over. I do.

Don't fret about mould
You might see a white furry film develop on the surface. It won't hurt you. Skim it off as soon as you see it.

CHOPPED SALAD PICKLE

MAKES A 1 LITRE JAR

This is the simplest ferment doing the rounds. And so pretty to boot.

1 teaspoon spices or herbs (chilli flakes, black or white peppercorns, bay leaf, dill seeds, fennel seeds, coriander seeds)

3 cups (450 g) chopped vegetables (cauliflower, courgettes, beans, beetroot, carrot, radishes, peppers, turnip, broccoli, red onion, spring onions)

2 cups (500 ml) water mixed with 1 tablespoon Himalayan pink salt

I use my pickle as I would gherkins – diced and added to mayo to make a tartare, or to a salsa for an extra boost.

Place the spices or herbs in the base of your jar. Arrange the chopped veggies in lovely layers, leaving 4 cm of room at the top. Pour in enough brine to cover, leaving 3 cm clear of the rim. Place a cabbage leaf or weight on top to submerge the veggies. Seal loosely (or cover with a cloth) and keep at room temperature for 2–7 days (the colder it is the longer it will take). You'll need to try it after the second day. Once it tastes tarty and the liquid is a bit fizzy, seal and transfer to the fridge where it will keep for several months.

If you use peppers in your pickle, use 1 tablespoon of salt for every cup (250 ml) water.

MAKE IT A CHARD STEM PICKLE:

Use 3 cups (300 g) chard or beetroot leaf stems sliced into 2 cm pieces, 1 small sprig of dill or thyme and ½ teaspoon each of chilli flakes, fennel seeds and coriander seeds and follow the recipe above.

Just a note: these stems can go mushy easily, so don't use whey. Also, try to make it during cooler periods and use 4 tablespoons of salt.

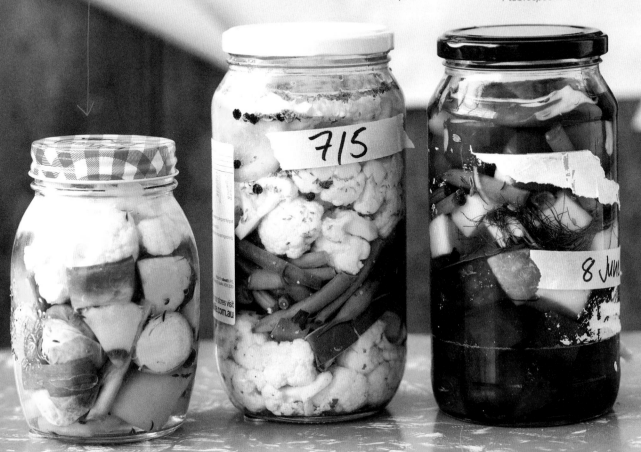

'BUCHA MUSTARD

(£0.62) to make at home
(£5.54) to buy

MAKES 1 JAR

As little as 1 teaspoon of mustard seeds will provide a potent injection of antioxidants and anti-inflammatory helpers selenium and magnesium. So goes the research. Ferment the little things with life-giving kombucha and the ante is upped that little bit more.

1 packet whole mustard seeds (brown or yellow)

Plain Kombucha (page 344) or use store-bought

Fill a glass jar (preferably broad-mouthed) with mustard seeds to about one-third full. Add enough kombucha to cover the seeds. Place the lid on loosely (or cover with a tea towel) to allow air to release, and leave on the kitchen worktop for 5–10 days (fewer days in summer). Check the seeds each day and add extra kombucha to ensure the seeds stay covered in a little liquid and remain moist. The seeds will swell and come to fill the jar – pretty fun to watch! Once they stop absorbing liquid, and you see bubbles forming, blend into a paste using a stick blender (if you've used a broad-mouthed jar, you can do this in the jar).

MAKE IT GARLICKY:
Add a clove or two before pouring on the kombucha.

MAKE IT COOLING FOR PITTA TYPES:
Add some coriander seeds before pouring on the kombucha.

Brown or yellow mustard?
In Ayurvedic parlance, mustard seeds increase Pitta (fire) while minimising Vata (air) and Kapha (earth and water). Brown mustard seeds are hotter and more pungent and potent. They are balancing for Kapha and Vata. Yellow seeds impart a milder, Dijon flavour and are better for Pitta types (also see the 'Make it cooling' variation).

Food Nerd Tip: Coconut oil turns from solid to liquid at 22°C. I use a jar of it to gauge my perfect ferment conditions!

SIMPLICIOUS SAUERKRAUT

MAKES 3–4 CUPS (ABOUT 850 ML)

In my previous books, I've shared a recipe that involves shredding and hammering and pushing and fussing a big ball of cabbage into submission. Since then I've got simplicious with my 'kraut. I'm rather happy with the far more elegant result.

Red cabbage makes a slightly sweeter and crunchier 'kraut.

1 small (or ½ large) white or red cabbage, cored, cut into wedges and rinsed

1 tablespoon caraway seeds

3 tablespoons Himalayan pink salt

Shred the cabbage in a food processor using the grater option (or use a hand grater . . . tedious!). Toss with the caraway seeds and salt in a big bowl and let it sit for 30 minutes. Spoon into a large jar (or several), pressing down as you go so the juices come to the top of the cabbage. Fill each jar, leaving 3 cm of room at the top. Place a weight on top (to help the juices rise), then seal loosely and keep at room temperature for 1–3 days. Transfer to the fridge where it will keep for several months.

MAKE IT YOUR OWN FLAVOUR:
Substitute the caraway seeds with mustard seeds, cumin seeds or white peppercorns.

MAKE IT A PINK SAUERKRAUT:
Replace half of the cabbage with 1–2 beetroots, scrubbed, and follow the recipe as above. (Oh, and use a red cabbage.)

Salt versus whey
Salt encourages the growth of local bacteria found on the vegetable itself, which is always best. It also slows and tempers the ferment process. Plus salt hardens the pectins in vegetables, giving them added crunch and a bitier flavour.

Whey produces a more rounded flavour in ferments than salt, but can also lead to slightly mushy vegetables, in part because it speeds up the ferment process.

I tend to use whey in winter, and in sauces, mayo and pesto. I use salt when the temperature is around 23°C or higher.

'BUT THE KITCHEN SINK' KIMCHI

MAKES ABOUT 8 CUPS (2 LITRES)

This is one of my favourite ferments. Mostly 'cos you can make huge quantities with minimal effort and then use it with gay abandon to boost casseroles and stews and toasties (page 84). Feel free to choose your own veggies (though cabbage is a staple). Beans and okra also work well.

12 radishes or 1 small daikon

2 carrots (orange, yellow or purple)

1 green apple

1 onion or ½ bunch spring onions, chopped

1 Chinese leaves, coarsely chopped (or ½ red cabbage, shredded)

1 bunch pak choi or ½ bunch kale, stems removed (or ½ bunch dandelion greens), coarsely chopped

5 cm knob of ginger or turmeric, finely chopped

5 cloves garlic, finely chopped

1–2 large red chillies, finely chopped or 1½ teaspoons chilli flakes

3 tablespoons fish sauce or dulse flakes (or a couple of tinned anchovies, chopped)

3 tablespoons Himalayan pink salt

Or you can use brussels sprouts, quartered

Grate the radishes or daikon, carrots, apple and onion or spring onions using a blender with a grater option (or use a grater) and place in a large glass or ceramic bowl. Add the remaining ingredients and, using your bare hands, massage and squeeze the mixture to release the juices. Cover with a tea towel and let it sit overnight.

The next day scoop into a large jar (or two smaller ones), leaving 5 cm clear at the top. Try not to leave much more than this – more air means more chance of the ferment going mouldy. And make sure the ingredients are completely submerged in liquid (if not, add a little water). Place a weight on top to submerge the veggies, put the lid on loosely and leave on the worktop (ideally at 20–22°C) for 2–3 days until it starts to fizz a little. Screw the lid on tight and store in the fridge for up to 3 months.

MY INDIAN KIMCHI

MAKES 4–6 CUPS (ABOUT 1–2 LITRES)

There are four reasons I wrap my turmeric-stained arms around this sweet-but-tangy mix-up of the Korean classic. Daikon boosts the digestive enzymes we need to break down fats, complex carbohydrates and proteins. It's also been shown to counteract the carcinogens in processed and fried foods, which is why it is traditionally served with tempura in Japan. Even better, when eaten with foods high in beta-carotene (um, like carrots!!) daikon improves the body's ability to absorb vitamin D. And, even betterer . . . When's the best time to make this little combo I've put together you may ask? Funnily enough, at the end of summer when carrots and daikon are at their peak . . . and just as we're heading into the darker months. Which is when our vitamin D levels drop. Oh, it's all such a beautiful thing!

800 g–1 kg carrots, peeled

1 daikon, peeled

5–7 cm knob of turmeric, peeled

2 large red chillies, finely chopped
(or 1 tablespoon chilli flakes)

2 teaspoons fenugreek seeds

2 teaspoons mustard seeds

3 tablespoons Himalayan pink salt
(in summer) or 1 tablespoon salt and
4 tablespoons Homemade Whey (page 46;
in winter)

I use salt to make kimchi because to get the best 'fizzy' vibe, the ferment needs to be slowed down a little. Of course, if your house is cooler than, say, 20°C, feel free to prod things and use a bit of whey and less salt.

Grate the carrots, daikon and turmeric (use the grater attachment on your blender or food processor) and place in a glass or ceramic bowl. Add the rest of the ingredients. Mix and let sit for 20 minutes to allow the salt (and whey, if using) to release the juices. If it's not looking juicy enough, use a mallet or pestle to 'massage' the veggies to release the juices.

Spoon into a large jar with a lid. Press down on the veggies so the juices rise up to cover them. Put a weight on top to submerge the veggies and put the lid on loosely. Allow to sit at room temperature for 3–5 days (1–2 weeks if you don't use whey) before sealing tightly and moving to the fridge, where it will last for up to 3 months

FIVE WAYS TO USE KIMCHI:

1. Toss it through a Crisp Bibimbap Skillet Pancake (page 250).

2. Make a Kimcheese Toastie (page 84).

3. Make Kimchi Instant Noodles (page 116).

4. Add kick to an Abundance Bowl (pages 126–37).

5. Make Leftovers Kimchi Soup (page 264).

½ SERVE VEG + FRUIT PER SERVE

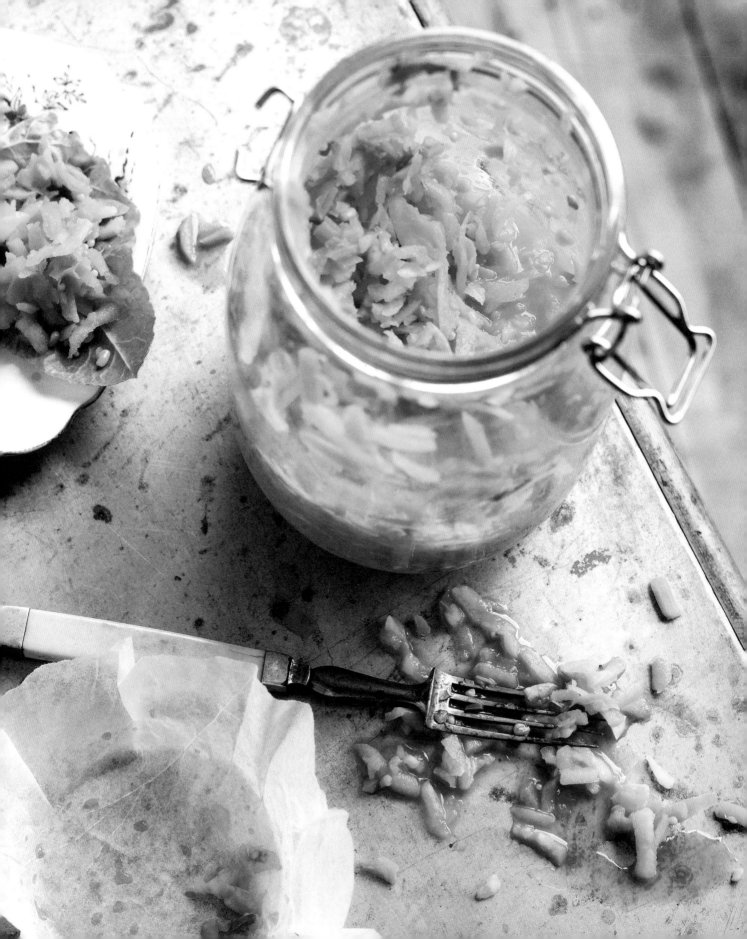

FIVE WAYS TO GET A GOOD DOSE OF TURMERIC PASTE:

1. Warming Golden Milk (page 81).
2. Golden Milkshake (page 81).
3. TMT Dressing (page 53).
4. My Gut-Healing Brew (page 87).
5. Thai Coconutty Cabbage (page 182).

Cumin also increases curcumin's bioavailability.

Be prepared to stain your blender doing this.

If you prefer (I do), you can use the leftover fermented turmeric from my Lemon and Turmeric Tonic-Ade (page 347) to make your paste. Whatever works for you.

If you can't find fresh turmeric, make this.

FERMENTED TURMERIC PASTE

MAKES 1 CUP (250 ML)

Turmeric is an Ayurvedic staple, long known to have anti-inflammatory, antibacterial and antifungal properties. Its active ingredient, curcumin, is also a rich source of antioxidants and is said to have anti-platelet properties that help protect against strokes and heart attacks. However, curcumin is not easily absorbed by the body *unless* you eat it with fat (it's fat-soluble), black pepper (the piperine in pepper ramps up the absorption by 2000%) or you ferment it. Herewith two recipes that ensure you get the full benefits from this amazing little root.

200 g fresh turmeric, peeled and roughly chopped

½ teaspoon organic freshly ground black pepper or cumin

¼–½ teaspoon sea salt

4 tablespoons Homemade Whey (page 46), plus extra to cover

Blend the turmeric to a smooth paste in a high-powered blender (or use a mortar and pestle). Stir in the pepper or cumin, salt and whey. Press into a jar and top with a little more whey so the turmeric is completely submerged. Cover with a lid and place in a cool, dark place for about 5 days or so, adding extra whey if required. Seal and store in the fridge for up to 6 months.

MAKE IT EASY TURMERIC PASTE:

4 tablespoons ground turmeric

¾ teaspoon finely ground black pepper

Place the turmeric and pepper in a saucepan with ½ cup (125 ml) water and bring to the boil over a medium heat. Reduce the heat and simmer, stirring vigorously, until the mixture forms a thick paste (about 5–7 minutes). Allow to cool, then transfer to a sealable jar. This will keep in the fridge for 2 weeks.

GOOD FOR YOUR GUTS GARLIC

MAKES 4 CUPS (1 LITRE)

Garlic has amazing properties and is particularly good for fighting off infections in the digestive tract and lungs, but it can be rough on your guts when eaten raw. Relate much? Fermenting famously fixes most things, including this issue. Plus, if you hate peeling garlic, then doing up a bunch of heads in one fell swoop makes a lot of sense. Note my nifty peeling trick, below.

6–8 heads garlic

1 teaspoon Himalayan pink salt

1 tablespoon Homemade Whey (page 46) or 1 teaspoon salt

1 teaspoon dried oregano or basil (optional)

1 bay leaf (optional)

Preheat the oven to 90°C (gas ¼). Place the garlic heads on a baking tray and bake for 1 hour or until the cloves begin to pop out of their skins. (Some ovens may take longer, but don't be tempted to crank the temp!) Cool a little, then simply pop the cloves from their skins, being sure to leave the ends intact.

Place in a 1 litre preserving jar with the rest of the ingredients and top with water, leaving 3 cm clear at the top. Seal loosely and leave on the worktop for 3–5 days (a little longer if you don't use whey). Then seal tightly and place in the fridge for 6 months. Best left for a couple of weeks before eating.

Be gentle with garlic
Avoid damaging the flesh of the garlic clove, especially the root end (don't cut it off). Any cuts will cause it to ferment unevenly and make the clove turn blue . . . which is nothing to be worried about; it's merely an amino acid reacting with the acid. All good. Just not pretty.

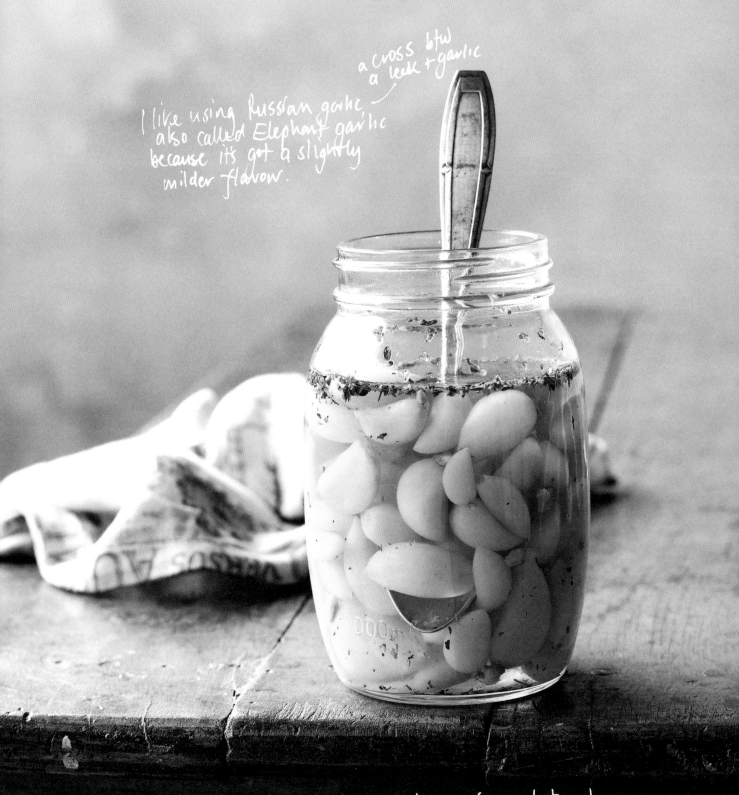

I like using Russian garlic, a cross btw a leek + garlic also called Elephant garlic because it's got a slightly milder flavour.

P.S. As you eat your ferment, transfer the remainder to a 'smaller' jar to reduce oxygen + thus spoilage.

KOMBUCHA

A fizzy-drink addict? Loved a sugar-laced iced tea in your past life? Let me introduce you to The 'Bucha. You might have seen kombucha-crazed kids parodied about town and rolled your eyes with the masses. Fair enough. It's kind of boundary-pushing stuff. But I'll try to ground it for us.

Kombucha is a slightly fizzy, fermented 'iced tea' made by adding a disgusting-looking creature called a SCOBY (short for 'symbiotic culture of bacteria and yeast') or 'mother' to a batch of brewed tea. This spongy, mushroomy thing activates and propels the drink (by eating sugar – yes, sugar!!) to become an 'alive' gut-healing beverage. With bubbles. And tang. Oh goodness, I know . . . Please don't leave me yet.

The stuff is brimful of probiotics and is a standout for digestive health. I bang on about it over at sarahwilson.com if you'd like to learn more. For now, know this much: countless studies have shown it can assist in the treatment of arthritis, depression, heartburn and candida. It's also great for liver detoxification, plus it improves pancreatic function and increases energy.

The sugar content of most fermented drinks here is about ½ tsp sugar for 100 ml of goodness.

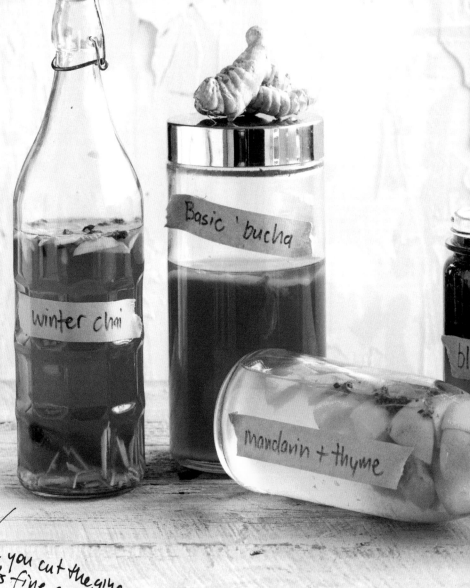

winter chai

Basic 'bucha

mandarin + thyme

bla

make sure you cut the ginger + other bits fine enough so they'll come back out.

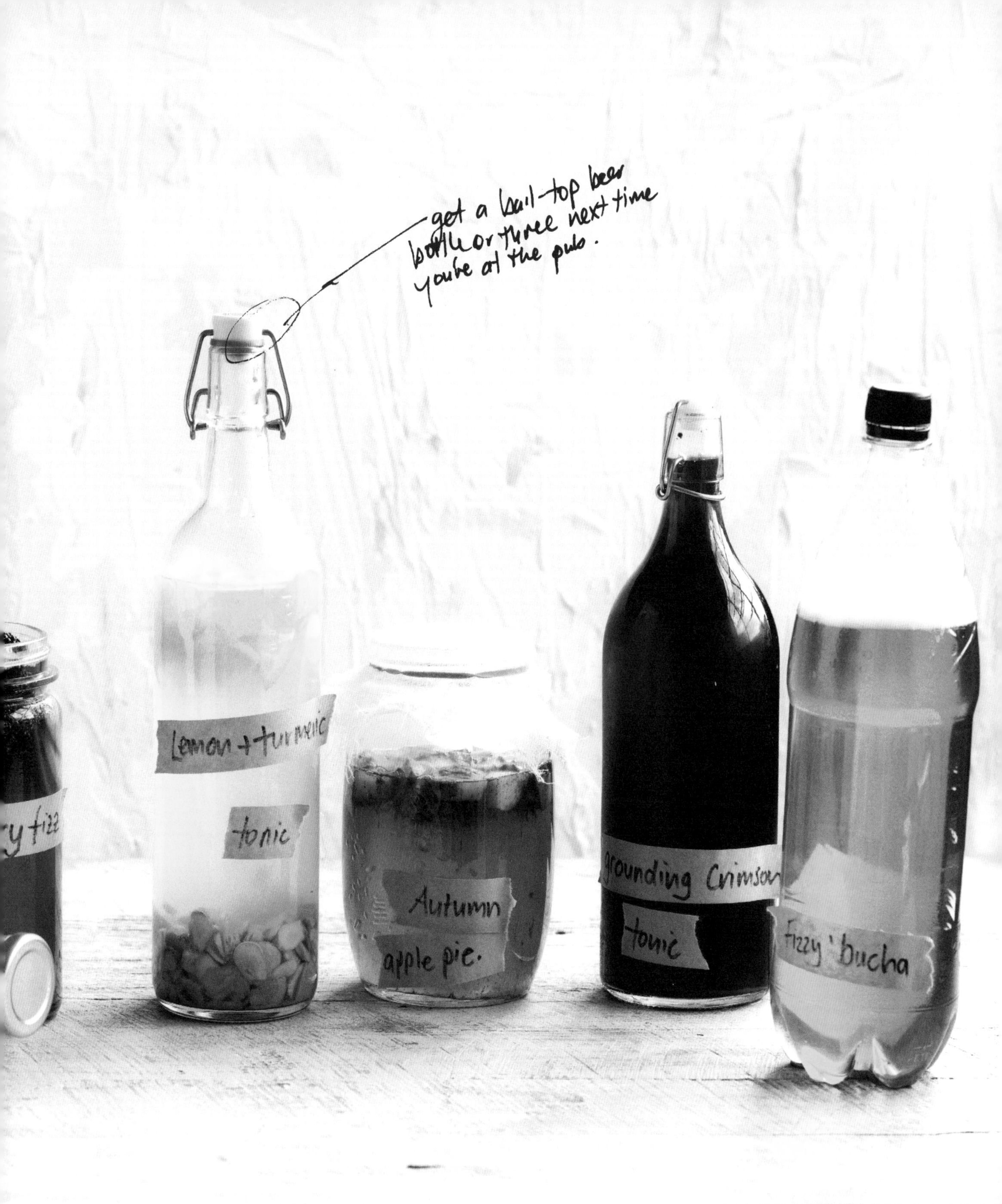

get a bail-top beer bottle or three next time you're at the pub.

Lemon + turmeric

tonic

Autumn apple pie.

grounding Crimson

tonic

Fizzy 'bucha

y fizz

£1.09 total cost
(£5.97 to buy the same amount
at a hipster supermarket)

Do you have to use sugar?

No. I'd read that honey doesn't work when making kombucha – the theory being that the honey's natural antibacterial agents kill the SCOBY. So I was a little concerned about using rice malt syrup instead of sugar. (Rice malt syrup is a fermented product and I pictured the different bacteria squabbling for attention in the bowl, eventually annihilating each other.) I chatted to various experts and Googled the bejesus out of the topic – no one had tried it. So I did. The result? Rice malt syrup maketh for a wonderful kombucha. You just have to leave it to ferment a day or two longer than its sugary cousin, and I think it does produce a slightly tarter brew. Which I kinda love.

Where does one obtain this SCOBY fellow?

This is the fun bit . . . You have to become part of a very cool witchy 'bucha community to get hold of one. SCOBYs can't be manufactured as such but are spawned from a 'mother' when one makes a batch of brew. Regular kombucha makers are always happy to give away a baby SCOBY.

How to drink the stuff

Straight from the fridge. About 100 ml (one-third of a glass) a couple of times a day. First thing in the morning before breakfast is fab (I have some before heading off for exercise and it's beautifully energising), so is after dinner as something of a digestive chaser. I like to team it with a dash of soda water for extra fizz.

Check out sarahwilson.com for details on finding one online.

PLAIN KOMBUCHA

MAKES ABOUT 3½ CUPS (850 ML)

4 tablespoons rice malt syrup, or sugar if you prefer

2 organic black tea bags (many say non-organic tea just doesn't work as well)

½ cup (125 ml) kombucha (from a previous batch or store-bought)

1 SCOBY

Sterilise a broad-mouthed glass or ceramic bowl or jug with boiling water. (It needs a wide opening to allow plenty of contact with oxygen.)

Combine the rice malt syrup or sugar in a saucepan with 1 litre of water and bring to the boil. Remove from the heat, add the tea bags, cover and allow to steep for 15 minutes. Remove the tea bags and pour the liquid into the sterilised container. Leave it to cool to around body temperature. Or cooler.

This is an important bit, okay? Hot tea will kill your mother!

Add the kombucha and then gently place the SCOBY on top (it may sink, but this is okay, says my mate Kate). Cover with a clean tea towel or muslin and leave to sit for 7–10 days (a week will be plenty in warm weather and/or if you use sugar). The temperature needs to be around 24–30°C.

If it's cool where you live, stick the bowl on top of the fridge.

At the end of 7–10 days, a 'baby' SCOBY will have formed on top of the 'mother'. Remove both SCOBYs, placing them in a glass container. Pour a little of the kombucha liquid onto the SCOBYs, then pour the rest into a 1 litre swing-top bottle (one with a hinged lid and rubber stopper), or a plastic soft-drink bottle, and refrigerate, ensuring you leave a 2–3 cm space at the top.

You could use one to start a new batch and give the other to a mate.

MAKE IT FIZZIER:

Get a little more fizz going by adding a dash of extra rice malt syrup or a little chopped fruit and securing the lid. Leave the bottle out at room temperature for an additional 2–4 days. The live yeast and bacteria will continue to consume the residual sugar from both the first fermentation, plus the extra dash you've just added. In the absence of oxygen (now that the whole thing is lidded), carbon dioxide is produced (and trapped), thus building up the fizz. (If you like a 'bucha with fizz, you may wish to use sugar instead of rice malt syrup in the fermenting stage. It fizzes faster.)

WINTER CHAI KOMBUCHA

3 cups (750 ml) Plain Kombucha
(see opposite)

5 cloves or cardamom pods

1 cinnamon stick, broken up

3 cm knob of ginger or turmeric,
cut into matchsticks

1 star anise

Place all the ingredients in a large jar with a
tight seal or a 1 litre swing-top bottle and let it
sit at room temperature for 3–4 days. You can
choose to strain the spices after 2 days and
rebottle, though I don't as I prefer the mixture
to become stronger with time.

**USE THE LEFTOVER
GINGER OR TURMERIC:**

Add it to smoothies.

AUTUMN APPLE PIE
KOMBUCHA

3 cups (750 ml) Plain Kombucha
(see opposite)

½ apple, cored and chopped

½–1 teaspoon Pumpkin Spice Mix
(page 45)

Place all the ingredients in a large jar with
a tight seal or a 1 litre swing-top bottle and
let it sit at room temperature for 3–4 days.
Strain the apple out after 2 days and rebottle,
if you wish, or leave it in so that the flavours
become stronger with time.

MAKE IT PUMPKIN PIE KOMBUCHA:

Add 4 tablespoons Pumpkin Purée (page 23)
instead of the apple. Toss in a bit of grated
ginger too.

SPRING STRAWBERRY
AND VANILLA KOMBUCHA

3 cups (750 ml)
Plain Kombucha (see opposite)

6–8 strawberries
(fresh or frozen)

1 vanilla pod, split, or ¼ teaspoon pure
vanilla extract (or make your own; page 45)

*Or use 2 leftover
vanilla pods when
you've used the seeds
for something else.*

Place all the ingredients in a large jar with a
tight seal or a 1 litre swing-top bottle and let it
sit at room temperature for 3–4 days. You can
choose to strain the strawberries and vanilla
pod out after 2 days and rebottle, if you like.

**USE THE LEFTOVER
FERMENTED STRAWBERRIES:**

Have them with yoghurt for dessert
or breakfast.

*Discomfort or
pain associated
with intestinal
gas may subside
soon after eating
4–6 strawberries.
I'm not exactly sure
why this works, but
it seems to give
quick relief for
some people.*

SUMMER PEACH
AND BASIL COLADA

3 cups (750 ml) Plain Kombucha
(see opposite)

1 large ripe peach, stone removed
and chopped

5 basil leaves

Place all the ingredients in a large jar with a
tight seal or a 1 litre swing-top bottle and let
it sit at room temperature for 3–4 days. Strain
out the peach and basil after 2 days and
rebottle if you like, or if you prefer a stronger
flavour, leave them in.

*when done, use the
fermented peach pieces in
a smoothie or atop yoghurt
for dessert.*

GUT HAPPY TONICS

Fiddly, witchy kombucha-making ain't for everyone. Forthwith, a bunch of super-simple probiotic drinks that cut out as much palaver as possible.

A few things to know about these tonic-y things

* Always make two batches back to back, re-using the remaining fruit and roots, adding another tablespoon of salt and leaving to ferment for the same period.

* Once you've done two batches, keep the fruits 'n' roots and eat them – they're lovely and activated!

* If it's winter, or if you're not keen on using so much salt, add 1–2 tablespoons of Homemade Whey (page 46) or some sauerkraut juice (page 337) or some leftover tonic from a previous batch and halve the salt.

* To increase carbonation, decant the tonic into a wine bottle and cork it, or into a recycled plastic soft-drink bottle and cap tightly. Leave at room temperature until you can see a rim of bubbles at the top of the wine bottle or until the plastic bottle bulges from CO_2 pressure build-up.

HARDCORE FLU TONIC

MAKES 1 JAR

This stuff is seriously potent and will fix the worst kind of man flu (and lesser variants). I gargle 1–2 tablespoons straight and then swallow several times a day. Again, I've kept the amounts loose. We'll work to proportions on this one. (PS: Don't fret; you really can't get it wrong.)

EQUAL PARTS FRESH:

garlic, peeled

onion, peeled

chilli (hot jalapeno is best)

ginger, unpeeled

turmeric, unpeeled

horseradish, peeled (optional)

PLUS:

apple cider vinegar

Place all of the ingredients except the vinegar in your blender and blitz. Add a dash of apple cider vinegar (enough to form a pourable slurry). Transfer to a jar large enough to three-quarters fill. Add a little more apple cider vinegar to your blender and swirl to capture any remaining slurry. Pour into the jar, leaving a 3 cm space at the top. Seal and shake. Leave on the worktop for 2–4 weeks, shaking daily (you might need to release the lid occasionally to prevent an explosion!). Strain into a swing-top bottle. Store in the fridge for 6 months (maybe even longer).

USE THE LEFTOVER FERMENTED VEGGIES AND SPICES:
These add umami flavour to a stew, soup or stir-fry.

GROUNDING CRIMSON TONIC

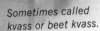

Sometimes called kvass or beet kvass.

MAKES ABOUT 1 LITRE

¾ cup (100 g) coarsely chopped beetroot

4 tablespoons chopped turmeric

1 tablespoon salt

Place all the ingredients in a 1 litre jar with a lid. Top with water, stopping 2 cm from the rim. Screw on the lid and leave on your kitchen worktop, shaking a few times a day, for 2–6 days, depending on the season (winter requires longer fermentation). Keep an eye on the bubbles. Once they start to appear, open the jar to release some of the CO_2 and have a taste. Strain, leaving the beets and turmeric in the jar along with enough liquid to cover them. Pour the rest of the tonic into a swing-top bottle and store in the fridge for up to 1 week.

USE THE LEFTOVER BEETROOT:
Add it to Abundance Bowls (pages 126–37) or mix it with yoghurt, with a sprinkle of apple cider vinegar or ground cumin as a side at dinner.

USE THE LEFTOVER TURMERIC:
Purée and keep in a jar in the fridge for up to 2 months and use in place of finely chopped turmeric.

LEMON AND TURMERIC TONIC-ADE

MAKES ABOUT 1 LITRE

½ cup (50 g) sliced turmeric or ginger, unpeeled

1 sliced lemon or lime, unpeeled

1 tablespoon rice malt syrup or sugar

1 tablespoon salt

Place all the ingredients in a 1 litre jar with a tight-fitting lid. Top with water, leaving a 2 cm space from the rim. Screw on the lid and leave on your kitchen worktop for 2–6 days, shaking a few times a day. How long you leave it will depend on the season (winter requires longer fermentation). Keep an eye on the bubbles. Once they start to appear, open the top to release some of the CO_2 and have a taste. (I brew mine a little longer than most – I like a tarty, less sugary flavour.) Strain into a 1 litre swing-top bottle and store in the fridge for up to 1 week.

USE THE LEFTOVER LEMON OR LIME:
Keep it in a clean jar in the fridge for 2 months and use with Sweet Persian Tagine (page 224) or in any recipe calling for lemon or lime zest.

APPLE AND BLACKBERRY CARDAMOM FIZZ

MAKES ABOUT 1 LITRE

½ cup (75 g) sliced apple, unpeeled

½ cup (75 g) pitted cherries or blackberries

1 tablespoon rice malt syrup or sugar

½ teaspoon ground cardamom

½ teaspoon ground cinnamon

Place all the ingredients in a 1 litre jar with a lid. Top with water, leaving a 2 cm space from the rim. Screw on the lid and leave on your kitchen worktop, shaking a few times a day, for 2–6 days, depending on the season (winter requires longer fermentation). Keep an eye on the bubbles. Once they start to appear, open the jar to release some of the CO_2 and have a taste. Strain into a swing-top bottle and store in the fridge for up to 1 week

MAKE IT A MANDARIN AND THYME FIZZ:
Use 1 cup (150 g) chopped mandarin (seeds removed, peel left on) and a few sprigs of thyme.

GUT-GIVING GUMMIES

Gelatine, a collagen powder made from the bones, hides and connective tissues of animals, is the gift our tired guts have been waiting for. This might be enough for you to give gelatine a go. If so, skip to my gummy recipes. If not, read on for the finer claims made of the stuff.

How to buy and eat gelatine

* Only get stuff made from pasture-fed cows. This is non-negotiable when you're eating the very gelatinous fibre of their being.

* The best stuff comes as a powder (as opposed to sheets and envelopes). 1 envelope granulated gelatine = 4 teaspoons powdered gelatine = 3 sheets of leaf gelatine.

* Start with ½–1 tablespoon per day and slowly increase to about 3–4 tablespoons a day.

* Since gelatine is a protein, it's important to eat it with fats to stimulate strong digestive juices and allow the body the fuel to use the protein properly.

* Get gelatine made from complete collagen, not collagen hydrolysate, to make these gummies.

* You can purchase bone gelatine via the The Kit (see page 5).

Gummies for insomnia? Eat one gummy before bed.

What you need to know about gelatine:

* It helps heal our tired gut linings by boosting acid production and restoring the mucosal lining.

* It reduces heartburn, ulcers and acid reflux by binding gut acids with the foods.

* It balances out meat intake. Muscle meats contain elevated levels of certain amino acids that can be inflammatory over time (you know those headlines about red meat being harmful?). Gelatine contains two anti-inflammatory amino acids, thus balancing, completing and complementing the other meat sources. This is particularly important for autoimmune sufferers.

* It helps your liver do its detox thing. Gelatine provides the amino acid glycine, which assists the liver in ridding toxins from your body.

* It boosts metabolism and can be used for weight loss.

* It's great for injury. It not only reduces inflammation, which can trigger pain receptors and cause stiffness in the joints, but it can also help repair small tears in the cartilage.

* And it helps with insomnia. Research has shown that taking glycine just before bed can actually enhance sleep quality, reduce daytime sleepiness and even improve memory.

Gummies for weight loss?

I don't advocate weight-loss obsessing, but if you're trying to curb late night eating try this: stop eating at least 3 hours prior to bedtime and consume at least 1 tablespoon of gelatine powder right before bed.

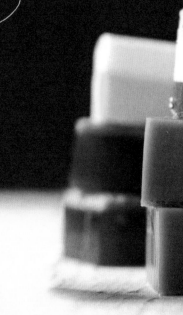

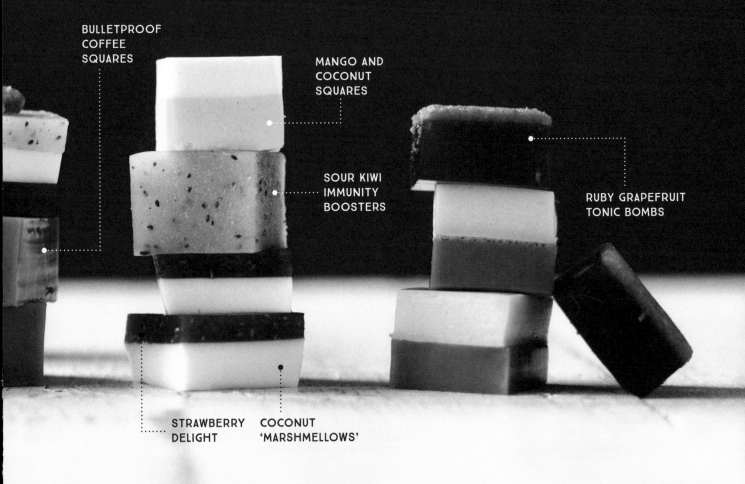

BULLETPROOF
COFFEE
SQUARES

MANGO AND
COCONUT
SQUARES

SOUR KIWI
IMMUNITY
BOOSTERS

RUBY GRAPEFRUIT
TONIC BOMBS

STRAWBERRY
DELIGHT

COCONUT
'MARSHMELLOWS'

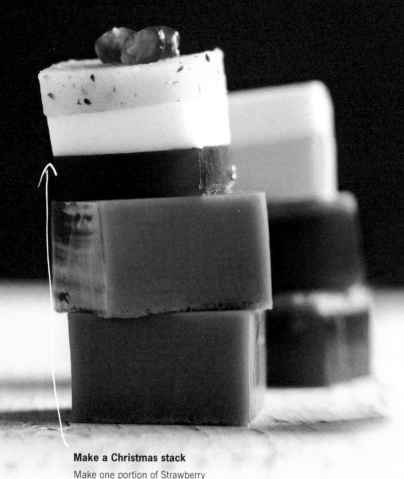

BASIC GELATINE GUMMIES

MAKE ABOUT 15

Use this basic recipe to make the delights that follow.

4½ tablespoons gelatine powder

1½ cups (225 g) chopped fruit or 1–1½ cups (250–350 ml) liquid

½ tablespoon rice malt syrup or 2 drops liquid stevia (optional)

'Bloom' the gelatine by stirring it into ⅓ cup (75 ml) cold water until dissolved. Let it sit for 5 minutes; it will expand and become 'rubbery'.

Heat the fruit or liquid and sweetener (and any spices or essences) in a small saucepan until it's almost boiling and the fruit has softened. Turn off the heat and add the bloomed gelatine (break the large blob into little blobby bits) and stir until dissolved, then use a stick blender to purée. Pour into moulds or a 10 × 15 cm square glass dish (or similarly sized plastic one – I use a lunchbox). Cool a little then place in the fridge to set for 1 hour. Cut into squares. Store in the fridge in an airtight container for up to 1 week.

LESS THAN ¼ TSP ADDED SUGAR PER SERVE

Make a Christmas stack

Make one portion of Strawberry Delight (see opposite) and pour into a slightly deeper dish. Allow to set for 1 hour, then add a layer of Coconut 'Marshmellows' (opposite) and a layer of Sour Kiwi Immunity Booster (opposite) allowing each layer to set. Top with some pomegranate seeds to make them special.

SOUR KIWI IMMUNITY BOOSTERS

In my obsessed reading on the subject, I came across gelatine devotees who think the acid in kiwi stops the gelatine from goobing correctly. I beg to differ. These things wobbled out a treat.

½ cup (125 ml) lemon juice

4 ripe kiwi fruit, peeled and chopped

2 tablespoons vitamin C powder (optional; added after the gelatine has been mixed in and the liquid has cooled a little)

Note: You'll need to use sweetener for this one . . . it's rather tarty. Also, feel free to use 5 tablespoons of gelatine.

COCONUT 'MARSHMELLOWS'

270 ml can coconut milk

(125 ml) cream

½ teaspoon pure vanilla extract
(or make your own; page 45)

pinch of sea salt

BULLETPROOF COFFEE SQUARES

½ cup (125 ml) black coffee

½ cup (125 ml) almond milk

¼ teaspoon pure vanilla extract
(or make your own; page 45)

MAKE IT A BUBBLE TEA:
Add bulletproof coffee squares
to a glass of cold milk.

STRAWBERRY DELIGHT

1 cup (150 g) strawberries

1 teaspoon rosewater

Add the rosewater to the gelatine.

MANGO AND COCONUT SQUARES

½ cup (75 g) chopped mango
(about ½ mango)

½ cup (125 ml) coconut cream or milk

juice of 1 lime

¼ teaspoon pure vanilla extract
(or make your own; page 45)

big pinch of cardamom powder

You're a vegan or veggo?
The best option would be to
use agar, derived from a
seaweed, although it doesn't
create the same 'creamy' texture,
nor does it possess the same
gut-giving gifts. It sets more
firmly than gelatine, so you'll
only need 1¼ tablespoons of
agar powder (though this varies
between brands). Although,
bearer of bad news and all,
if you take any kind of vitamin
capsule or eat commercial
gummy bears or snake lollies,
um, you're eating beef gelatine,
albeit inferior stuff.

GREEN JUICE DETOX JELLIES

1½ cups (350 ml) green smoothie
of your choice

2 scoops of green powder (optional)

If using the green powder, add after
the gelatine has been mixed in, once
the liquid has cooled a little.

PROBIOTIC BERRIES 'N' CREAM CHEWS

½ cup (75 g) frozen blueberries,
strawberries or raspberries

½ cup (125 ml) coconut cream

3 probiotic capsules (optional)

If using probiotic capsules, add them
after the gelatine has been mixed in,
once the liquid has cooled a little.

RUBY GRAPEFRUIT TONIC BOMBS

1 ruby grapefruit or 2 blood oranges,
peeled, pith and pips removed, chopped

½ cup (125 ml) Grounding Crimson Tonic
(page 347)

Add the tonic after the gelatine has
been mixed in, once the liquid has
cooled a little.

VANILLA PEACH KOMBUCHA GUMS

3 peaches, peeled (if you want,
I don't) and chopped

½ cup (125 ml) kombucha

¼ teaspoon pure vanilla extract
(or make your own; page 45)

Add the kombucha after the gelatine
has been mixed in, once the liquid
has cooled a little.

SIMPLICIOUS SPROUTS IN A JAR

↓ ↓ ↙
5p = total cost
↗ ↑ ╲ £1.85 to buy in a packet

This recipe pares the sprouting caper back to basics –
no fancy sprouting kits required.

The deal with sprouts

Un-sprouted beans, grains, nuts and seeds (BGNSs) contains enzyme inhibitors that prevent them from growing until the conditions are just right for germination. These anti-nutrients hinder our own enzymes from digesting them, blocking our ability to absorb their goodness. BGNSs also contain phytic acid (mostly in the bran) to deter bugs from munching them. Problem is that this acid binds to minerals making them unavailable for absorption in our intestines.

But! Soaking and sprouting de-activates the bothersome acids and inhibitors, making the BGNSs far more digestible and absorbable, saving (indeed, boosting) our bodies' enzymes for other things. They turn the little buggers into living things, making a bunch of vitamins and minerals in the process.

The depletion of our bodies' enzymes is, in fact, the ageing process. So . . . eating sprouts slows down the ageing process!

3–5 tablespoons raw legumes, seeds and/or nuts of your choice

dash of apple cider vinegar or lemon juice

Place the legumes, seeds or nuts and apple cider vinegar or lemon juice in a large, wide-mouthed jar and cover with water. Place a piece of muslin, cheesecloth or nylon cloth over the mouth and secure it with a rubber band. Leave to soak for 12 hours or overnight.

In the morning, drain (pouring the water through the cloth). Rinse and drain again (your cloth is still on!) and then leave the jar inverted at an angle out of direct sunlight – on your dish rack is a great idea. Repeat this rinse and drain business twice a day for the next day or three until your sprouts have tails.

Ensure your beloved sprouts are completely drained after the final rinse and store in an airtight container in the fridge for several days.

Keep your sprouts spritely by rinsing and draining as often as possible.

MAKE IT A MIXED BAG:
Combine a number of legumes in one jar, ensuring you use legumes that take the same amount of time to sprout. Lentils, mung beans and chickpeas is a good combo.

MAKE IT HEALTHIER:
Do the final drain in a sun-lit position to allow the chlorophyll and carotenes to develop.

MAKE IT LAST LONGER:
Remove the mould-attracting hulls before the final rinse (dump in a bowl and cover in water so the hulls rise to the surface), and drain. Rinsing them daily once you've refrigerated them will also see them last up to 1 week.

FIVE WAYS TO USE YOUR SPROUTS:

1. Sprinkle on top of or mix into a salad.
2. Blend into a smoothie or shake (mung bean sprouts are great for this).
3. Add to a stir-fry just before serving.
4. Make **Indian Sprouts Raita**: Mix 2 handfuls of sprouts with 1 cup (200 g) full-fat organic plain yoghurt, a handful of chopped mint and 1 teaspoon ground cumin. Chill for 1 hour. Done.
5. Add sprouts that are 'turning' to soups and stews in the final 5 minutes of cooking.

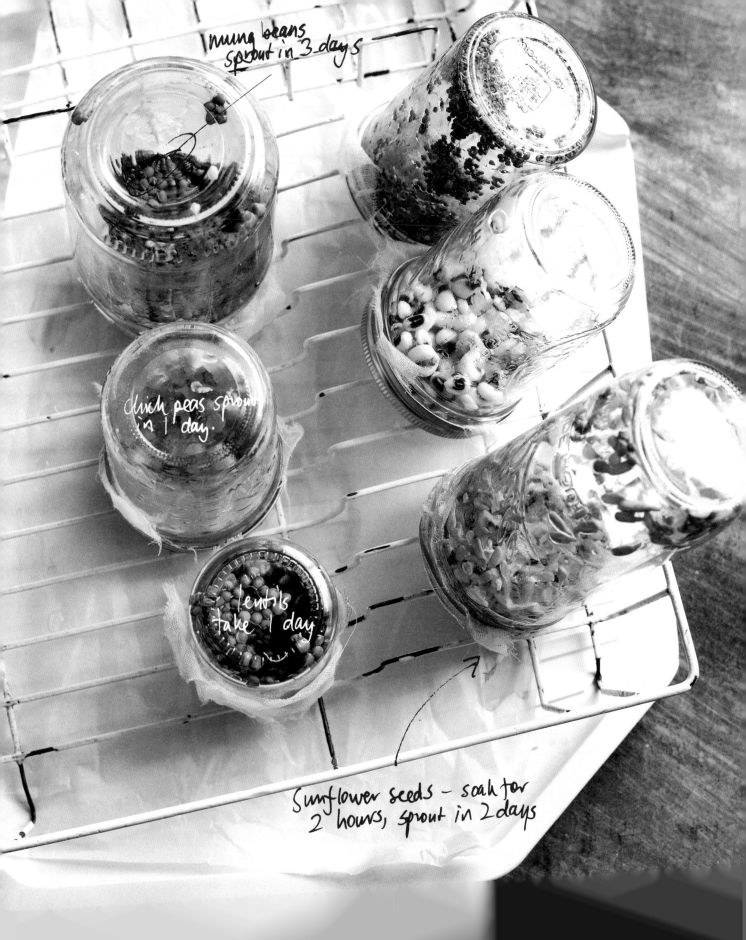

mung beans
sprout in 3 days

chick peas sprout
in 1 day.

lentils
take 1 day

Sunflower seeds - soak for
2 hours, sprout in 2 days

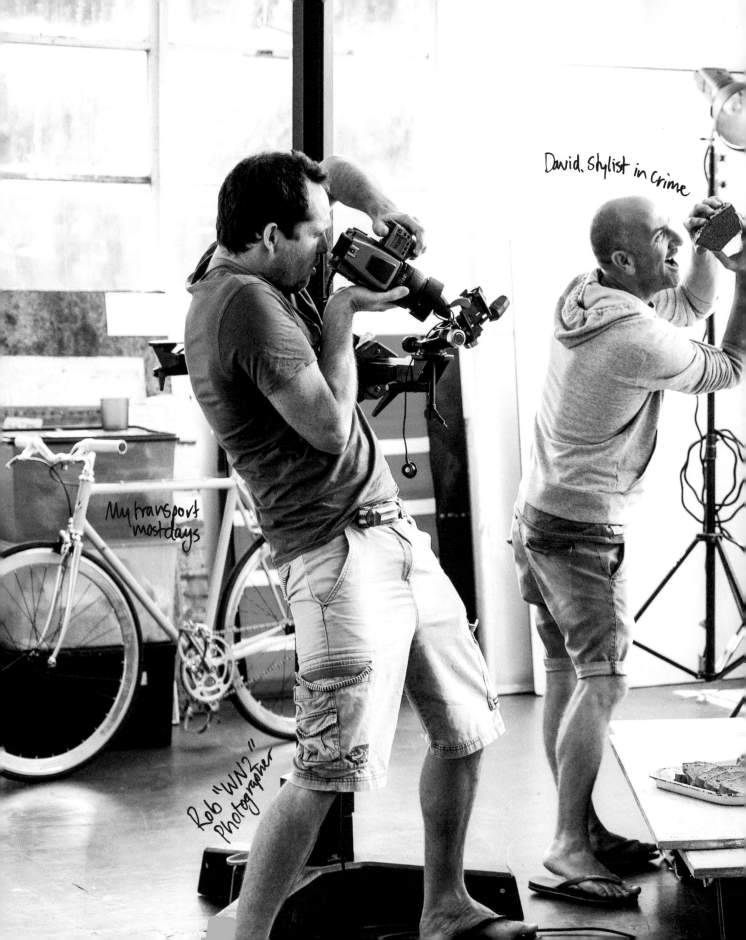

David, Stylist in Crime

My transport mostdays

Rob "WN2" Photographer

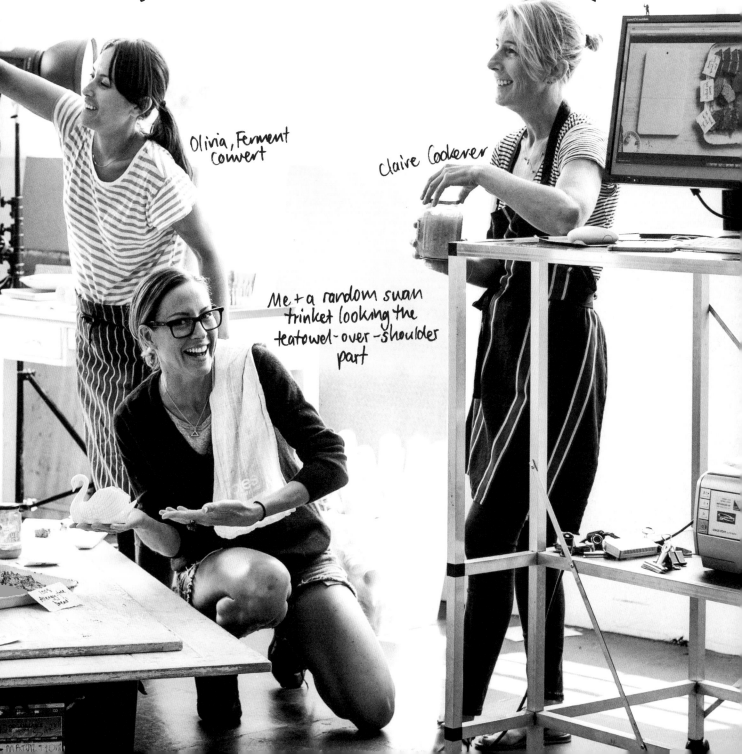

A TIDY LITTLE SHOPPING LIST

Forthwith a list of common ingredients I keep on hand and the versions I recommend.

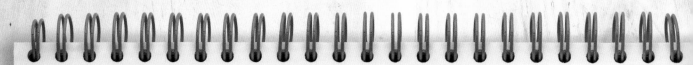

☐ **Apple cider vinegar:**
Organic, raw, unpasteurised with a 'mother' (a cloudy floater at the bottom).

☐ **Buckwheat:**
I buy organic, unhulled buckwheat and make my own activated buckwheat groats (page 27).

☐ **Cacao powder:**
Raw, unprocessed cocoa powder. It's much higher in anti-oxidants and minerals and has a richer taste. But feel free to use the processed version if that's all you have.

☐ **Canned beans:**
I much prefer to soak and cook dried ones, but I still keep a few cans of chickpeas and lentils for convenience. Choose organic beans in BPA-free cans and drain and rinse them well. I always cook them for a while (in whatever dish I've added them to); see page 28 for reasons why.

☐ **Capers:**
In salt is best. Vinegary ones are, well, vinegary and lose their caper-y taste. Worried about the salt intake? Rinse them first. Personally, I use their saltiness to season a dish so that I don't need to add any extra salt. Finely chopped they become a 'caper salt'.

☐ **Chia seeds:**
Non-GMO and sustainably farmed black or white.

☐ **Coconut (shredded and flakes):**
Check for added sugar/preservatives.

☐ **Coconut cream:**
Organic, full-fat, virgin, sustainably sourced in a BPA-free can if you, um, can-can. And you don't need to buy coconut milk – just thin out the cream with water to make 'milk'. *A little trick from Megan Y. in the office*

☐ **Coconut oil:**
Choose unrefined, organic, cold-pressed, virgin oil with the lowest carbon miles possible. I look out for brands that come in a re-usable glass jar.

☐ **Curry paste:**
Go for versions that contain recognisable ingredients and the least (preferably no) added sugar.

☐ **Dairy:**
Always use full-fat butter, milk, cheese and yoghurt. Low-fat dairy products usually contain a lot of added sugar to make up for the loss of flavour and texture. The sugar content should be no more than 4.7 g per 100 g (this is all lactose; anything more is added sugar).

☐ **Gelatine:**
Look for regular bone gelatine (not hydrosolate) from a company that raises pasture-fed or grass-fed animals. Make sure it contains no high fructose corn syrup or artificial colours. Head to The Kit to get hold of some.

☐ **Kimchi:**
When I buy it (I often make my own) it's raw (unpasteurised) and found in the chilled section. If it's in the aisle it's been vinegared or had preservatives added. Obtainable from Asian supermarkets and online.

☐ **Kombucha:**
When I buy it (rather than make my own) I get the brand with the least amount of sugar. *1.8g/100ml is my benchmark*

☐ **Miso:**
Fermented, not dried. I use red miso in this book. If you have white miso, double the quantity listed in the recipe.

☐ **Nut butters:**
Always choose sugar-free, salt-free versions. Better still, make your own from raw, unsalted and activated nuts (see iquitsugar.com).

☐ **Olive oil:**
Always choose extra-virgin to ensure the oil has been produced by a simple pressing of the olives without the use of chemicals or temperature treatments. Look for small producers who cold-press their olives. Save the best stuff for drizzling, not cooking.

☐ **Olives:**
Good-quality ones in olive oil. Best if they're not pitted (they keep their flavour). See my olive pitting trick on page 170.

☐ **Peanut butter:**
Choose organic. Why? See page 17.

❑ **Protein powder:**
I recommend whey protein powder. The whey needs to be cold-pressed and sourced from grass-fed cows, chemical — and hormone-free. Also make sure the powder has no artificial flavourings or preservatives, no sugars or sweeteners and no bulking agents or thickeners. If you're vegan, look for a pea-based protein powder that's 100% natural pea protein isolate.

❑ **Quinoa:**
White, red, black or a mix of all three. Try to source non-GMO, sustainably farmed versions (see page 27).

❑ **Rice malt syrup:**
This is made from fermented brown rice. Go for versions that list only brown rice and water as the ingredients.

❑ **Salt:**
I use pure rock salt or sea salt (processed table salt lacks many of the minerals found in rock and sea salt). Himalayan rock salt is a good choice (especially for fermenting; see page 334) as it contains a full spectrum of 84 minerals and trace elements.

❑ **Sauerkraut:**
Really easy to make yourself (page 337). If you're purchasing, choose raw (unpasteurised) from the chilled section (if it's in an aisle, it's likely to be full of vinegar and sugar – check the label.) Also try to buy locally – the bacteria will be more beneficial.

❑ **Sesame oil:**
Dark (toasted) or light (regular, untoasted). Always choose organic and cold-pressed. The darker, toasted variety has a distinct flavour and fragrance more suited to Asian dishes in particular.

❑ **Spices:**
Mustard seeds, fenugreek, coriander seeds, cumin seeds and ground cumin, dill seeds, black peppercorns, ground turmeric, cinnamon sticks, ground nutmeg, star anise and ground allspice make a good core stash. I also use these spice mixes a lot: garam masala, five-spice and Ras el Hanout (see recipe on page 45). If you're buying ground spices, look for small packets (they go stale easily), avoid the glass jars at the supermarket (they've probably been on the shelf for a year or two) and, if possible, buy spices whole and grind them yourself using a mortar and pestle.

❑ **Stevia:**
This sweetener is made from the leaves of the *Stevia rebaudiana* plant and comes in granulated, powdered or liquid form. I prefer the liquid (2–4 drops are equivalent to 1 teaspoon sugar), 'cos it suits my whole 'minimise the sweet stuff' principle.

❑ **Tahini:**
Organic and hulled or unhulled. I prefer unhulled for cooking, but hulled is best for drizzling or spreading (the flavour is not as strong).

❑ **Tamari:**
This is a fermented, wheat-free version of soy sauce. It should contain no sugar.

❑ **Tinned tuna:**
Much cheaper than fresh fish and more likely to be wild-caught, with higher levels of anti-inflammatory omega 3 fatty acids. Always opt for 'pole-and-line' varieties. Pole-and-line fishing is much more selective than the standard method which scoops up and kills every creature within reach. It also allows for a more sustainable rate of fishing. Choose brine or springwater versions; in-oil versions only if it's 100% olive oil (most aren't). For a full rundown of the best brands see The Kit.

❑ **Turmeric paste:**
Make your own (see page 340) or look out for it in a jar. I've found it in a few speciality stores, generally preserved in apple cider vinegar.

❑ **Yoghurt:**
Full-fat, organic, unflavoured with live cultures (no stabilisers, gums or inulin).

A note on bottled drinks
I actively avoid bottled drinks for sustainability reasons. The carbon miles from the packaging and distribution of a single-use product doesn't stack up. And don't get me started on bottled water (click over to sarahwilson.com if you want to read my rant).

IQS nutritionist Kate c shared this one!

SUBSTITUTIONS AND FIXES

A few tips on finding alternatives and taking shortcuts when you're creating your simplicious flows.

SUBSTITUTIONS

Whenever I list a homemade ingredient in a recipe (stock, cream cheese, spice mixes, pesto, sauces and dressings) please know that you can substitute store-bought versions. Just make sure you check the labels for added sugar, crappy oils etc.

CAKE ↔ MUFFINS

All cakes can be turned into cupcakes or muffins and vice versa. Just bake the cake version 5–10 minutes longer (and use a log/loaf tin rather than a round tin).

CHEESE

I use quite a bit of hard cheese in my recipes (parmesan, cheddar and mature cheddar). If you're sensitive to cow's milk, you might be able to tolerate goat's or sheep's cheese. Please also feel free to substitute Homemade Cream Cheese (page 46) with an organic, store-bought version.

COCONUT FLAKES / ACTIVATED GROATIES ↔ OATS

Toasted coconut flakes and Activated Groaties (page 27) are great for making crumbles or cake bases that usually call for oats.

EGGS ↔ CHIA SEEDS

A great technique if you have vegan friends coming over or if you've clean run out of eggs. Can be used for baking and dishes where an egg is used for thickness and binding (see Flours, below).

1 egg = 1 tablespoon chia seeds + 4 tablespoons water (mix and let sit for 15 minutes)

FERMENT BRINE ↔ APPLE CIDER VINEGAR ↔ AGED KOMBUCHA

Use interchangeably in dressings, for braising, deglazing and for your morning digestive shot.

FLOURS

It's fine to use grain-based white flours interchange-ably in baking (wheat, gluten-free wheat, oat flour, spelt etc), but nut flours and other naturally gluten-free flours require some tweaking to reduce crumbliness and you may have to experiment to get the texture you like. The following flour substitutes are for 1 cup (125 g) of wheat flour:

Almond meal/flour: ½ cup (50 g) + 1 beaten egg + 1 tablespoon arrowroot

Coconut flour: ⅓ cup (40 g) + 2 beaten eggs + ⅓ cup (75 ml) coconut milk (or water)

Buckwheat flour: just under 1 cup (120 g) (or use ½ cup (60 g) buckwheat flour + ½ cup (45 g) oat or 75 g brown rice flour – you get a similarly dense product, often darker in colour and with less rise)

Rice flour: just over ¾ cup (120 g) + just under 4 tablespoons arrowroot or other thickener (or 1 cup (160 g) rice flour + 1–2 beaten eggs)

GARLIC

1 clove Good for Your Guts Garlic (page 340) = 1 clove garlic

HERBS

Soft herbs can be used interchangeably:
parsley ↔ mint ↔ basil ↔ coriander.
Ditto spriggy herbs: rosemary ↔ thyme ↔ sage ↔ oregano.

MEATBALLS / SAUSAGES ↔ MINCE

When a recipe calls for mince, simply mush up some Basic Meatballs (page 144) or brown sausages for 1–2 minutes, remove the skins, cut into chunks and continue cooking, breaking them up further. When a recipe calls for meatballs, use sausages cut into chunks. (Make sure they are good-quality with plenty of meat in them.)

MILK ↔ COCONUT MILK

When a recipe calls for milk, you can use dairy milk (from cows, sheep or goats), nut milk (watch out for added sugar, or make your own) or coconut milk (full-fat, organic and cold-pressed – the ingredients on the can should read: 'coconut, water').

RED MISO ↔ WHITE MISO

Double the quantity if using white miso.

SEEDS

I use these interchangeably for salads, Abundance Bowls (pages 126–137) and cakes, breads and muffins: pumpkin seeds ↔ sunflower seeds ↔ sesame seeds.

SPICE MIXES

Pumpkin Spice Mix (page 45)**:** 1 heaped tablespoon ↔ 3 teaspoons ground cinnamon + 1 teaspoon ground nutmeg (or 2 teaspoons ground cinnamon + 1 teaspoon ground nutmeg + 1 teaspoon ground allspice)

Ras el Hanout (page 45)**:** This North African spice mix varies from region to region and can have more than 30 different spices. The alternatives I give throughout the book also vary, depending on what other spices are in the dish. If you're looking to create your own flavour bomb, the following spices make a good base: ground cumin, turmeric, coriander seed, paprika and cinnamon (in equal amounts). Then you can add in (at 4:1) some ground cardamom, allspice, cayenne pepper or nutmeg.

STOCK

All of my recipes call for homemade stock – it's a key ingredient in my simplicious flows – but feel free to use a store-bought version if you're happy that it contains no added sugar, dodgy oils or ingredients you don't recognise.

SWEETENERS

Rice malt syrup: Use in place of sugar or honey, roughly in a 1:1 ratio. Some people say it is not as sweet as honey or sugar, but I beg to differ, and I tend to put less of it in my recipes than many others would. Perhaps it's because my tastebuds have shifted!

Stevia: Stevia is 300 times sweeter than sugar and has a liquorice-y aftertaste that some people take a while to get used to. If you use granulated stevia, be aware that it is bulked out with other ingredients (enabling people to use it 1:1 as a sugar replacement). Check the label, as some manufacturers add sugar alcohols, maltodextrin, lactose, cellulose powder and silicone dioxide (among other things).

1 cup (200 g) granulated stevia ↔ 1 teaspoon liquid stevia

1 tablespoon granulated stevia ↔ 6–9 drops liquid stevia

1 teaspoon granulated stevia ↔ 2–4 drops liquid stevia

1 teaspoon pure powdered stevia ↔ 1¾ teaspoons liquid stevia

TURMERIC

1 tablespoon Fermented Turmeric Paste (page 340) ↔ 1–2 tablespoons grated fresh turmeric ↔ a 3–5-cm knob of fresh turmeric ↔ 1 teaspoon ground turmeric

VANILLA

1 teaspoon Never-Ending Vanilla Extract (page 45) ↔ 1 teaspoon pure vanilla extract ↔ ¼ teaspoon pure vanilla powder

QUICK FIXES

To thicken sauces and stews: Add chia seeds or arrowroot (tapioca), 1 teaspoon at a time, until desired goobiness is reached.

To thin a sauce or gravy: Toss in a frozen stock cube (see page 24). If it's a sweet recipe or has Thai-style flavours, use a cube of frozen coconut water or coconut milk.

To bulk out a meal: Add red lentils – they lend creaminess to soups and casseroles, plus lots of fibre. Add to the pot at least 15–20 minutes before serving.

To sweeten a sauce: Add Pumpkin Purée (page 23).

To add saltiness: Throw in a tinned anchovy or three; the oil or brine from a can of tuna or jar of olives; some capers (preserved in salt); a pinch of dulse flakes or a tablespoon or two of sauerkraut brine.

YOUR DEFINITIVE GUIDE TO SUGAR AND SAFE SWEETENERS

For the next time you're at a dinner party + you get DRILLED about your silly sugar diet!

Q So, you quit sugar; do you mean all sugar?

A Not quite. I quit fructose. But we mostly get our fructose from everyday table sugar (sucrose), which is 50% fructose. Besides, 'I Quit the Fructose Component of the Sucrose Molecule' doesn't really translate.

Q Why is fructose nasty, then?

A It goes like this: fructose is the only food molecule on the planet with no corresponding hormone in the brain that tells us when we've eaten enough of it – we have no 'off switch' for the stuff. Which means we overeat it. And so we can drink a mega cup of Coke or eat a family pack of lollies and not even feel 'full'. Worse, studies show it stimulates appetite, making us eat more of everything. Worse still, research shows it's more addictive than heroin and cocaine.

Fructose is also the only food molecule not metabolised by our cells; instead it's mostly metabolised in the liver, where it's turned into fat – the worst kind – visceral fat that settles around the vital organs. It also forms triglycerides, uric acid and free radicals.

The upshot of this domino-ing situation? Excess sugar consumption is now strongly linked to non-alcoholic fatty liver disease, obesity and diabetes. And much more. (Head to The Kit (see page 5) to read more.)

But why would we evolve this way? To be obsessed by fructose, addicted to it, programmed to binge on it and store it as fat? Well, 10,000 years ago fructose was very rare (a few bitter berries, the occasional beehive), so it made evolutionary sense to hunt it down and gorge on it – precisely because it was such a great source of instant energy! This was a boon back when famine or wildebeest could strike at any time . . . not so much now, right?

Q But sugar is natural!

A Sure; although, *so is arsenic and petroleum*. What's unnatural is how much of the stuff we're eating. Just 100 years ago we ate less than 1 kg a year, now we eat 60 kg a year of added sugar. Dis-as-ter.

Q Surely you're not saying we shouldn't eat fruit?

A Nope. When I refer to 'added sugar', it doesn't include *whole* fruit. Fruit *juice* and *dried* fruit, however, are counted as added sugar – without the fibre and the water you're left with concentrated sugar. When doing my 8-Week Programme we cut out all sugar including fruit for 4 weeks so that our bodies can recalibrate and we can 'retrain' our palate. Then whole fruit is reintroduced.

Q How much should I be eating?

A Ha. This is interesting. For years I have been saying that 6–9 teaspoons of added sugar a day (3 teaspoons for kids) is about the amount our bodies can handle. Now the World Health Organization has advised the Exact. Same. Amount. It also includes fruit juice as 'added sugar' (though doesn't mention dried fruit). Go figure!

Q So, what exactly does 6 teaspoons of sugar look like?

A The World Health Organization announced in March 2015 that sugar consumption should be 5–10% of total energy intake (roughly 6–9 teaspoons of sugar per day), preferably less. This includes the sugar in honey, syrups and fruit juice, but doesn't include the sugars naturally present in fresh fruit, vegetables, milk and cheese. I've been saying this for yonks! (Note that I also count dried fruit as added sugar, though some people don't.)

6 TEASPOONS OF SUGAR EQUALS...

1¼ SULTANA & APRICOT SNACK PACK

⅔ OF A CAN OF COKE

½ A BOTTLE OF APPLE JUICE

1 SINGLE-SERVE TUB OF LOW FAT STRAWBERRY YOGHURT

2 BLOCKS OF 85% DARK CHOCOLATE

Q **Gosh, am I eating too much sugar?**

A Not sure. This is how you work it out:

1. Look at the sugar content in the 'per serve' column on your label (not the 'per 100 g' column).

2. Divide that quantity (it's in grams) by 4 (1 teaspoon is about 4 g of sugar) to get the rough number of teaspoons.

3. For dairy products, remember to subtract the first 4.7 g per 100 g (which is lactose). For example, if the serving size is 50 g, 2.3 g is lactose.

4. Double or triple the serving amount if you tend to eat more, as I do. Be realistic!

Q **What sweetener do you use, then?**

A **Stevia:** a natural sweetener derived from the leaves of the *Stevia rebaudiana* plant. It's 300–450 times sweeter than sugar. I use it in liquid form (you can get it granulated or powdered).

Rice malt syrup: a natural sweetener made from fermented, cooked rice and a blend of complex carbohydrates, maltose and glucose. It is relatively slow-releasing so does not dump on the liver as much as pure glucose.

Q **So I can eat as much of the 'safe' sweetener as I want, then?**

A Nope. To live sugar-free successfully I suggest minimising all sweeteners. The science now shows that even rice malt syrup, stevia and artificial sweeteners can cause blood-sugar spikes and mess with the reward centre in our brains – continuing the sugar addiction.

Q **What about artificial sweeteners?**

A Studies have shown that artificial sweeteners are correlated with a host of health complications. The body poorly ingests sugar alcohols like sorbitol and isomalt. Instead they end up in our bloodstream and feed the bacteria in our large intestine. Studies have also shown that artificial sweeteners can cause weight gain, contribute to diabetes, lead to cancer and muck up our gut microbiome.

Q **What about honey; it's natural, surely!?**

A Sugar cane could equally be described as natural. Regardless, our bodies don't really care where the fructose comes from.

Dates: 30% fructose (total sugar content 60%)
Honey and maple syrup: 40% fructose
Agave: 70–90% fructose
Coconut sugar/nectar/syrup: 38–49% fructose

Be aware: I try to reference studies that are as close to 'gold standard' as possible. However, nutritional science is rarely 'gold', being frequently conducted on rats (not humans), and neither controlled nor randomised.

Hopefully the above rant will set the pesky doubter straight. You're welcome!

AYURVEDA 101

A traditional Indian healing system, Ayurveda is more than 5000 years old. It gave us yoga and meditation, and Buddhism stemmed from it 3000 years ago. Ayurveda says we're made up of three doshas (energy types) – Vata, Pitta and Kapha. Each of us is a combination of all three doshas, but we generally have one that dominates. When our dominant dosha is out of balance, we get wobbly and unwell.

Vata types are lanky, flighty and easily excited, and they hate the cold. Their dominant force is wind, so they do not like sitting idle, preferring to seek constant action. When out of balance, Vatas often experience problems with digestion and malabsorption, get anxious and distracted, and suffer insomnia.

For Vatas to stay in balance, they need warm, 'sweet', mushy foods to bring them back down to earth – stews, soups, sweet potato and spices such as cinnamon, ginger and cardamom. And to slooooow down.

Vatas love sugar! It provides temporary stimulation, but adds to the flightiness. Not good.

Pitta types have a medium but strong build and possess great concentration, but they can also be angry and judgemental. Their force is fire, so when out of balance Pittas can get 'hot under the collar'. They don't tolerate summer well.

For Pittas to stay in balance, they need cooling foods, such as salads. They should avoid chillies and hot spices.

Pittas love a greasy burger. Pitta peeps tend to go for alcohol, meat and fatty, salty, sour or spicy foods, which make them more intensely driven. Not good.

Kapha types have a 'thick' frame, oily skin, strong teeth and thick hair. They also have a slow metabolism and pace. Kaphas are earthy types (their force is earth and water) and when out of whack they can become heavy and phlegmatic and require firing up.

For Kaphas to stay in balance, they need stimulating spices, such as pepper, chilli and cumin and aerobic exercise.

Kaphas love doughnuts and meat pies. They search out sugary, salty, dairy-based or fatty foods, which reinforce their natural lethargy. Not good.

Whatever your dosha, balancing Vata is key.

This is because when our Vata gets over-stimulated, it can throw all our doshas out of whack. And so the recipes in this book mostly work to pacify Vata energy. Thus:

- Warming, slow-cooked foods 'sweetened' with cinnamon, ginger and cardamom are great.
- Fewer ingredients are best (simplicious!). Lots of flavours are hard to assimilate. When a recipe requires a big bunch of different ingredients, we cook them for a while as a one-pot meal so they have time to 'get to know each other'.
- Foods high in nutrients can also be tough to digest, so simple combinations of these are best.
- For more, head to The Kit (see page 5).

FYI: I'm a vata-pitta, with a fair bit of deranged vata going on! :-)

VERY FREQUENTLY ASKED QUESTIONS ALL IN ONE SPOT

Q **CAN I DRINK ALCOHOL WHEN I QUIT SUGAR?**

A **Yup. Sort of.**

Wine: Contains minimal fructose. How so? It's the fructose in the grapes that ferments to become alcohol, leaving red wine low in sugar. It can contain very low levels of residual sugar – less than 1 g per litre in the case of dry reds. White wine contains more residual sugar and should be avoided.

Sparkling wine (champagne): Bubbles retain quite a lot of the sugar (fructose). Avoid.

Spirits: Dry spirits like gin, vodka and whisky contain little or no fructose.

Beer: Doesn't contain fructose. The sugar in beer and stout is maltose, which we can metabolise fine.

Dessert wine: A stack of sugar remains unfermented. Don't touch the stuff.

Q **CAN I EAT CHOCOLATE?**

A **Well, yes. But it depends what kind.**

Homemade chocolate: If you make it with raw cacao powder, which is less than 1% sugar, and coconut oil (and perhaps a little rice malt syrup) it is fructose-free. Great! This is how I eat my chocolate.

Store-bought plain chocolate: The majority is made with cocoa (the refined version of cacao containing fewer nutrients) that comprises less than 50% of the ingredients (the other 50% is largely sugar). It also often contains bad oils and additives (look for versions that use cacao butter not vegetable oil). However, there are now varieties with 85% cocoa. This means that a 100 g block will contain a total of 15 g or 3.5 teaspoons of sugar. And if you eat just a couple of squares (say, 20 g) it equates to about ¾ teaspoon of sugar – not that much.

Q **CAN I EAT FRUIT?**

A **Yes, please do.**

NB: I count ½ banana and ½ mango (and other high-fructose, often tropical, fruits) as 1 serve.

Fruit can contain a fair whack of sugar – up to 3 teaspoons a piece. So I advise keeping to 1–2 serves a day, steering your way to low-fructose fruits like kiwi fruit, blueberries, raspberries and honeydew melon, and never eating grapes (unless you can stick to just a few at a time). On my 8-Week Programme I advise cutting out fruit from Week 2 to Week 6 so that your body can properly recalibrate and your tastebuds can regroup.

Q **SHOULD I QUIT CARBS WHEN I QUIT SUGAR?**

A **I wouldn't. Do one thing at a time.**

Quitting sugar is a big undertaking and one that will require your focus and willpower. Once you have mastered quitting sugar and if you feel a desire to do so, try cutting carbs for about 4–6 weeks and see if it suits YOUR body. Don't get caught up in what everyone else is doing. Experiment and learn for yourself – it's the only way to truly know if something works for you.

head to The Kit for the full shopping list. (see page 5)

TEN DAYS OF DINNER FOR FOUR
(REQUIRING ONLY THREE COOK-UPS!)

Here's how to use cook-ups to extend things further. Feel free to draw up your own version on your own fridge planner, inserting other bulk cook-ups and secondary dishes.

PS: I've designed this to allow for flexibility – you can use leftover cooked veggies and meat, or meat and veggie scraps. As you clear the fridge out, you can make a quick trip to grab a head of broccoli or a bag of beans. It's the ultimate perpetual meal!

SUNDAY: Chicken Pot au Feu (page 214) *Reserve the leftover veggies, chicken and stock.*

1

MONDAY: The ~~Fish~~ Chook That Got Away Pie (page 261) made with chicken and veggies from last night. *While the oven is on, feel free to roast some more veggies at the same time (see page 23) to use later in the week.*

2

TUESDAY: Sweet Potato, Miso and Sage Soup (page 244) with Poached Egg Floaters (page 245) made with Sunday's chicken stock.

3

WEDNESDAY: The Cheapest Stew Ever (page 212) made with brisket in a slow cooker and served as a veggie soup with a few beef cubes on top. *Reserve most of the beef and 2 cups (500 ml) stock.*

4

just crank the temp to 200°C (gas 6) once your pie is out.

THURSDAY: Last Night's Dinner With An Egg Stuck In It (page 256) made with leftover roasted veggies from Monday and some of the brisket from Wednesday. Serve with steamed greens and peas and any leftovers from the previous week.

5

FRIDAY: Fridge-Door Tonnato (page 254) made with the remaining leftover brisket from Wednesday and an egg or two. *Boil up the whole dozen eggs while you're at it.*

6

SATURDAY: Jerk Pork Shoulder Roast (page 222) made in the oven. *Roast some extra roots at the same time (page 23).*

7

SUNDAY: Baked Stuffing Loaf (page 305) made with last night's roast veg and served with steamed greens or green salad.

8

MONDAY: 'Pizza' Bread and Butter Crumble (page 262) made with leftover Pulled Pork from Saturday and greens. Throw in a spare boiled egg or three.

9

TUESDAY: Vegan Whatchagot Quiche (page 260) made with whatever veggies you have left, or Green Scraps Shakshouka (page 248) if you also have some uncooked eggs that need to be used.

Now, repeat . . . 10

A MINDFUL LEFTOVERS INDEX

By leftovers I'm referring not only to the peels, stalks, cores, scraps, bones, skin and pan juices left behind after cooking, but also the veggies at the bottom of the crisper that you bought up and forgot about – or indeed any ingredient that you need to use up to avoid waste.

GENERAL INDEX Page numbers in *italics* refer to photographs.